DIGESTIVE DISEASES - RESEARCH AND CLINICAL DEVELOPMENTS

MOTOR DYSFUNCTION, ETIOLOGY AND PATHOGENESIS OF GALLSTONES

DIGESTIVE DISEASES – RESEARCH AND CLINICAL DEVELOPMENTS

Additional books in this series can be found on Nova's website under the Series tab.

Additional e-books in this series can be found on Nova's website under the e-book tab.

DIGESTIVE DISEASES - RESEARCH AND CLINICAL DEVELOPMENTS

MOTOR DYSFUNCTION, ETIOLOGY AND PATHOGENESIS OF GALLSTONES

SHING-MOO HUANG

New York

For permission to use material from this book please contact us:
Telephone 631-231-7269; Fax 631-231-8175
Web Site: http://www.novapublishers.com

Library of Congress Cataloging-in-Publication Data

Library of Congress Control Number: 2013941188

ISBN: 978-1-62808-296-8

Published by Nova Science Publishers, Inc. † New York

Contents

Preface

This book adheres to strict scientific principles and is designed to explore the whole aspect of gallstone disease from the micro world of the genetic profiles, basic metabolisms of bile lipids in cholesterol gallstone patients, to the macro world of clinical triple defects of gallstone patients. It is especially suitable for medical professionals: internists, surgeons, residents, nurses and medical students, and for collection by libraries. This book deals with motor dysfunction in calculous gallbladders as well as reactive oxygen species in relation to gallstone formation. Etiology and pathogenesis of pigment, calcium carbonate and intra-hepatic gallstones are also discussed.

Volume II deals with motor dysfunction in calculous gallbladders as well as reactive oxygen species in relation to gallstone formation. Etiology and pathogenesis of pigment, calcium carbonate and intra-hepatic gallstones.

Shing-Moo Huang, M.D., Ph.D., F.A.C.S.
Division of General Surgery, Department of Surgery,
Chung Shan Medical University Hospital, Taichung, Taiwan, Republic of China
Institute of Medicine, Chung Shan Medical University

Correspondence to be sent: Dr. Shing-Moo Huang,
3-2th floor, No. 76, Ren-Yee Street,
South District, Taichung city, 402 Taiwan,
Tel.: 886-4-22850527
Fax: 886-4-2406 9842.
E-mail: shingmooeel@yahoo.com.tw

Chapter I

Motor Dysfunction in Calculous Gallbladders

Abstract

Background: The aims of this study were to compare the gallbladder volume among gallstone patients with acute cholecystitis, chronic cholecystitis, contracted gallbladders and non-gallstone subjects and to compare the gallbladder ejection fractions between gallstone patients with chronic cholecystitis and normal subjects.

Materials and methods: Between October 1, 2007 and June 30, 2009, we measured fasting gallbladder volume from gallstone patients with acute cholecystitis ($N = 99$), chronic cholecystitis ($N = 85$) and non-gallstone subjects ($N = 240$) by computerized tomography. We measured the fasting and postprandial gallbladder volume of 65 patients with gallstones and chronic cholecystitis and 53 healthy subjects by abdominal ultrasonography. We then calculated the gallbladder ejection fractions.

Results: The average fasting gallbladder volume in gallstone patients with acute cholecystitis ($N = 99$), chronic cholecystitis ($N = 85$) and non-gallstone subjects ($N=240$) was 57.00 ± 41.20, $28.77 \pm 15.00cm^3$ and $16.77 \pm 15.75cm^3$, respectively. The average fasting gallbladder volume was larger in gallstone patients with acute cholecystitis than that in chronic cholecystitis ($P < .0001$). The fasting gallbladder was larger ($39.96\pm20.83cm^3$ vs. $23.30\pm12.88cm^3$, $P = .000$, 2.9E-9) and the average gallbladder ejection fraction was lower (34.6 ± 10.6 %, $N=65$, vs. 53.3 ± 24.9 %, $N=53$, $P < .0001$) in gallstone patients with chronic cholecystitis as compared to those in non-gallstone and normal subjects.

Conclusion: We find gallstone formations are associated with poorer gallbladder contractility and larger gallbladder volume in gallstone patients as compared to non-gallstone and normal subjects. Gallbladder volume increases as acute cholecystitis progresses and gallbladder decompression is mandatory to prevent gangrene and/or empyema.

I. The Pathophysiologic Significance of Gallbladder Volume - Changes in Gallstone Diseases [1]

Gallbladder volume (GBV) can reflect clinical and therapeutic implications, physiologic and functional status and possibly pathophysiologic mechanisms of gallstone diseases. In 1880, Courvoisier and Terrier's law stated that large painless, palpable gallbladder was mostly due to malignant obstruction of the bile duct. [2] In 1963, Maingot found tensely swollen, tenderly palpable gallbladder in acute cholecystitis was due to stone impaction in the cystic duct. [3] In 1989, Masclee noted in one third of patients with cholesterol gallstones increased gallbladder volume and delayed emptying were present at the postprandial phase. [4-6]. In 2000, Portincasa demonstrated in a comparative study that patients with cholesterol gallstones showed significantly larger fasting volume and postprandial volumes of gallbladders than controls and patients with pigment stones at each time point during a 2-hour study period. [7] He proposed that larger GBV predisposed to bile stasis.

However, the differences and changes of GBV among different age groups in non-gallstone subjects and their correlations with the formation of gallstones were not reported in the previous literature. Also, the correlations between GBV changes in different stages in the pathophysiologic development of acute cholecystitis in gallstone patients were not clear. Furthermore, we wished to investigate the possible reciprocal correlation between GBV and GB contractibility.

The aims of this study were to compare the gallbladder (GBV) among gallstone (GS) patients with acute cholecystitis, chronic cholecystitis, contracted gallbladders and non-gallstone subjects; also, to compare between GS patients with chronic cholecystitis and non-gallstone subjects in different age periods and with different genders. Furthermore, in order to investigate the correlations of GBV changes and the development of gallstones, we further investigated the differences of gallbladder (GB) contractility between GS patients with chronic cholecystitis and normal subjects.

Methods

Between October 1, 2007 and September 30, 2008, 99 gallstone (GS) patients with acute cholecystitis, 85 GS patients with chronic cholecystitis and 5 patients with contracted GB admitted to Chung Shan University Hospital undergoing cholecystectomy were recruited in this study.

Diagnostic Criteria

Acute cholecystitis. The clinical imaging findings of acute cholecystitis in ultrasonography of abdomen include thick gallbladder wall greater than 3 mm, stones present in gallbladder, distended GB with pericholecystic fluid and sonographic Murphy's sign with tenderness over the GB from the ultrasound transducer. The pathological features of acute cholecystitis include leukocytes infiltration throughout the tissues, local flattening and denuded mucosal folds and tissue edema. If untreated or treated late, localized region of necrosis (gangrene) or abscess formation (empyema) can be found.

Chronic cholecystitis. The pathological features of chronic cholecystitis include subserosal fibrous tissues, lymphocytes, plasma cells, macrophages found beneath the columnar epithelium and Rokitansky-Aschoff sinus in the muscular layer.

Contracted GB

Contracted gallbladders (GB) are known to result from long-standing chronic cholecystitis. Anatomic characteristics about contracted gallbladders include severe adhesions and complete coverage by greater momentum, severe pericholecyst fibrosis, thickening of gallbladder walls (usually thicker than 5 mm), loss of elasticity, obscure anatomy at triangle of Calot, dense adhesions to duodenum, transverse colon and common hepatic duct and small GBV (usually smaller than 10 ml.).

Non-gallstone controls. Next, we randomly chose 240 patients receiving abdominal CT examinations for non-gallstone reasons between July 1, 2008 and July 31, 2008 as non-gallstone controls.

Demographic data. The age, gender, associated diseases and previous operations undergone of all patients and normal subjects were recorded.

The procedures undergone, the preoperative CT GB diameters measurements, direct GB diameters measurements and direct saline-filling GBV measurements in patients of gallstones with acute and chronic cholecystitis were also recorded. So were the CT measurements of non-gallstone controls recorded. The GBV were calculated from GB lengths and short axis diameters by the equation shown below.

GBV measurements and calculations. We measured the lengths and short axis diameters of the fasting GB of these patients from their preoperative computerized tomography (CT) films, measured the lengths and short axis diameters directly after their removal in the operating room and recorded their lengths and short axi diameters measured by the pathologist postoperatively. We then calculated the GBV according to the equation:

GBV (cm^3) = $4/3 \times \pi \times r1 \times r2 \times r3/\cos\theta$, where r1, r2 and r3 represent the three greatest radii of the GB ellipsoid and θ is the angle between the z-axis of the gallbladder and the z-axis of the transverse cross sectional CT imaging.

We also measured directly the GBV after the gallbladders were removed. After withdrawing the GB bile with a syringe, the volume of normal saline injected into the intact gallbladders was added to the volume of GB stones measured after opening of the GB walls. Comparing the GBV obtained by direct measurement and calculations of the various techniques, correction factors for different measuring methods were obtained to modify the calculated GBV, thus minimizing the measurement bias.

Rationale for GBV equation [8]

The gallbladder is a pear-shaped organ located under the liver that stores bile. It can be approximated to an ellipsoid. The volume of an ellipsoid can be obtained as follows: [9]

Claim Area for ellipse is π r1 r2 : Given an ellipse $x^2/r1^2 + x^2/r2^2 = 1$

Since an ellipse is symmetric to x-axis and y-axis,

Area $= 4\int_0^{r1} r2(\sqrt{1- x^2/r1^2})\, dx = 4r2/r1\int_0^{r1}(\sqrt{r1^2- x^2})\, dx$

(Let $x = r1\mathrm{Sin}\theta$, then $dx = r1\mathrm{Cos}\theta d\theta$, where $-\pi/2 \leqq \theta \leqq \pi/2$)

$= 4r2/r1\int_0^{\pi/2}(\sqrt{r1^2- r1^2\sin^2\theta})\, r1\cos\theta d\theta = 4r1r2\int_0^{\pi/2}\cos^2\theta d\theta$

$= 4r1r2\int_0^{\pi/2}1/2(1 + \cos 2\theta)d\theta = 2\, r1r2\, [\theta+1/2\sin^2\theta]_0^{\pi/2} = \pi\, r1r2$

=> For a slice of ellipse of the ellipsoid parallel to the yz-plane, the radius parallel to the z-axis is $g(z) = r1(\sqrt{1 - z^2/r3^2})$

Similarly, its radius parallel to the y-axis is $h(z) = r2(\sqrt{1 - z^2/r3^2})$

Thus, the volume V of the ellipsoid $= \int_{-r3}^{r3}\pi\, g(z)\, h(z)dz$

$= \int_{-r3}^{r3}\pi\, r1(\sqrt{1 - z^2/r3^2})\, r2(\sqrt{1 - z^2/r3^2})dz$

$=\pi\, r1\, r2\int_{-r3}^{r3}(1 - z^2/r3^2)\, dz =\pi\, r1\, r2\, [z - z^3/3r3^2]_{-r3}^{r3}$

$= 4/3\pi\, r1r2r3$ #

Correction factors for GBV

θ. Since the gallbladder does not always lie in the same plane on, the measured GBV is corrected by multiplying a correction factor 1/cos θ, where θ is the angle between the z-axis of the gallbladder and the z-axis of the transverse cross sectional CT imaging and 0 degree ≦θ < 90 degrees.

c = 0.82 ± 0.40 (N = 65)

: CT measurement correction factor = $\dfrac{\text{Direct measurement calculated GBV}}{\text{CT measurement calculated GBV}}$

p = 0.85 ± 0.42 (N = 65)

Pathology measurement correction factor = $\dfrac{\text{Pathology measurement calculated GBV}}{\text{Direct measurement calculated GBV}}$

s = 0.88 ± 0.36 (N = 65):

Sueh-Ding correction factor = $\dfrac{\text{Direct injection measurement GBV}}{\text{Direct measurement calculated GBV}}$

Direct measurement GBV = (s, Sueh-Ding correction factor) Direct measurement calculated GBV x 0.88

u = 0.90 (N = 65):

$$\text{US measurement correction factor} = \frac{\text{Direct measurement calculated GBV}}{\text{US measurement calculated GBV}}$$

US: ultrasound

Direct injection measurement
GBV = Direct measurement calculated GBV x s
= CT measurement calculated GBV x cs (cs = 0.72= 0.82 x 0.88)
= US measurement calculated GBV x us (us = 0.79 = 0.9 x 0.88)

Sub study on gallbladder contractility

In order to investigate and compare the GB contractility between patients with gallstones and chronic cholecystitis and normal subjects to investigate the possible reciprocal correlation between GBV and GB contractibility, the authors designed and conducted a subsequent second study. Between October 1, 2008 and June 30, 2009, the authors measured the fasting and postprandial GBV of 65 patients with gallstone and chronic cholecystitis and 53 healthy subjects by abdominal ultrasonography.

Study protocol. Subjects came to the hospital after an overnight fast. They were reminded the night before the study not to eat or drink after supper. Their adherence to this instruction was confirmed by means of a history. Gallbladder size was determined in the fasting state. The subjects then drank a standard liquid meal with a total 420 kcal – 30% as fat, 15% as protein, and the rest as carbohydrate. The postprandial GB size was measured and the GBV calculated 90 minutes after the meal.

Ultrasound Technique

The abdominal sonography was performed by the same investigator (S.M.H.) with techniques modified from the literature [10.5] The hand-held transducer was placed in a sagittal longitudinal projection in the right-upper quadrant and rotated until the largest longitudinal dimension of the gallbladder was obtained on the oscilloscope screen. Then image was frozen, measured by electronic calipers and photographed. The transducer was then rotated 90 degrees and the largest short axis through the gallbladder was obtained. Occasionally deep inspiration was required but all patients were successfully examined. We used three dimensions – length, lateral and antero-posterior diameters to calculate the GBV and modified empirically as the above descriptions.

The ejection fractions (EF) of the GB were calculated by the following equation:

$$\text{EF (\%)} = \frac{\text{Fasting GBV (ml.) - Postprandial GBV (ml.)}}{\text{Fasting GBV (ml.)}} \times 100$$

Statistics. We compared the GBV measurements and patient age with Student's unpaired *t*-test and use Chi square test to compare the gender differences. $P < .05$ is considered statistically significant.

Results

Demographic Data

We found male predominance in acute cholecystitis group and female predominance in chronic cholecystitis group: M/F = 53/46 and 32/53 respectively ($P = .04$ by Chi square test). There was no gender difference between patients in the chronic cholecystitis group and the non-gallstone group (M/F = 32/53 vs. 117/123. $P = .10$).

There was no age difference among patients in the acute cholecystitis group, the chronic cholecystitis group and the non-gallstone group (57 ± 17 years, 53 ± 15 years and 54 ± 18 years, $P = .09$ and .64, respectively).

Associated diseases and previous operations undergone of all patients and normal subjects included cerebral vascular accident (3), diabetes mellitus (4), pneumonia (1), hyperlipidemia (1), hypertensive cardiovascular diseases (5), s/p exploratory laparotomy (2) and coronary artery disease (5) in the GS with acute cholecystitis group; diabetes mellitus (5) and manic-depressive psychosis (1) and s/p gastrectomy/vagotomy (2) in the GS with chronic cholecystitis group; and liver tumor (2), liver cysts (5), diabetes mellitus (9), hypertensive cardiovascular diseases (10) and s/p exploratory laparotomy (5) in the non-gallstone group.

The fasting GBV in GS patients with acute cholecystitis (N = 99), chronic cholecystitis (N = 85) , contracted GB (N = 5) and non-gallstone subjects (N = 240) was 57.00 ± 41.20 cm^3, 28.77 ± 15.00cm^3, 6.15 ± 2.52 cm^3 and 16.77 ± 15.75cm^3, respectively (Figure 1.1.1, Table 1.1.1). The average fasting GBV was larger in GS patients with acute cholecystitis than that in chronic cholecystitis (P < .0001). In turn, the average fasting GBV was larger in GS patients with chronic cholecystitis than that in non-gallstone subjects (P < .0001) (Figure 1.1.2).

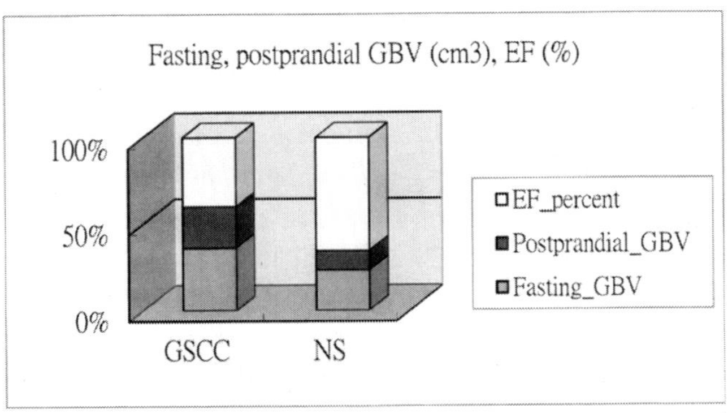

Figure 1.1.1. Histogram of the mean fasting, postprandial gallbladder volume and ejection fraction in gallstone patients with chronic cholecystitis and normal subjects, measured by abdominal ultrasonography. GBV: Gallbladder volume; EF: Ejection fraction; GSCC: Gallstones with chronic cholecystitis; NS: Non-stone.

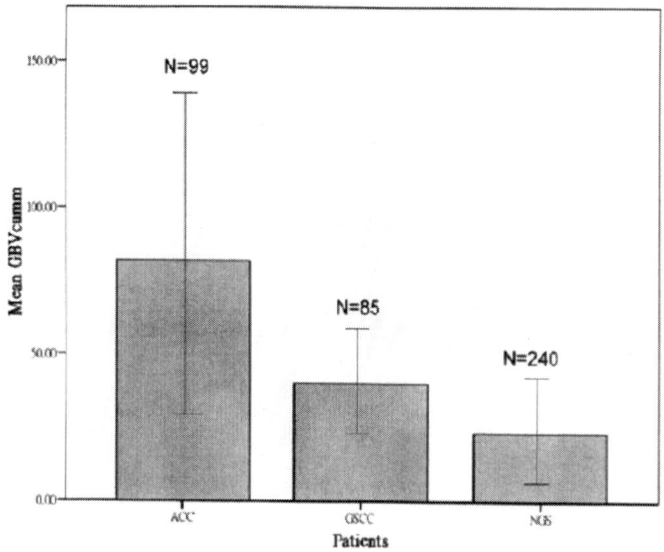

Figure 1.1.2. Histograms of gallbladder volume (mean and standard deviation, cm^3) in gallstone patients with acute cholecystitis, chronic cholecystitis and non-gallstone patients. *P*-value between acute and chronic cholecystitis: < .0001. *P*-value between chronic cholecystitis and non-gallstone patients: < .0001. GBV: gallbladder volume.

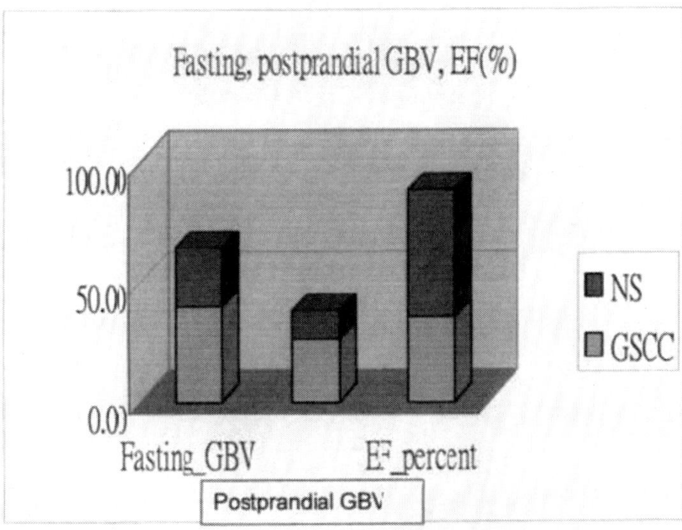

Figure 1.1.3. The histogram of the mean fasting, postprandial GBV and EF in GS patients with chronic cholecystitis and normal subjects measured by abdominal ultrasonography. GBV: gallbladder volume, EF: ejections, GS: gallstone.

In non-gallstone subjects, there was significant differences in the fasting GBV between two age groups, i.e., Age ≦ 20 vs. 20 <Age≦40 (6.33 ± 2.75 cm^3, N=9 vs. 16.84 ± 4.04 cm^3, N=35, *P*=.0070) and 40 <Age≦60 vs. 60 <Age≦80. (15.12 ± 7.55 cm^3, N=106 vs. 19.83 ± 9.99 cm^3, N=81, *P* < .0003) (Table 1.1.2). The fasting GBV had a tendency to increase with age. In compatibility with this tendency, the occurrence of gallstone with chronic cholecystitis also increase with age (*P* = .0027 by Fisher's exact test, Table 1.1.2).

There was no gender difference in the fasting GBV (M vs. F = 16.35 ± 8.56 cm^3, N = 113 vs. 17.14 ± 9.93 cm^3, N=127, *P* = .53).

Table 1.1.1. Demographic data and GBV in GS patients with acute, chronic cholecystitis, contracted GB and non-gallstone subjects

Variables Diagnosis	M/F	Mean age (years)	Mean GBV (cm3)(N)	Standard deviation (cm3)	*P-value* *(95% CI†)*
Acute Cholecystitis	53/46	*** 57±17	57.00 (99)	41.20	.0004 * (7.73 to 26.35)
Chronic Cholecystitis	32/53	53±15	28.77 (85)	15.00	< .0001 ** (8.14 to 15.86)
Contracted GB	1/4	44±21	6.15 (5)	2.52	
Non-gallstone	39/41	54±18 (240)	16.77 (240)	15.75	

P-values *: between GBV of acute and chronic cholecystitis,
**: between chronic cholecystitis and non-gallstone subjects,
*** :between gender of acute and chronic cholecystitis, = .04. †: 95% confidence internal of GBV difference. GBV: gallbladder volume. GS: gallstone, GBV: gallbladder volume, GS: gallstone.

Table 1.1.2. Demographic data and GBV in GS patients with acute, chronic cholecystitis, contracted GB and non-gallstone subjects

Variables Diagosis	Mean age (years)	Mean GBV (cm3)(N)	Standard deviation (cm3)	*P-value* *(95% CI†)*
Age ≦ 20	0	6.33 (9)	275	.007 **
20 <Age≦40	15	16.84(35)	11.04	.30
40<Age≦60	42.5	15.12 (106)	7.55	.0003***
60 <Age≦80	42.5	19.83 (81)	9.99	.76
80 <Age	0	18.73 (9)	10.32	

P-values *: = .0027 by Fisher's exact test, **:between Age ≦ 20 and 20 <Age≦40 ***: between 40 <Age≦60 and 60 <Age≦80, GBV: gallbladder volume.

In the second sub study, there was no gender or age difference (M/F: 24/41 vs. 25/27, *P = .20) (52 ± 15 years, N=65 vs. 54 ± 18 years, N=53, P = .51)*. The average fasting GBV in patients with gallstone and chronic cholecystitis was 31.44 ± 16.46 cm^3 and the average postprandial GB volume was 20.50 ± 6.20cm^3. The average GB ejection fraction of patients with gallstone and chronic cholecystitis was 34.6 ± 10.6 % (N=65) . The average fasting GBV in normal subjects was 19.22 ± 11.30cm^3 and the average postprandial GBV in normal subjects was 9.03 ± 3.63 cm^3. The average EF of normal subjects GB was 53.3 ±24.9 % (N=53). The differences in the average fasting, postprandial GBV and ejection fractions were statistically significant (all three *P's were* < .0001) (Figure 1.1.3, Table 1.1.3).

So were the differences of GBV between fasting and postprandial states in patients with gallstone and chronic cholecystitis and normal subjects statistically significant (all two *P's were* < .0001).

Table 1.1.3. The mean fasting, postprandial GBV and EF in GS patients with chronic cholecystitis and normal objects measured by abdominal ultrasonography

Variables	fasting mean GBV±SD (cm3)(N)	postprandial mean GBV±SD (cm3)(N)	EF±SD (%)(N)
GS with			
Chronic	31.34±16.46†	20.50±6.20 †	34.6±10.6
Cholecystitis	(65)	(65)	(65)
Normal subjects	19.24±11.30‡	9.03±3.63‡	53.3±24.9
	(53)	(53)	(53)
P-value	< .0001*	< .0001**	< .0001***
(95%CI)	(6.93 to 17.47)	(9.56 to 13.48)	(11.9 to 25.5)

P-values *: between fasting GBV of chronic cholecystitis and normal subjects, **: between postprandial GBV of chronic cholecystitis and normal subjects, ***: between ejection fractions of chronic cholecystitis and normal subjects, † *P*-Value < .0001, 95%CI: 6.62 to 15.26, ‡ *P*-Value < .0001, 95%CI: 6.98 to 13.44, CI: confidence interval, GBV: gallbladder volume. GS: gallstone, SD: standard deviation, EF: ejection fraction.

Discussion

Male predominance in acute cholecystitis group might suggest higher threshold for pain in male patients, resulting in delayed treatment.

Our study shows the fasting GBV grows in two age periods in the life of non-gallstone subjects, i.e., from age 20 to 40 years and 60 to 80 years, especially the former period. In compatibility with this, the occurrence of gallstone with chronic cholecystitis reaches its plateau between 40 and 80 years of age (from 15% to 42.5% in gallstone patients before 40 to after 40 years of age, $P = .0027$, Table 1.1.2).

Gallbladder is a hollow visceral elastic organ. Its actual maximal fasting volume under *in vivo* physiologic condition is difficult to measure. Measuring methods include *in vivo* ultrasonography, nuclear scintigraphy, computerized tomography and *in vitro* post-cholecystectomy saline-filling measurement. HIDA-scan scintigraphy is seldom used clinically except to demonstrate cystic duct obstruction in acute cholecystitis patients, due to its isotope radioactivity. On the other hand, *in vitro* post-cholecystectomy saline-filling measurement is the most accurate gold standard for measuring GBV. In contrast, abdominal ultrasonography is the most convenient examination for obtaining the measurements of GBV, although the accuracy and precision, most of the time, depends greatly on individual experiences of the operator. CT represent more uniform, constantly used and easier methods as diagnostic tool for GS diseases and for measuring the GBV. These are the reasons why the authors adopted abdominal ultrasonography, CT and *in vitro* post-cholecystectomy saline-filling measurement in the present study.

GBV can reflect clinical and therapeutic implications, physiologic and functional status and possibly pathophysiologic mechanisms of gallstone diseases. The clinical and therapeutic implications of increased GBV in malignant obstruction of the bile duct and cystic duct obstruction in acute calculous cholecystitis lie in their different aetiology. In malignant obstruction of the bile duct the obstruction was insidious and slow as the tumor grows. By the time the painless jaundice appears, a non-tender dilated GB is usually palpable over the patient's right upper quadrant abdomen and percutaneous transhepatic cholangiographic drainage (PTCD) is usually required before surgery is planned. In contrast, in the case of acute calculous cholecystitis, the dilatation of GB is due to stone trapped in the spiral valve of Heist causing obstruction of the cystic duct. The onset of painful dilatation of the GB is acute as caused by the stone irritating the GB mucosa and the pressure exerted by the dilated GB on the visceral nerve endings distributed over the entire GB wall. Early dilatation of the GB due to undrained mucus secretions also predispose to compromised local blood circulation to the mucosa and the GB wall, leading to impaired mucosa physiologic function of absorbing water and electrolytes which further aggravates the GB dilatation, reaching usually up to 3.4 fold of normal GB volume. The vicious cycle coupled with chemical irritation by lysozyme, cytokines and chemokines sometimes causes gangrene and/or perforation in about 15 % and 1.5% of acute calculous cholecystitis respectively.[3] When combined with the presence or absence of bile duct dilatation, GB dilatation can reflect the location of lesions and level of obstruction. In other words, if bile duct and GB are both dilated, the lesion site of obstruction probably lies below the insertion of cystic duct into the CBD. When the bile duct is dilated but not the GB, the obstructive lesion may well lie above the cystic duct insertion.

In our study, the fasting GBV was largest in GS patients with acute cholecystitis (Table 1.1.1) implicating the need for preoperative or intraoperative drainage/aspiration for decompressions for local GB wall necrosis (gangrene), abscess and even perforations are associated with further increase in GBV (Table 1.1.4). It is possible that GB decompressions might prevent gangrene/ empyema, perforation and make it easier to manipulate the GB during cholecystectomy.

Table 1.1.4. Comparison of GBV between acute cholecystitis only group and gangrene (or abscess) group

Variables	GBV±SD	*P-value (95% CI*
GS patients	(cm3)(N)	
Acute Cholecystitis Only	53.19±33.80 (87)	.002 (12.28 to 52.66)
Gangrene (or abscess)	84.66±26.32 (12)	

P-values *: between GBV of GS patients with acute cholecystitis only and with GS patients with acute cholecystitis and gangrene (or abscess), CI: confidence interval, GBV: gallbladder volume. GS: gallstone, SD: standard deviation.

Contracted gallbladders are known to result from long-standing chronic cholecystitis and have the smallest GBV in this study. Anatomic characteristics of contracted gallbladders include severe adhesions, severe pericholecyst fibrosis, thickening of gallbladder walls (usual thicker than 5 mm) and loss of elasticity, obscure anatomy at triangle of Calot. These characteristics make them difficult challenges when performing a safe laparoscopic cholecystectomy.

The fasting GBV was larger in GS patients with chronic cholecystitis than that in non-gallstone subjects (28.77 ± 15.00 cm^3 , N = 85 vs. 16.77 ± 15.75, N =240, *P* < .0001), indicating possible pathophysiologic mechanisms of weaker GB contractility in GS patients with chronic cholecystitis confirmed in our second study. In 2000, Portincasa proposed that larger gallbladder volume predisposed to bile stasis [7].

Weaker GB contractility in GS patients with chronic cholecystitis might provide a suitable micro-milieu for cholesterol monohydrate micro-crystals to grow into larger gallbladder stones by preventing them to be expelled from the gallbladder lumen when gallbladder contracts in response to cholecystokinin secreted from duodenum I cells stimulated by proteins and lipids in ingested food [10].

The gallbladder performs many physiologic functions, namely absorption and secretion of water and electrolytes, control of the content and concentration of bile [11-13].

In our second study, the authors measured fasting and postprandial GBV of 65 patients with gallstone and chronic cholecystitis and 53 healthy subjects by abdominal ultrasonography and calculated the GB ejection fractions of patients with gallstone and chronic cholecystitis and healthy subjects. The average GB EF of patients with gallstone and chronic cholecystitis was lower than that of the healthy subjects (34.6±10.6 %, N=65 vs. 53.3±24.9 %, N=53). The difference in the EF was statistically significant (*P* < .0001).

The developmental stages of acute cholecystitis. From our observations on the GBV changes during the development of acute cholecystitis from chronic inflammatory state, we hypothesize that there are three stages for acute cholecystitis based on GBV changes and pathologic changes. These correspond to the three stages of severity of acute cholecystitis proposed by Miura et al. [13] at the *Tokyo International Consensus Meeting* in 2007. In the early clinical stage of acute cholecystitis, which correspond to the mild (grade I) severity in the Tokyo consensus meeting, the mechanical effect of cystic duct obstruction causes increase in GBV (from averaging 28.77 ± 15.00 ml, N = 85. to 54.16 ± 35.17 ml., N = 44, *P* < .0001). No acute inflammatory leukocytes infiltrations but chronic inflammatory reactions like presence of subserosal fibrous tissues, lymphocytes, plasma cells, macrophages infiltraions beneath the columnar epithelium and Rokitansky-Aschoff sinus in the muscular layer are present as revealed by pathological examinations. It comprised about 44.4% (44/99). Early laparoscopic cholecystectomy is suggested by the Tokyo guidelines.. In the second stage of development, corresponding to the moderate severity (grade II) stage of the Tokyo guidelines, the GBV does not change significantly (52.20 ±32.40 ml., N = 43 vs. 54.16 ± 35.17 ml., N = 44, *P* = .79). However, pathologic findings of acute immunoreactive and inflammatory responses appear in the GB sections. These include leukocytes infiltration throughout the tissues, local flattening and denuded mucosal folds and tissue edema. It comprised about 43.4% (43/99). Early laparoscopic or open cholecystectomy is suggested by the Tokyo guidelines. If a patient has serious local inflammation making early cholecystectomy difficult, then percutaneous or operative drainage of the gallbladder is recommended. Elective cholecystectomy can be performed after improvement of the acute inflammatory process. If the condition goes untreated or unresolved, the late complicated stage ensues. which corresponds to the severe *(grade III)* organ dysfunction stage of the Tokyo guidelines.

In this stage, GBV further increases (84.66 ± 26.32 ml., N = 12, vs. 53.19 ± 33.80 ml., N = 87, *P* = .002, Table 1.1.4). Besides the pathologic findings of acute immunoreactive and inflammatory responses, local GB wall necrosis (gangrene), abscess and even perforations occur. Organ dysfunctions appear. It comprised about 12.2% (12/99). Appropriate organ support in addition to medical treatments necessary for patients with organ dysfunction as suggested by the Tokyo guidelines Management of severe local inflammation by percutaneous gallbladder drainage and/or cholecystectomy is needed. Biliary peritonitis due to perforation of the gallbladder is an indication for urgent cholecystectomy and drainage. Elective cholecystectomy may be performed after improvement of the acute illness by gallbladder drainage [14].

In our study, the GS patients with chronic cholecystitis had either cholesterol or pigment stones, which comprises 42.9% and 36.8%, respectively from our previous study. [15] Among them, 77.6% (66/85) of the patients had GBV larger than the average non-gallstone GBV, while 43.5% (37/85) had GBV larger than the average GS patients with chronic cholecystitis group GBV. The proportion of increased gallbladder volume is higher than that reported by Masclee. There is a likelihood that patients with pigment GB stones have a higher proportion of increased gallbladder volume and weaker GB contractility.

Zhu found the amount of GB cholecystokinin (CCK) receptor is lower in patients with gallstones who have poor gallbladder contraction. [16] Choi found that FGF15 knockout mice displayed a GB completely devoid of bile and administration of recombinant FGF15 or FGF19 restored the GBV. [9, 17] Whether GS patients with poor GB contraction and increased GBV have lower amount of GB CCK receptor and/or lower FGF 19 gene expression is worth future investigation.

There is a limitation to this study, i.e., the GS patients were not sub grouped into cholesterol and pigment stones. Therefore, the findings of Msclee(4-6) and Portincasa(7) could not be investigated in this study.

In conclusions, we find gallstone formations are associated with poorer gallbladder contractility and larger fasting and postprandial gallbladder volume with lower gallbladder ejection fractions in gallstone patients as compared with those in non-gallstone and normal subjects. Also, gallbladder volume increases as acute cholecystitis progresses and gallbladder decompression is mandatory to prevent gangrene and/or empyema.

II. Coordinate Regulation of Gallbladder Motor Function in the Gut-Liver Axis [9]

Gallstones are one of the most common digestive diseases with an estimated prevalence of 10%-15% in adults living in the western world, where cholesterol-enriched gallstones represent 75%-80% of all gallstones. In cholesterol gallstone disease, the gallbladder becomes the target organ of a complex metabolic disease. Indeed, a fine coordinated hepatobiliary and gastrointestinal function, including gallbladder motility in the fasting and postprandial state, is of crucial importance to prevent crystallization and precipitation of excess cholesterol in gallbladder bile. Also, gallbladder itself plays a physiopathological role in biliary lipid absorption. Portincassa et al. present a comprehensive view on the regulation of gallbladder motor function by focusing on recent discoveries in animal and human studies, and discuss the role of the gallbladder in the pathogenesis of gallstone formation.

Gallstones are one the most common gastrointestinal diseases that require hospitalization in the western world as reported by Everhart et al., [18] and this is a true health burden as suggested by Sandler and Portincassa et al. [14, 19, 20] with enormous costs estimated at 6.5 billion dollars each year in United States reported by Sandler and Shaffer et al. [20, 21] Because life expectancy and the incidence rate of obesity are both rising worldwide reported by Haslam et al., [22] the incidence rate of gallstones may increase, often in the context of the "metabolic syndrome" proposed by Grundy [23] The estimated prevalence of gallstones is 10%-15% in the general population of developed countries. In the United States, approximately 20 million to 25 million adults have gallstones. The burden of the disease is highest (60%- 70%) in American Indians followed by Hispanics of mixed Indian origin. In contrast, the rate is lowest (less than 5%) in Asian and African populations as reported by Shaffer. [21] The prevalence is intermediate (10%-15%) in Caucasians in developed countries. In Europe, the Multicenter Italian Study on Cholelithiasis (MICOL) ultrasonographic survey, which was performed across Italy including 29,000 subjects aged 30-69 years, reported an overall prevalence rate of 18.8% and 9.5% in women and men, respectively reported by Attili et al. [24] Major risk factors for the development of gallstones have been better identified over the past years and include age, female sex, some genetic polymorphisms within a background of a complex genetic disorder, pregnancy, obesity and rapid weight loss on low caloric diets or following bariatric surgery, delayed small intestine transit time, liver cirrhosis, hemolytic anemia, increased serum triglycerides, metabolic syndrome, terminal ileal resection, reduced physical activity, and some medications (for example, estrogens and oral contraceptives, octreotide, clofibrate, and ceftriaxone) as reported by Everhart, Shaffer, Stolk and van Erpectum et al. [18, 21, 25, 26]. The gallbladder is deemed as the end-organ of gallstone disease, and a defective gallbladder motility has been strongly linked to the formation of gallstones and particularly of cholesterol-enriched stones (approximately 75%-80% of all gallstones in Western countries) reported by Sherlock and Portincassa et al. [12, 27] Abnormal gallbladder motility has been documented in humans in both the fasting and postprandial state as recorded by Greaves and Niebergall-Roth et al. [28, 29]. Additionally, an abnormal gallbladder motor function has also been reported in subjects at high risk of gallstone formation (total parenteral nutrition, very low calorie dieting, treatment with somatostatin analogs). As a consequence, the pathophysiology of gallbladder motility is seen with growing interest, where a complex interplay exists between factors involving the content of the gallbladder lumen, the intrinsic ability of the gallbladder smooth muscle to contract, and extrinsic neurohormonal factors. Recently, major new developments have been obtained concerning the molecular mechanisms driving gallbladder dynamics. Of note, the identification of fibroblast growth factor 19 (FGF19) as the hormonal signal responsible for gallbladder distension represents a formidable step forward in the understanding of gallbladder modulation in the context of the gut-liver axis identified by Choi. [17] The exploitation of these innovative theoretical attainments is just beginning, with potential implications for future pharmacological approaches. This review will offer the most recent insights into the mechanisms implicated in the regulation of gallbladder motor function and in the pathogenesis of gallbladder dysmotility by focusing on both basic and clinical aspects. Features concerning the clinical setting, *in vitro* studies, and the role of luminal, parietal, and neurohormonal factors will be highlighted.

Physiology and Pathophysiology of Gallbladder Contraction

In the interdigestive phase, bile is stored and concentrated in the gallbladder before being actively expelled in the duodenum in response to food intake. In the intestine, bile plays a key role in lipid digestion and absorption. Because of the importance of timely bile delivery in the intestine for the physiology of the digestive system, both interprandial and postprandial gallbladder motility are regulated by complex mechanisms involving the interplay of neural, humoral, and paracrine factors as found by Pauletzki and Portincassa et al. [7, 30] These mechanisms participate in the multiorgan regulatory function operating between intestine and liver, which defines the gutliver axis. Several substances and receptors as suggested by Otsuki [31] mediating either contraction or relaxation of the gallbladder are involved in this complex scenario. In patients developing cholesterol gallstones, a disrupted interdigestive gallbladder emptying is present due to a poor integration with the intestinal migrating motor complexes reported by Stolk et al. [28] Also, in the postprandial phase, increased gallbladder volume and delayed emptying have been documented in about one-third of patients with cholesterol stones by Greaves and Stolk et al. [4-6, 29, 32] Although the presence of cholesterol-supersaturated bile is considered the *primum movens* of cholesterol gallstone disease, alterations of gallbladder motility, which often anticipate the formation of cholesterol gallstones, favors the formation and growth of stones by multiple, interconnected mechanisms. Impaired gallbladder emptying prolongs the residence time of concentrated gallbladder bile, with the result that more time is available for nucleation and crystallization of cholesterol crystals from supersaturated hepatic bile, and less cholesterol crystals can be ejected into the duodenum. Among humoral factors, the most relevant impact for gallbladder contraction and relaxation is currently attributed to cholecystokinin and the recently identified FGF19, respectively.

Cholecystokinin

Cholecystokinin (CCK) is one of the most important circulating gastrointestinal hormones involved in gallbladder motility first reported by Maselli et al. [33] In healthy subjects, the ingestion of a standard fat-containing meal induces gallbladder emptying up to 80% of the fasting gallbladder volume by stimulating CCK secretion from the duodenal I cells. CCK influences gallbladder muscular tone mainly in the postprandial state suggested by Portincassa and van Berge-Henegouwen, [34] principally through specific CCK-1 receptors proposed by Portincassa et al., [35] by a complex mechanism leading to smooth muscle contraction and relaxation elucidated by Schneider and Upp et al. [36, 37] *In vitro* evidence suggests that changes of CCK-receptor number/ expression and of processes governing signal transduction play a key role in the determination of the motility dysfunction observed *in vivo* reported by Wang and Miyasaki et al. [38, 39] In a recent integrated *in vivo* and *in vitro* study, it was shown that the amount of gallbladder CCK receptor is lower in patients with gallstones who have poor gallbladder contraction compared with that in both healthy subjects or a subgroup of patients with gallstones who have well-contracting gallbladders. Moreover, gallbladder ejection fraction has been positively correlated with the density of CCK receptors on gallbladder smooth muscle cells by Choi et al. [16] Further, it has been demonstrated that, whether on chow or a lithogenic diet, mice with deletion of CCK-1 receptor (*Cck-1r*) present larger gallbladder volumes (predisposing to bile stasis), significant retardation of small intestinal transit times (resulting in increased cholesterol absorption), and increased biliary cholesterol secretion rates by Ding et al. [40] This scenario facilitates nucleation, growth, and agglomeration of cholesterol monohydrate crystals. In fact, these sequences of events result in a significantly higher prevalence of cholesterol gallstones in the CCK-1 receptor knockout mice. Interestingly, it has been found that some polymorphisms in the CCK-1R gene are associated with gallstone formation in humans by Grundy. [41] Interestingly, a recent observation suggests that density of CCK-1 receptors on gallbladder smooth muscle cells is significantly decreased in patients with the combination of gallstones and diabetes mellitus compared to those with only gallstones by Inagaki et al, [42] thus underlining the possibility that cholesterol gallstone disease is an associated condition of the metabolic syndrome, which is studied by Afdhal. [23]

Fibroblast Growth Factor 19

It has been recently shown that in response to bile acid, the distal small intestine secretes FGF15 in mice (human ortholog FGF19), a hormone required for gallbladder filling. As identified by Coi [17] The role of FGF19 in the endocrine regulation of the gut-liver axis was first identified in the regulation of hepatic bile acid synthesis in response to intestinal bile acid concentrations as found by Inagaki et al. [43] After being actively absorbed in the distal ileum, bile acids activate the nuclear receptor farnesoid X receptor (FXR) as reported by Modica et al., [44] which in turn promotes the expression of FGF19. FGF19 is a circulating hormone, secreted in the portal circulation and active in the liver, where it binds to FGF receptor 4 (FGFR4), and ignites a metabolic cascade which results in inhibited bile acid synthesis. The effect is mediated by the atypical nuclear receptor small heterodimer partner (SHP), which inhibits gene expression of 7α-hydroxylase (CYP7A), the rate-limiting enzyme for bile acid synthesis s reported by Goodwin and Lu et al. [45, 46] Compelling new evidence now extends the physiological role of FGF19 in the gut-liver axis to include endocrine control of gallbladder motility. FGF15 knockout mice display a gallbladder completely devoid of bile, in the absence of any impairment of gallbladder histology, bile flow, and interprandial or postprandial CCK release. In parallel, administration of recombinant FGF15 or FGF19 doubles gallbladder volume of wild-type mice, and restores gallbladder volume in FGF15 knockout mice at levels just as high as that of the wild-type. Although the mechanism for this effect is not completely solved, the relaxation induced by FGF15/FGF19 is likely dependent on increased production of cyclic adenosine monophosphate (cAMP), which antagonizes the effect of CCK. The ability of FGF15/FGF19 to actively mediate gallbladder relaxation is conserved in FGFR4 knockout mice. Apparently, this receptor does not mediate the effects of FGF15/FGF19 on the gallbladder reported by Choi et al. [17] Gene expression profiling demonstrates high levels of FGFR3 in the gallbladder, thus suggesting this receptor as the top candidate to mediate the effects of FGF19 also reported by Choi et al. [17] Further, the identification of different isoforms of FGFRs in additional anatomical districts of the enterohepatic system (that is, bile duct and the sphincter of Oddi) holds the promise for new exciting discoveries on the role of FGF19 in the endocrine regulation of digestive physiology. Also, Portincassa et al. believe that the tissue specificity for different receptors of the same hormone might be of future pharmacological relevance. These studies demonstrate that gallbladder filling is actively regulated by an endocrine pathway and suggest a postprandial timing mechanism that controls gallbladder motility. After the ingestion of a meal, CCK secretion would induce gallbladder contraction and provide the adequate concentration of duodenal amphipathic bile acids, which directly contribute to solubilization and absorption of cholesterol, fat, and fat-soluble vitamins. Once bile acids arrive at the terminal ileum, they regulate the FXR-induced production and the secretion of FGF15 (or the human ortholog FGF19), which now signals back to the gallbladder in order to guide its refilling and prepare the target organ for the next meal. Future studies are needed to clarify if this regulatory network would also act as the ileal brake of the digestion, possibly ending postprandial pancreatic secretion and regulating gastric emptying.

Neuronal Control

Apart from humoral factors, gallbladder motility is under control of neuronal stimuli. The gallbladder is innervated by both sympathetic and parasympathetic (vagal) terminations reaching the smooth muscle and interconnecting with noradrenergic nerve cells. Ganglia, connected with both sympathetic and parasympathetic terminations, are distributed throughout the three layers of the gallbladder tissues (subserosal, myenteric, and mucosal plexuses) and provide intrinsic innervations as elucidated by Sutherland. [47] Ganglia represent the site of complex modulatory interactions influencing muscle and epithelial cell function as demonstrated by Mawe et al. [48] CCK may also be active presynaptically within ganglia to increase acetylcholine release from vagal terminals also found by Mawe et al. [48] During fasting and in the early postprandial phase, gallbladder motility is also under the control of neural cholinergic pathways mediated by muscarinic receptors reported by Stengel and Yegen et al., [49, 50] which, if stimulated, invariably involve myosin light-chain phosphorylation reported by Parkman et al. [51] Because neural pathways also govern gallbladder motility, the presence of autonomic neuropathy might affect gallbladder motor function in several conditions and be a further factor predisposing an individual to gallstone formation. In diabetic patients, a link between autonomic neuropathy and impaired gallbladder motility has been suggested as suggested by Shaw, Palasciano, Burgstaller and others. [52-59] Patients with chronic functional constipation as suggested by Altomare et al.., [60] and gastrointestinal motility is defective at various levels, including at the gallbladder as indicated by Altomare et al. (61) A pathophysiological link between autonomic neuropathy and gallbladder motility has also been observed in patients with chronic alcohol abuse reported by Wedmann et al. (62) or chronic liver diseases reported by Chaudhry and Oliver et al. [63, 64] It has been proposed that autonomic neuropathy contributes to (pigment) gallstone formation in patients with advanced liver cirrhosis (Child class C), who indeed show a high prevalence of both gallstone disease and autonomic neuropathy as reported by Chawla et al. [65] Also, in a recent study from Portincassa et al.'s group, 86% of adult patients with thalassemia major had abnormal tests of sympathetic and parasympathetic system and, in these subjects, positive tests for autonomic neuropathy tended to correlate with abnormal gallbladder motility reported by Portincassa et al. [66]

Conditions Associated with Impaired Gallbladder Motility

Impaired gallbladder motor function has been also documented as a complication in a number of diseases. Such conditions include patients who develop pigment gallstones as suggested by Carey and Trotman et al. [67, 68] as a consequence of chronic hemolysis, that is, sickle hemoglobinopathy as reported by Everson et al., [69] and adults with liver cirrhosis as suggested by Attili, Li and Pompili et al. [70-72] and α-thalassemia major reported by Portincassa et al. (66) Patients with nonhemolytic black pigment stones may also exhibit some degree of gallbladder motility defects, although these are less, compared with patients with cholesterol stones as reported by Portincassa et al. [7] Other conditions can be found as part of the so-called "metabolic syndrome" as reported by Grundy, [23] inflammatory bowel diseases or celiac disease, spinal cord injury, total parenteral nutrition, and gastrectomy. Certain medications can worsen gallbladder motility and increase the predisposition to gallstone formation as reported by van Erpectum et al. [27]. In acromegaly patients, the use of the long-acting octreotide formulation resulted in the increase of fasting gallbladder volume, severe inhibition of postprandial cholecystokinin release, and gallbladder emptying (all changes associated with gallbladder stasis and high risk of gallstone formation) as reported by Lee et al. [73] In these patients, the motility defects of the gallbladder and intestine during octreotide therapy are associated with increased cholesterol saturation in bile as reported by Pereira et al.; [74] potential prophylactic therapies for gallstones might therefore include prokinetics and/or hydrophilic ursodeoxycholic acid.

Bile Composition and Gallbladder Motility

At present, gallbladder motility defects observed in patients with gallstones are mainly interpreted as secondary events related to cholesterol supersaturation. Nucleation of solid cholesterol monohydrate crystals from supersaturated bile leads to the precipitation of the sterol, absorption by the gallbladder wall as suggested by Giananni et al., [75] and ensuing incorporation into the smooth muscle sarcolemma. Excessive incorporation of cholesterol inside gallbladder smooth muscle cells would then trigger biochemical alterations, resulting in impaired motility of the organ (see below). In addition, at the moment, there is no direct evidence that the impaired gallbladder motor function observed in cholelithiasis associated with metabolic disorders, as diabetes, obesity, or insulin resistance, is the primary event; rather, also in these conditions, gallbladder dyskinesia is likely the result of systemic impaired lipid metabolism and altered biliary lipid composition. The pathophysiological scenario could be that of a vicious cycle: an impairment of biliary lipid composition causes cholesterol supersaturation and precipitation. Following epithelial absorption, cholesterol is incorporated into the sarcolemma of gallbladder smooth muscle cells, causing contraction defects and gallbladder relaxation. The impairment of gallbladder motor function delays gallbladder emptying, and this alteration increases contact time of precipitated cholesterol with the mucosa, leading to additional cholesterol absorption and more extensive muscular damage as reported by Chen and Behar et al. [76, 77] Bile contains also plant sterols (campesterol, sitosterol) and oxysterols that may play a role in the pathogenesis of chronic inflammation of the gallbladder. Complex relationships exist between bile compositions and gallbladder motor function, because different patterns of postprandial gallbladder emptying can regulate bile compositions as reported by Stolk et al. [5] Conversely, luminal biliary lipids and/or proteins can influence gallbladder smooth muscle contractility as reported by Portincassa et al. [37] Because of the importance of biliary lipid composition for the pathogenesis of gallbladder motor dysfunction and gallstone disease, the biochemical and biophysical events driving lipid physiology in the gallbladder have been the object of intense research.

Molecular Mechanisms Controlling Lipid Absorption in the Gallbladder Epithelia. In addition to its active role in absorbing water, the gallbladder wall is also capable of absorbing significant amounts of cholesterol from bile. In healthy subjects, this mechanism might keep biliary cholesterol saturation within physiological ranges by absorption of excess cholesterol as reported by Ginanni et al. [75] Interestingly, the absorptive capacity of gallbladder mucosa is not limited to cholesterol, but also includes bile acids and phospholipids as reported by Ginanni and Corradini et al. [75, 78] *In vitro* experiments performed in isolated, intra arterially perfused gallbladder suggest that the human gallbladder displays preferential absorption for cholesterol and phospholipids, whereas bile acid absorption capacity is significantly smaller. In addition, *in vitro* evidence suggests that the gallbladder epithelium is also capable of the active efflux of cholesterol through both the apical and the basolateral membranes as reported by Lee et al. [79] At a molecular level, the identification of the proteins involved in the processes of cholesterol absorption and secretion has taken advantage of the progresses made regarding the mechanisms responsible for cholesterol transport in liver and intestine. Indeed, gallbladder epithelia and enterocytes of the proximal gut express similar molecular mechanisms regulating cholesterol absorption. A coordinated interplay between different lipid transport proteins might exist, because the net cholesterol absorption in the gallbladder, as in the gut, probably depends on the interaction between scavenger receptor class B type I (SR-BI), Niemann-Pick C1-like 1 (NPC1L1), ABCG5-ABCG8, and ABCA1 activities. Two of these proteins are potential candidates for mediating active cholesterol absorption: SR-BI and NPC1L1. In 1998, SR-BI was suggested as the protein responsible for intestinal cholesterol absorption by Hauser et al. [80] SR-BI had been isolated 5 years earlier Calvo and Vega et al. [81] and later identified as the high-affinity receptor for circulating high-density lipoprotein (HDL) by Acton and Labonte et al., [82, 83] and a high-affinity cholesterol binding protein on intestinal brush-border membrane vesicles by Labonte et al. [83] Nevertheless, the importance of SR-BI for intestinal cholesterol absorption has been challenged by the finding of unaltered intestinal cholesterol absorption in SR-BI knockout mice reported by Mardones et al. [84] Also, an accelerated lipid absorption has been observed in mice overexpressing SR-BI reported by Bietrix et al. [85] SR-BI is present in gallbladder epithelial cells, where it localizes on the apical membrane and may participate in the process of cholesterol absorption, because its expression has been found to be reduced in conditions of cholesterol hypersecretion reported by Johnson and Miquel et al. [86, 87]However, the translational value of these findings is still controversial, because gallstone formation and gallbladder wall cholesterol content do not correlate with SR-BI expression levels in experimental models of diet-induced cholelithiasis performed by Miquel et al. [87] Identified and characterized in 2000 by Davies et al., [88] NPC1L1 was later proposed as the protein mediating intestinal cholesterol absorption at the brush-border membrane of the enterocyte reported by Altmann et al. [89] Although NPC1L1 is expressed only in the intestine and gallbladder in mice, NPC1L1 is present at high levels in liver and intestine in humans indicated by Altmann et al. [89] The recent generation of transgenic mice with selective overexpression of NPC1L1 in the liver has proven the role that this protein plays in restraining excessive biliary cholesterol secretion, by actively reabsorbing cholesterol at the hepatocyte canalicular membrane reported by Temel et al. [90] Given the species differences between humans and mice, it is fascinating to speculate that NPC1L1 in mouse gallbladder fulfills the same role as human NPC1L1 in the liver. The involvement of NPC1L1 in gallstone disease has not yet been established, but theoretically its loss of function would favor gallstone formation by increasing the amount of biliary cholesterol. Ezetimibe is a drug that reduces intestinal cholesterol absorption in hypercholesterolemic patients, probably via inhibition of NPC1L1 as reported by Spencer. [91] In the near future, the impact of ezetimibe therapy upon hepatic and gallbladder handling of cholesterol and on gallstone disease needs to be evaluated. Regarding the process of cholesterol efflux, the role of ATP-dependent binding cassette (ABC) transporters appears critical; these transport proteins are located both on plasma and intracellular membranes, and are responsible for active, energy-dependent transport of molecules across biological membranes. The heterodimer ABCG5/ ABCG8 is responsible for cholesterol secretion into bile at the canalicular side of the hepatocyte, and also for apical secretion of cholesterol in the intestinal lumen at the brush border membrane of the enterocyte as repoted by Yu et al. [92, 93] By simultaneously enhancing biliary secretion and restraining intestinal absorption, ABCG5/ABCG8 play a critical role in enhancing fecal cholesterol disposal. Mutations of either ABCG5 or ABCG8 result in sitosterolemia, a genetic syndrome characterized by excessive accumulation of cholesterol and phytosterols in the body reported by Berge et al. [94] ABCG5/ABCG8 are expressed in human gallbladder epithelial cells, where they could act to limit excessive cholesterol absorption suggested by Repa et al. [95] *In vitro* evidence generated in canine gallbladder epithelial cells suggests that ABCG5/ABCG8 are localized intracellularly in basal conditions, but are shuttled on the apical membrane in conditions of cholesterol overload suggested by Repa et al. [95]

The translocation is triggered by activation of the oxysterol liver X receptors (LXRα and LXRβ), which are nuclear receptors activated by increased intracellular levels of oxysterols and responsible for the upregulation of genes that limit cholesterol overload, including cholesterol effluxers ABCG5/ABCG8 reported by Lawn et al. [96] ABCA1 is yet another ABC transporter involved in cholesterol trafficking. In the circulation, ABCA1 mediates the transfer of intracellular cholesterol and phospholipids to circulating HDL reported by Bodzioch et al. [97] ABCA1 is mutated in Tangier disease, a clinical condition characterized by nearly absent plasma levels of HDL and increased cardiovascular mortality reported by Brooks-Wilson, Rust and Erranz et al. [98-100] Although confocal imaging proves the basolateral localization of ABCA1 in gallbladder epithelial cells, the role of ABCA1 in gallbladder needs further investigation as suggested by Lee et al. [79] Both human and mouse gallbladder epithelia also expressed megalin, which is a protein able to mediate the endocytosis of numerous ligands, including HDL/apolipoprotein A-I (apoA-I). Bile acids and a lithogenic diet are able to strongly increase the expression of megalin, thus supporting a pathophysiological role of megalin in gallstone pathogenesis reported by Erranz et al. [101] Lastly, several other transporters are present in the epithelial cells of the gallbladder, including the bile acid transporters apical sodium-dependent bile acid transporter (ASBT) reported by Chignard et al. [102] and organic anion transporting polypeptide (OATP-A) reported by Dray-Charier et al., [103] cystic fibrosis transmembrane conductance regulator (CFTR) reported by Dray-Charier et al., [104] multidrug resistance 1 (MDR1), and anion exchanger 2 (AE2) reported by Scoazec et al. [105] The eventual contribution of these proteins in the development of gallstone disease is, at the present time, purely speculative.

Intraluminal Cholesterol

Defective lipid absorption in the gallbladder has been reported in patients with cholesterol gallstones reported by Corradini et al. [78]. Nevertheless, the cholesterol-absorbing capacity of the gallbladder wall might induce excess membrane accumulation of cholesterol in the muscular layer. In fact, gallbladder muscle from patients with cholesterol stones displays an increased mole ratio of membrane cholesterol/phospholipid and decreased membrane fluidity. The increased cholesterol content in gallbladder smooth muscles results in either defective contractility suggested by u, Guarino and Chen et al. [77, 106, 107] and/or relaxation reported by Behar and Chen et al. (108, 109) Interestingly, similar to what is observed in arterial myocytes during atherogenesis reported by Chen et al., [110] proliferative modifications of smooth muscle cells have also been reported in gallbladder smooth muscle exposed to excess cholesterol reported by Portincassa et al., [29] depicting a form of gallbladder hypertrophic leiomyopathy.

The presence of bile supersaturated with cholesterol is thus a condition predisposing to impaired receptor–G protein activation and reduced gallbladder contractility reported by Chen, Guarino, Jenning and Stolk et al. [77, 111-114] Isolated gallbladder smooth muscle cells from patients with cholesterol gallstone show greater dysfunction in response to CCK than smooth muscle cells from gallbladders of patients with pigment stones distinguished by Portincassa et al. [29] Also, excess cholesterol could contribute to reduced gallbladder contractility by affecting calcium channel activity, whereas potassium-channels and chloride-channels are not affected as suggested by Chen and Xu et al. [77, 115] These abnormalities may be corrected by removing the excess cholesterol from the plasma membranes, at least in the *in vitro* model of isolated gallbladder smooth muscle cells by Chen et al. [77] Of note, a recent study on patients with gallstones who were treated with ursodeoxycholic acid before cholecystectomy suggests that, after bile acid administration, an improvement of gallbladder muscle contractility is associated with a decreased cholesterol content in the plasma membranes of muscle cells by Chen et al. [106]

Intraluminal Bile Acids

Bile acids are able to relax the smooth muscle. Increased biliary/serum concentration of more hydrophobic bile salts (for example, deoxycholate) might lead to impaired gallbladder smooth muscle contractility reported by Xiao et al, [116] probably by an effect on intramural neurons indicated by van de Heijning et al. [117] In an animal model (guinea pig), incubation of isolated gallbladder smooth muscle cells with a hydrophobic taurochenodeoxycholic acid causes muscle cell dysfunction by inducing formation of H_2O_2 (activation of NADPH and xanthine oxidase). This leads to lipid peroxidation and activated cytosolic phospholipase A2 (cPLA2) to increase prostaglandin E2 (PGE2) production and, ultimately, to increased free-radical scavengers through protein kinase C (PKC), and mitogen-activating protein kinase (MAPK) pathway as illustrated by Dopico et al. [118] In contrast, the more hydrophilic ursodeoxycholate seems to prevent the deoxycholate- dependent impairment of smooth muscle contractility, as demonstrated by *in vitro* studies of gallbladder smooth muscle strips in an animal model by Dopico et al. [118] and from patients with gallstones demonstrated by Xiao and Wang et al. [116, 119] The relaxing mechanism of bile acids might also involve their ability to enhance $Ca2^{+}$-activated K^{+} (BKCa) channel activity in smooth muscle cells, as demonstrated by patch-clamp studies by Wilhelmi et al. [120]

Intraluminal Mucin

Intraluminal mucin also plays an important role in cholesterol gallstone formation and, as demonstrated by a recent animal study by Gustafsson et al., the increased gallbladder epithelial mucin encoded by mucin gene 1 (MUC1) strongly influences cholelithogenesis by impairing gallbladder motility in mice transgenic for the human *MUC1* gene, through an increased cholesterol absorption by the gallbladder wall, [121] a lithogenic mechanism completely different from the gel-forming mucins. Therefore, it is possible that inhibiting the secretion and accumulation of not only the gel-forming mucins but also the epithelial mucins in the gallbladder may prevent the formation of cholesterol gallstones. In fact, decreased MUC1 mucin in the gallbladders of mice with disrupted *Muc1* gene reduces susceptibility to cholesterol gallstone formation as suggested by Wang et al. [40] In addition, expression levels of the gallbladder *Muc5ac*, a gel-forming mucin gene, are significantly reduced in *Muc1$^{-/-}$* mice challenged to the lithogenic diet. Consequently, cholesterol crystallization and gallstone formation are drastically retarded. This finding suggests that there may be gene-gene interactions between *Muc1* and *Muc5ac*, which might influence mucin secretion and accumulation in the gallbladder. Elevated concentration of mucin suggested by Brotschi et al. [122] and its marker hexosamine by Hemming et al. [123] have been measured in bile of patients with cholesterol crystals and stone, therefore opening the speculative hypothesis that changes in bile viscosity secondary to soluble mucin content in bile, could also influence gallbladder emptying. Overall, these results suggest that the epithelial mucin genes may influence gallbladder mucin accumulation by regulating expression and function of the gel-forming mucin genes.

Gallbladder Wall Inflammation

Substances involved in inflammation processes can strongly influence gallbladder contractility as reported by Jennings, Martinez-Cuesta, O'Riordan, Trevisani and Kano et al. [124-129] Increased proportion of arachidonyl-phosphatidylcholine species (PLA2 activity, PGE2), as a marker of gallbladder mucosal inflammation and mucin concentrations, are found in the animal model fed a lithogenic diet in Marschetta et al.'s experiment. [130] Mice susceptible to gallstone formation show, after the lithogenic diet, an altered gallbladder histology associated with impaired motility and reduced concentrating function as proposed by Xiao et al. [131, 132] Prostaglandins are produced during the inflammatory process in the gallbladder and they induce relaxation of gallstone-containing gallbladders; these mediators might therefore be a determinant of the impaired gallbladder motility by Greaves et al. [133] Studies on human gallbladder tissues have shown that CCK-induced smooth muscle contraction via the CCK-1 receptor pathway is modulated by prostaglandins in the healthy state. This modulation disappears in gallstone-containing gallbladders, but the excessive serotonin release in advanced cholecystitis normalizes the CCK-induced contraction as indicated by Trevisani et al. [127] Several animal studies by Al-jiffry, Morschetta, Dopico and Alcon et al. demonstrate a strong interplay between factors such as inflammation, oxidative stress, and cytotoxic bile salts, and impaired CCK effect during cholesterol gallstone formation. [118, 130, 134, 135] In humans, the administration of ursodeoxycholic acid (a more hydrophilic and less cytotoxic bile acid) has been demonstrated to play a role in decreasing chronic gallbladder inflammation in patients with cholesterol gallstones, with better *in vitro* contractility to CCK and other mediators, such as acetylcholine and KCl reported by Wang and Chen et al. [106, 119] The mechanism of action of ursodeoxycholic acid might include decreased biliary cholesterol saturation, decreased incorporation of cholesterol molecules into smooth muscle plasma membrane, and decreased inflammatory mediators such as arachidonyl-phosphatidylcholine species and PLA2 reported by Bird et al, [136] and markers of oxidative stress suggested by Chen et al. [106].

Studies of Gallbladder Motor Function

Gallbladder Contractility In Vitro

The ability of the gallbladder smooth muscle to contract in the absence of extrinsic neuroendocrine control and/or effects of bile composition/intraluminal content can be effectively studied *in vitro* with isolated smooth muscle cells and smooth muscle strips obtained from animals and patients following cholecystectomy. The whole gallbladder has also been studied in animal models by Portincassa et al. [37] Similarly to what is seen *in vivo*, the contractile function of gallbladder smooth muscle cells of cholesterol gallstone patients is abnormal *in vitro*, as shown by several tensiometric studies by Huang, McKirdy, Xiao and Xu et al. [29, 35, 51, 77, 112, 114, 128, 130, 137-149] Gallbladders containing cholesterol stones show a defective muscular contractility as reported by Trevisani, Lindaman and Portincassa et al. [29, 38, 76, 77, 107, 127, 141, 150] and/or relaxation as reported by Behar and Chen et al. [108, 109] This latter phenomenon seems to parallel the decreased gallbladder refilling observed *in vivo* which, in turn, can increase the tendency toward cholesterol crystal precipitation and aggregation into macroscopic stones indicated by Jazrawi et al. [151] The potassium K(ATP) channels seem to play an important role for gallbladder smooth muscle relaxation indicated by Bird et al. [139].

Gallbladder Motility in a Clinical Setting

Real-time abdominal ultrasonography provides key information about the morphology and content of the gallbladder including the features of the wall (thickness) and of the content (that is, anechoic bile, sludge, solitary or multiple stones, polyps, neoplasms). This method is noninvasive, highly accurate, and widely available demonstrated by Portincassa et al. [18, 152]. The study of gallbladder motor function, nevertheless, requires repeated measurements of the gallbladder volume at different time points after meal ingestion, as markers of fasting gallbladder volume, postprandial gallbladder emptying and refilling ability, and, indirectly, of cystic duct patency as suggested by Portincassa, Everson and Festi et al. [152-154] Biliary scintigraphy, although providing information on gallbladder emptying, refilling, and cystic duct patency, does not allow the study of gallbladder morphology and requires use of radiation reported by Jaseawi and Pomeranz et al. [4, 151, 155] Afterward, a negative feedback exists between intraduodenal bile and CCK release reported by Palasciano et al. (156) The impaired gallbladder emptying which may anticipate the formation of cholesterol gallstones prolongs the residence time of concentrated gallbladder bile, provides more time for nucleation and crystallization of cholesterol crystals from supersaturated bile, and lessens the amount of nucleated cholesterol crystals that can be ejected into the duodenum. Microscopic cholesterol crystals are evolved through aggregation and growth into macroscopic stones with assistance of mucin gels. A subgroup of patients with cholesterol gallstones have defective gallbladder emptying and refilling by Jasrawi et al. [151] and increased fasting gallbladder volume by Huang, Stolk, Portincassa and Pauletzki et al. [1, 5, 28, 29, 32] In the fasting state, the fluctuations of gallbladder volume is under the subtle control of the fasting gastrointestinal hormone motilin as reported by Portincassa et al. [157] Finally, from a clinical point of view, the evaluation of gallbladder motility is also important in the decision-making for patients symptomatic for gallstones. In a recent study, an efficient gallbladder motility in patients with gallstones represented a risk factor for the development of biliary pain as indicated by Colecchia et al. [158]. By contrast, oral ursodeoxycholic acid increases gallbladder residual volume and reduces the percentage of gallbladder emptying, without affecting the rate of biliary symptoms in the highly symptomatic patient by Forgacs and Venneman et al. [159, 160] Conclusions and Future Perspectives.

The gallbladder plays an essential dynamic role if one thinks that liver bile—a solute highly enriched in cholesterol and lipids—is accumulated, mixed, concentrated in the gallbladder, and secreted intraduodenally during fasting and in the postprandial status. The results of integrated *in vivo* and *in vitro* studies in humans and in animal models depict a complex scenario in which subtle mechanisms govern gallbladder motility. Mechanisms include hormonal and extrinsic neuroendocrine factors, bile composition, biliary cholesterol saturation, and intrinsic gallbladder smooth muscle contractile properties with receptorial/postreceptorial features. These mechanisms are directly coordinated via regulatory mechanisms finely tuned in the gut-liver axis. The gallbladder motility abnormalities observed in patients with gallstones are considered mainly secondary rather than primary events. Although some well-known metabolic risk conditions for gallstone disease such as diabetes, obesity, and insulin resistance may be associated with impaired gallbladder motility, there is no direct evidence that in a subgroup of individuals with these conditions impaired gallbladder motility is the main factor involved in gallstone formation. Longitudinal clinical studies are needed to address this intriguing issue. Understanding the pathogenesis of gallbladder motor-dysfunction leading to gallstone formation could be fostered by wide integrated *in vivo* and *in vitro* studies of gallbladder function, in particular at a molecular and genetic level. These studies would eventually provide a better strategy for the treatment and prevention of cholesterol gallstones.

III. Identification of a Hormonal Basis for Gallbladder Filling [17]

The cycle of gallbladder filling and emptying controls the flow of bile into the intestine for digestion. Choi et al. show that fibroblast growth factor-15, a hormone made by the distal small intestine in response to bile acids, is required for gallbladder filling. These studies demonstrate that gallbladder filling is actively regulated by an endocrine pathway and suggest a postprandial timing mechanism that controls gallbladder motility.

The gallbladder stores and concentrates bile during fasting and, in response to feeding, releases it into the small intestine to facilitate digestion. The hormone cholecystokinin (CCK), which is secreted from the proximal duodenum, is the major determinant of gallbladder emptying. Although several neuroactive chemicals and second messengers are proposed to contribute to gallbladder filling, it is not known whether endocrine hormones regulate this process as raised by Shaffer and Pozo et al. [161, 162] Fibroblast growth factor-15 (FGF15) is a hormone that has a central role in the feedback regulation of bile acid synthesis in the liver reported by Inagaki et al. [43] FGF15 is made by the ileum, where its expression is induced by bile acids acting through the farnesoid X receptor by Li et al. [163] Examination of mice lacking Fgf15 revealed that their gallbladders were almost devoid of bile. Histology on gallbladders from Fgf15$^{-/-}$ mice showed the presence of normal gallbladder epithelium. Thus, Choi et al. tested whether administration of Fgf15 or its human ortholog, FGF19, affects gallbladder volume. Choi et al. injected fasted Fgf15$^{-/-}$ and wild-type mice with recombinant Fgf15 or FGF19, and measured gallbladder volume 15 min later. Both Fgf15 and FGF19 caused a 410-fold increase in gallbladder volume in Fgf15$^{-/-}$ mice and a 2-fold increase in wild-type mice. There was no effect of Fgf15 on bile flow rate in either wild-type or Fgf15$^{-/-}$ mice. FGFs mediate their biological actions by binding to transmembrane FGF receptors (FGFRs), which in mammals are encoded by four genes recorded by Ornitz. [164] Choi et al. measured Fgf15 and Fgfr mRNA levels by real-time quantitative PCR in the gallbladder, the common bile duct and the sphincter of Oddi, which regulates the flow of bile from the bile duct into the duodenum. Whereas Fgf15 was abundantly expressed in the ileum, no Fgf15 mRNA was detected in the liver, gallbladder, common bile duct or sphincter of Oddi by Ornitz and Li et al. [163, 164] These data suggest that Fgf15 produced in the small intestine functions as a hormone to stimulate gallbladder filling. In the liver, Fgf15 acts through Fgfr4 to repress bile acid synthesis by Inagaki et al. [43] Notably, Fgfr4$^{-/-}$ mice have reduced gallbladder volume, [164] although the phenotype is not as pronounced as that seen in the Fgf15$^{-/-}$ mice [Figure 1a,b). These data together with our finding that FGF19 administration increased gallbladder volume in Fgfr4$^{-/-}$ mice indicate that other Fgfr proteins contribute to the actions of Fgf15 in the gallbladder. In fact, all four Fgfr mRNAs were detected in the gallbladder, with Fgfr3 mRNA levels being the highest. Fgfr3 mRNA was also abundant in the common bile duct and the sphincter of Oddi, suggesting a key role for Fgfr3 throughout the biliary tract. FGF19 has comparable activity on all four FGFRs in in vitro mitogenicity assays by Zhang et al. [165] Choi et al. measured plasma CCK concentrations to determine whether changes in this hormone account for the empty gallbladders in Fgf15$^{-/-}$ mice. Postprandial CCK concentrations were lower in Fgf15$^{-/-}$ mice compared to wild-type mice, [17] demonstrating that changes in CCK concentrations are not responsible for the empty gallbladder phenotype. To further examine the relationship between Fgf15 and CCK, Choi et al. injected the two hormones either alone or together into wild-type mice, and measured the gallbladder volume. As expected, CCK reduced gallbladder volume. A 70-fold molar excess of Fgf15 completely blocked contraction of the gallbladder caused by CCK. Cyclic nucleotides relax gastrointestinal smooth muscle and are implicated in gallbladder filling reported by Inagaki and Kline et al. [43, 166] Choi et al. examined the effect of Fgf15 on cyclic AMP (cAMP) and cyclic GMP (cGMP) concentrations in the gallbladder in the presence and absence of CCK. CCK caused a marked decrease in the concentration of cAMP in the gallbladder. Co-administration of Fgf15 reversed this effect. Further, FGF19 caused a substantial increase in gallbladder cAMP concentrations in Fgf15$^{-/-}$ mice. Fgf15 had no effect on cGMP concentrations in either the presence or absence of CCK. To further examine the relationship between cAMP levels and gallbladder volume, Choi et al. injected Fgf15$^{-/-}$ mice with forskolin, which stimulates cAMP production. Forskolin caused an increase in gallbladder volume and cAMP concentrations that was comparable to that caused by FGF19 while only modestly increasing bile flow and not changing hepatic cAMP concentrations. To determine if FGF19 has direct effects on gallbladder smooth muscle, Choi et al. conduct tensiometry experiments with isolated gallbladders. Both FGF19 and forskolin caused relaxation of CCK-induced gallbladder contraction. Taken together, the data indicate that Fgf15 and FGF19 stimulate gallbladder filling at least in part by causing a cAMP-dependent relaxation of gallbladder smooth muscle. Nevertheless, these experiments do not rule out that Fgf15 and FGF19 also cause gallbladder filling through other mechanisms involving effects on the nervous system and the sphincter of Oddi. In summary, Choi et al.'s data demonstrate that FGF15 is an essential component of a postprandial feedback loop that stimulates gallbladder filling. Moreover, they suggest a mechanism for the temporal regulation of gallbladder motility. During feeding, CCK secreted from the duodenum causes gallbladder contraction and the release of bile into the duodenum, which facilitates digestion and suppresses further CCK secretion exemplified by LeMorte and Pauletzki et al. [167, 168] After traversing the small intestine, bile acids induce FGF15 synthesis in the ileum, which stimulates gallbladder refilling. Thus, the differential expression and regulation of CCK and FGF15 in the small intestine controls the periodicity of gallbladder emptying and filling. Consistent with this model, people with Crohn's disease or ileocecal resection have lower fasting gallbladder volumes. These individuals also have an increased prevalence of gallstone disease. Because impaired gallbladder motility is a key factor in the formation of gallstones suggested by Wang et al., [67, 169, 170] strategies to modulate FGF19 signaling may prove useful in the treatment of this common disease. Finally, the opposing actions of FGF15 and CCK on the gallbladder raise the possibility that FGF15 will inhibit the effects of CCK on other physiological processes including gastric emptying, pancreatic enzyme secretion and food intake.

IV. Effect of Gallbladder Hypomotility on Cholesterol Crystallization and Growth in CCK-Deficient Mice[171]

Wang et al. investigated the effect of gallbladder hypomotility on cholesterol crystallization and growth during the early stage of gallstone formation in CCK knockout mice. Contrary to wild-type mice, fasting gallbladder volumes were enlarged and the response of gallbladder emptying to a high fat meal was impaired in knockout mice on chow or the lithogenic diet. In the lithogenic state, large amounts of mucin gel and liquid crystals as well as arc-like and tubular crystals formed first, followed by rapid formation of classic parallelogram-shaped cholesterol monohydrate crystals in knockout mice. Further, three patterns of crystal growth habits were observed: proportional enlargement, spiral dislocation growth, and twin crystal growth, all enlarging solid cholesterol crystals. At day 15 on the lithogenic diet, 75% of knockout mice formed gallstones. Nevertheless, wildtype mice formed very little mucin gel, liquid and solid crystals, and gallstones were not observed. Wang et al. conclude that lack of CCK induces gallbladder hypomotility that prolongs the residence time of excess cholesterol in the gallbladder, leading to rapid crystallization and precipitation of solid cholesterol crystals. Furthermore, during the early stage of gallstone formation, there are two pathways of liquid and polymorph anhydrous crystals evolving to monohydrate crystals and three modes for cholesterol crystal growth. Physical-chemical studies of biliary lipids have clearly shown that in bile, cholesterol is solubilized as a mixture of simple and mixed micelles as well as vesicles, all in a dynamic equilibrium as suggested by Wang et al. [172] Although this equilibration process starts after hepatic secretion of bile and continues in the biliary tree, the nucleation and crystallization of cholesterol molecules occurs predominantly in the gallbladder when cholesterol concentrations reach supersaturation. It has been found that gallbladder biles in some normal subjects and in patients with cholesterol gallstones are often supersaturated with cholesterol s proposed by Carey and Holzbach et al. [173, 174] Further, the precipitation of solid plate-like cholesterol monohydrate crystals from supersaturated bile is the first irreversible physical-chemical step in the formation of cholesterol gallstones as indicated by Holan and Sedaghat et al. [175, 176] Clinical studies have observed that cholesterol monohydrate crystals could be detected in fresh duodenal bile samples by Marks, Susann and Neoptolemos et al. [177-179] Also, aggregated cholesterol monohydrate crystals embedded in mucin gel could often be observed by ultrasonography as biliary sludge, as confirmed by polarizing light microscopy in human gallbladder biles that are obtained after cholecystectomy by Lee and Ko et al. [180-182] It has been established that gallbladder stasis is an important prerequisite for gallstone formation because cholesterol is often nucleated into solid monohydrate crystals when cholesterol supersaturation in gallbladder bile reaches beyond a limit, as well as cholesterol crystal growth and aggregation are accelerated by pro-nucleating proteins such as mucins suggested by Portincassa et al. [9] However, little was known about how abnormal gallbladder motility influences crystallization and growth of excess cholesterol in gallbladder bile. Cholecystokinin (CCK) is a gastrointestinal hormone that is produced and secreted by intestinal I cells. It has been found that a significant increase in plasma concentrations of CCK occurs after ingestion of a meal or fat, which can induce a significant contraction of the gallbladder as indicated by Ivy and Schjoldager et al. [183, 184] A defective gallbladder motility has been strongly linked to the formation of gallstones by Potincassa et al, [18] and abnormal gallbladder motility has been observed both in vivo and in vitro in subgroups of cholesterol gallstone patients by Portincassa et al, [29] as well as in gallstone-free subjects under several conditions such as pregnancy, obesity and diabetes. This, in turn, might represent a significant pathophysiologically relevant stimulus predisposing to gallstone formation suggested by Portincassa et al. [9] As a result, a growing interest is focused on the lithogenic effect of gallbladder hypomotility as a key trigger condition. A CCK-deficient mouse model has been established by a gene targeting strategy in mouse embryonic stem (ES) cells as reported by Lacourse et al. [185] Because CCK can enhance gallbladder contraction by acting as an agonist at CCK-1 receptor, deletion of the *Cck* gene could result in a defective gallbladder motility. By using this unique mouse model, Wang et al. systematically investigated the effect of dysfunctional gallbladder motility on cholesterol crystallization and growth during the early stage of cholesterol gallstone formation. In Wang et al.'s studies, they found that the lack of CCK impaired gallbladder motility function, enlarged gallbladder size, and enhanced cholesterol crystallization mostly by prolonging the residence time of excess cholesterol in the gallbladder lumen. All of these changes promoted cholesterol crystal growth and gallstone formation. Wang et al. further observed that during the early stage of gallstone formation, there are two pathways of the liquid and the polymorph anhydrous crystals evolving to solid plate-like cholesterol monohydrate crystals, as well as three modes for cholesterol crystal growth.

In the materials and methods section, the CCK knockout (KO) mice were generated by using a gene targeting strategy in which of lacZ reporter gene was inserted into the mouse *Cck* gene, resulting in a null mutation as reported by Lacourse et al. [185] As a result, the CCK KO mice produced no functional CCK peptide fragments. All of the mice studied in these experiments were genotyped by PCR analysis of tail DNA to determine their genotype. Male CCK KO and wild-type (WT) mice on a pure C57BL/6J genetic background were studied. All mice were provided free access to water and the normal rodent chow diet containing trace (<0.02%) amounts of cholesterol (Harlan Teklad F6 Rodent Diet 8664, Madison, WI). During the cholesterol crystallization and gallstone studies, mice at 8–10 weeks old were fed a lithogenic diet containing 1% cholesterol, 0.5% cholic acid and 15% butter fat for 15 days. All procedures were in accordance with current National Institutes of Health guidelines and were approved by the Institutional Animal Care and Use Committee of Harvard University (Boston, MA).

Gallbladder Contraction Study

To explore whether gallbladder motility function was impaired due to loss of *Cck* gene expression, fasting and postprandial gallbladder volumes were measured in mice (n=8 per group) fed the lithogenic diet for 15 days. To study fasting gallbladder size, mice were fasted overnight but had free access to water. After weighing, mice were anesthetized with an intraperitoneal injection of 35 mg/kg pentobarbital (Abbott Laboratories, North Chicago, IL). Laparotomy commenced at 9:00 AM and was performed under sterile conditions through an upper midline incision. During laparotomy, the gallbladder was clearly exposed and its size was measured with a micro-caliper. Gallbladder volumes were calculated using the following formula, assuming an ellipsoid shape of the organ reported by Everson et al. [153]

$$\text{Gallbladder volume } (\mu\text{L}) = \text{length (mm)} \times \text{width (mm)} \times \text{depth (mm)} \times \pi/6$$

To determine gallbladder emptying function in mice (n=4 per group) in response to a high fat meal, a PE-10 polyethylene catheter was inserted into the duodenum during laparotomy. The duodenal catheter was externalized through the left abdominal wall and connected to an infusion pump (Kent Scientific, Litchfield, CT). Following completion of all surgical procedures, gallbladder size was immediately measured with a micro-caliper and gallbladder volumes were calculated using the above-mentioned formula. Then, mice were intraduodenally infused with corn oil (i.e., a high fat meal) or 0.9% NaCl (as a control) at 40 μL/minute for 5 minutes. At 30 minutes after the duodenal infusion, postprandial gallbladder volume was measured with a micro-caliper again. Gallbladder emptying function was determined by a difference in gallbladder size before and after the duodenal infusion of corn oil.

Collection of Gallbladder Bile and Microscopic Studies

Before (day 0) and at 6, 9, 12 and 15 days on the lithogenic diet, a cholecystectomy was performed in overnight fasted mice (n=4 per group) after anesthesia. Fresh gallbladder bile was immediately examined according to the methods described previously by Wang et al. [186]. After microscopic analysis, fresh gallbladder bile was harvested and stored at −20°C for lipid studies. In brief, the entire gallbladder bile was placed on a glass slide at room temperature (~22°C) and observed without a cover slip using a polarizing light microscope and phase contrast optics.

After a small hole was made in the fundus of gallbladder, bulk bile dribbled by gravity and mucin gel was pressed out digitally with the assistance of a 24 gauge needle. These fresh bile samples were examined by microscopic analysis for the presence of mucin strands, liquid and solid crystals, and sandy and true gallstones as reported by Wang et al. [186] Mucin was observed as non-birefringent amorphous strands. Arc-like and tubular crystals (assumed to be metastable transitional forms of anhydrous cholesterol being hydrated to cholesterol monohydrate crystals), plate-like cholesterol monohydrate crystals, as well as small, aggregated and fused liquid crystals were defined according to previously published criteria Wang et al. [186, 187].

Sandy stones were irregularly shaped, and easily disintegrable agglomerates of cholesterol monohydrate crystals surrounded by mucin gel. As visualized under the microscope, individual cholesterol monohydrate crystals projected clearly from the edges of sandy stones, and grossly they displayed a yellow color. True gallstones were hard, ball-like objects, and light yellow in color with smooth curved surfaces. Because of scattered and absorbed light, they were opaque, and black in color when observations were made with polarizing light microscopy. The images of cholesterol monohydrate crystals and gallstones were analyzed by a Carl Zeiss Imaging System with an AxioVision Rel 4.6 software (Carl Zeiss Microimaging GmbH Göttingen, Germany).

Lipid Analyses

Biliary phospholipid was measured as inorganic phosphorus by the method of Bartlett. (188) Cholesterol was determined using an enzymatic assay. Total bile salt concentration was measured enzymatically by the 3α-hydroxysteroid dehydrogenase method reported by Turley and Dietschy. [189] Gallstones were washed, air dried at 22°C, and the cholesterol content (wt/wt) was determined by HPLC reported by Wang et al. [186] Cholesterol saturation index (CSI) of pooled gallbladder biles was calculated from critical tables Carey [190] established for taurocholate, the predominant bile salts in mouse bile on the lithogenic diet. Relative lipid compositions of pooled gallbladder biles (n=4 per group at each time point) were plotted on condensed phased diagrams appropriate to their mean total lipid concentrations as illustrated by Wang et al. [187]

For graphic analysis, the phase limits of the micellar zones and the crystallization pathways were extrapolated from model systems developed for taurocholate at 37°C also by Wang et al. [187]

Statistical Method

All data are expressed as means ± SD. Statistically significant differences among groups of mice were assessed by Student's *t*-test, Mann-Whitney U-tests, or Chi square tests. If the F-value was significant, comparisons among groups of mice were further analyzed by a multiple comparison test. Analyses were performed with a *Super ANOVA* software (Abacus Concepts, Berkeley, CA). Statistical significance was defined as a two-tailed probability of less than 0.05.

In the results section, on the chow diet (i.e., at day 0), fasting gallbladder volumes were significantly ($P<0.01$) larger in CCK KO mice than in WT mice. The gallbladder wall was thin and transparent. Macroscopic and light microscopic examination of gallbladder biles showed no evidence of mucin gel, solid and liquid crystals, or gallstones in both CCK KO and WT mice. Concerning postprandial gallbladder sizes in mice in response to the high fat meal, as expected, duodenal infusion of 0.9% NaCl did not induce gallbladder emptying. It was observed that a significant portion of the gallbladder bile ($P<0.05$) emptied out in CCK WT mice in response to the high fat meal. However, it was not the case in CCK KO mice, suggesting that gallbladder emptying function was impaired due to the deletion of the *Cck* gene in mice. Concerning fasting gallbladder sizes as functions of days on the lithogenic diet, before feeding the lithogenic diet (day 0), gallbladders of CCK KO mice were approximately twice the sizes in CCK WT mice. Further, in CCK KO mice, gallbladder size increased significantly after 6 days when cholesterol crystallization and growth developed. This increase in gallbladder size paralleled the elevated CSIs in bile, and changes in these parameters were much more noticeable in CCK KO mice compared with CCK WT mice. Overall, in the lithogenic state, CCK KO mice still displayed dramatically enlarged gallbladders compared with CCK WT mice.

Physical-Chemical Analysis of Gallbladder Biles

Concerning the relative biliary lipid compositions in pooled gallbladder biles from mice fed chow (day 0) and the lithogenic diet for 15 days, of note is that the CSI value reached supersaturated at 9 days on the lithogenic diet in CCK KO mice, 6 days earlier than that in CCK WT mice. For the purposes of illustration, a truncated phase diagram (Figure 1.4.1) for pooled gallbladder biles was created according to the average total lipid concentration (~8.0 g/dl). The one-phase micellar zone at the bottom is enclosed by a solid curved line. Above it, two solid lines divide the two-phase zones from a central three-phase zone. Based upon the solid and liquid crystallization sequences present in bile, the left two-phase and the central three-phase regions are divided by dashed lines into Regions A to E. Figure 1.4.1 shows that during lithogenic diet feeding the relative lipid compositions of pooled gallbladder biles progressively shifted upward and to the right of the phase diagrams in both CCK KO and WT mice. This shift was caused by absolute and relative increases in cholesterol concentrations, a relative increase in phospholipid concentrations, and a relative decrease in bile salt concentrations. In CCK KO mice, the relative biliary lipid compositions at day 0 and 6 days plotted within the one-phase micellar zones, whereas by day 9 lipid compositions plotted above the micellar zone.

By phase analysis, these biles were predicted to be composed of two or three phases, namely saturated micelles, solid cholesterol crystals, and/or liquid crystals, exactly as what Wang et al. observed by microscopy. Because in CCK KO mice between 9 and 15 days the relative lipid composition of gallbladder bile passed through crystallization pathway B, anhydrous cholesterol crystals (i.e., arc-like and tubular crystals) appeared besides cholesterol monohydrate crystals.

In contrast, during lithogenesis, the relative lipid compositions of pooled gallbladder biles in CCK WT mice directly entered crystallization pathway C from the one phase micellar zone. Thus, Wang et al. did not find anhydrous cholesterol crystals in these biles.

Accordingly, as predicted from model bile systems, liquid crystals invariably preceded cholesterol monohydrate crystals during crystallization.

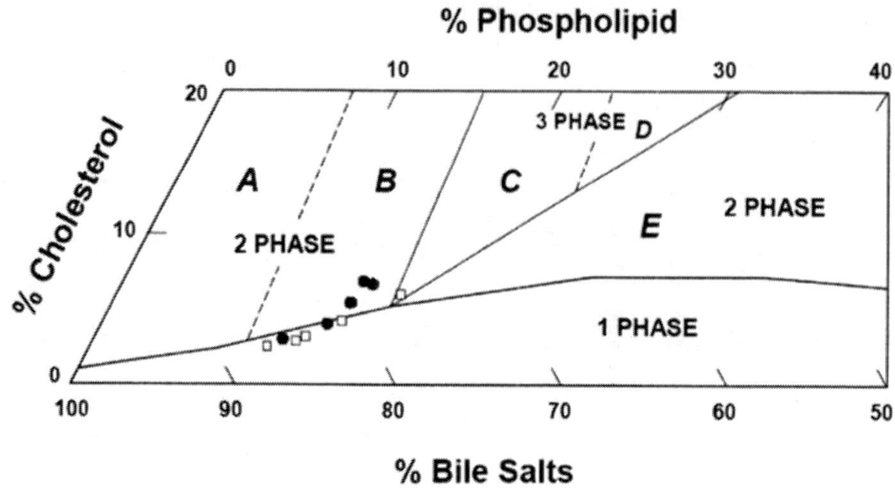

Figure 1.4.1. The relative lipid compositions of pooled gallbladder biles from CCK KO and WT mice at each time point are plotted on condensed phase diagrams for average total lipid concentrations (~8.0 g/dL) of the bile samples (from Table 1). The one-phase micellar zone at bottom is enclosed by a solid curved line. Above the micellar zone, two solid lines divide the two-phase zones from a central three-phase zone. Based upon the solid and liquid crystallization sequences present in the biles, the left two-phase and central three-phase regions are divided by dashed lines into Regions A to E. With passage of time, the relative lipid compositions of gallbladder bile shift upward and to the right in both CCK KO and WT mice. Only the lipid compositions of biles in CCK KO mice pass through Region B. In contrast, the lipid compositions of bile in CCK WT mice enter crystallization pathway C directly from the one-phase micellar zone. Black symbols represent CCK KO mice and white symbols are for CCK WT mice. Wang et al. Page 15 *Biochim Biophys.*

Morphology of liquid and solid crystals Concerning representative photomicrographs of mucin strands, habits of solid cholesterol crystals, and optical textures of liquid crystals and gallstones, mucin gel appeared as non-birefringent amorphous strands. In CCK KO mice, arc-like crystals were occasionally detected and they were short curved rods. Tubular crystals were found and often appeared to fracture at their ends producing classic plate-like cholesterol monohydrate crystals and frequently with a notched corner. As proposed from model bile studies by Wang et al., [187] liquid crystals were denoted as small, when minimally sized, non-birefringent, and scattered; aggregated, when non-birefringent with particles of 1– 5 μm diameter; and fused, when birefringent with focal conic textures and greater than 0.5–1 μm in size. These liquid crystals mainly in the aggregated form were found in some of the gallbladder bile samples. Typical plate-like cholesterol monohydrate crystals were 79.2° and 100.8° angled parallelograms, often with a small notched corner. These crystal forms observed by polarizing light microscopy were the same as those found in model and human biles and in human cholesterol gallstones as well as in animal models of cholesterol gallstones including prairie dogs, squirrel monkey and mice. Sandy stones were surrounded by mucin gel and exhibited individual cholesterol monohydrate crystals projecting from their edges. It is well established that true gallstones showed typical round contours and black centers as visualized under the microscope. Concerning effect of mucin gel on cholesterol nucleation and crystallization, of special note is that very tiny solid cholesterol crystals were often found first within the mucin gel. Also, numerous small single classic plate-like cholesterol monohydrate crystals embedded in mucin gel were detected. These observations were consistent with the concept that mucin gel is a strong pro-crystallizing agent acting as a matrix accelerating cholesterol nucleation and crystallization in bile as reported by Wang et al. [172].

Patterns of Cholesterol Crystal Growth

It has been observed from human studies that gallbladder hypomotility is an important risk factor for the formation of cholesterol gallstones as reported by Wang et al. [9] Although the bile stasis induced by the hypofunctioning gallbladder provides the time necessary to accommodate nucleation and crystallization of crystals and growth of gallstones within the mucin gel, little is known about how abnormal gallbladder motility influences crystallization and precipitation of excess cholesterol in bile. With this unique mouse model with gallbladder contractile dysfunction due to the deletion of the *Cck* gene, the effects of gallbladder hypomotility on cholesterol crystallization and growth during the early stage of gallstone formation were investigated systematically. Concerning the three modes of crystal growth habits as observed in CCK KO mice on the lithogenic diet, the first mode of crystal growth habits is: proportional enlargement patterns, which made solid cholesterol crystals larger in one direction – length and width. Also, two other predominant crystal growth habits were found. One was spiral dislocation growth: the pyramidal surface containing numerous growth spirals nucleated by a screw dislocation and the other was twin crystal growth: the crystals growing upright and perpendicular to the surface. These observations on cholesterol crystal growth habits are consistent with these as found in model bile systems by Toor and colleagues. [191]. All of these crystal growth habits induced solid cholesterol crystals enlarged in size.

Sequences of Cholesterol Gallstone Formation

To explore whether gallbladder hypomotility influences the sequences of gallstone formation, Wang et al. observed cholesterol crystallization and gallstone formation in CCK KO and WT mice for 15 days with the feeding of a lithogenic diet. Figure 7.4.2 shows crystals and liquid crystals in arbitrary number in the cholesterol crystallization sequence from fresh mouse gallbladder bile as functions of days on the lithogenic diet. At day 6, a layer of mucin gel adherent to the gallbladder wall was observed in all CCK KO mice, and some aggregated and fused liquid crystals were found in a few CCK KO mice. At day 9, anhydrous cholesterol crystals such as arc-like and tubular crystals were detected, and some tubular crystals fractured at the end to produce classic plate-like cholesterol monohydrate crystals. In addition, aggregated and fused liquid crystals were found more frequently within mucin gel, suggesting a more rapid evolution of crystallization. Classic plate-like cholesterol monohydrate crystals were present principally within gel-containing bile. Gradually, individual cholesterol monohydrate crystals were enlarged in size by means of the three modes of cholesterol growth habits. At day 12, solid cholesterol monohydrate crystals were consolidated by mucin gel as agglomerates. Also, soft and fragile amorphous sandy stones were surrounded by mucin gel, with individual cholesterol crystals projecting from the edges. At day 15, 75% of CCK KO mice formed true gallstones that exhibited rounded contours and black centers due to light scattering/absorption. In contrast, the crystallization and growth of cholesterol monohydrate crystals, as well as the development of gallstones, were greatly delayed in CCK WT mice. At day 15, 25% of CCK WT mice on the lithogenic diet formed solid cholesterol monohydrate crystals, but not sandy stones or true gallstones.

In the discussion section, in the normal physiological state, the gallbladder contracts frequently throughout the day. Between meals, the gallbladder stores and concentrates bile secreted from the liver and its average fasting volume is approximately 35–50 mL in healthy human subjects reported by Palasciano et al. [55] while following the meal, it discharges a variable amount of bile, which depends on the degree of neuro-hormonal stimulation including the CCK stimulus Ivy and Schjoldager et al. [29, 183, 184] Clinical investigations have found that abnormalities in gallbladder contractile function in response to exogenously administered CCK have been observed principally in patients with cholesterol gallstones by Pomeranz and others et al., [29, 76, 155] and an intermediate degree of gallbladder motility defect, in the absence of enlarged fasting gallbladder and any gallbladder inflammation, has been found also in patients with pigment gallstones by Portincassa et al. [7] In addition, dysfunctional gallbladder motility has been reported in gallstone-free subjects under several conditions such as patients with obesity and/or diabetes, and subjects on total parenteral nutrition by Wang, Portincassa, Roslyn, Kodama, Stampfer and others et al. [9, 192-198]. Further, slow emptying and increased volume of the gallbladder, as measured by ultrasonography, occur during pregnancy and during administration of oral contraceptives, two conditions that predispose to the formation of gallstones as reported by Ko et al. [199] Thus, the lithogenic actions of gallbladder hypomotility need to be further investigated. In Wang et al.'s studies, they investigated the effect of gallbladder hypomotility on cholesterol crystallization and growth in CCK KO mice vs. WT mice. Wang et al. found that the absence of the gastrointestinal hormone CCK resulted in impaired gallbladder contractile function, and enlarged fasting and postprandial gallbladder volume, and consequently these changes accelerated cholesterol crystallization and growth and promoted gallstone formation. These results indicated that gallbladder hypomotility is an important risk factor for the formation of cholesterol gallstones. Hence, the CCK-deficient mice provided an excellent animal model for the study of cholesterol gallstone formation as influenced by the gallbladder stasis mechanisms. In addition, it has been found that CCK peptides are potent stimulants of gallbladder contraction and of sphincter of Oddi relaxation for coordinating regulation of bile flow entering the duodenum for the digestion and absorption of intestinal lipids. Due to the absence of CCK, the motor function of sphincter of Oddi could be impaired in CCK KO mice. It was not excluded that defective function of sphincter of Oddi may have an effect on gallstone formation in CCK KO mice. Wang et al. also explored whether gallbladder hypomotility has an effect on evolutionary sequences of cholesterol crystallization and gallstone formation. This is not easily achieved in humans although investigators have attempted to study the physical-chemical phase separation sequences in bile before and during gallstone formation among obese patients who ingested a very low calorie diet or were undergoing weight reduction after gastric-bypass surgery by Marks, Shiffman and Broomfield et al. [200-202] Wang et al. found that in the lithogenic state, evolutionary sequences of gallstone formation were characterized by the initial accumulation of mucin gel, followed by the appearances of liquid crystals and/or anhydrous cholesterol crystals and classic plate-like cholesterol monohydrate crystals, and then agglomerated cholesterol crystals, sandy stones, and true gallstones (Figure 1.4.2), which were identical in appearance in all gallbladders of CCK KO mice. These sequences were in agreement with results of investigations in other animal models of cholesterol gallstones, such as the prairie dog by holzbach and Lee et al. [203, 204] and the gallstone-susceptible C57L mouse harboring *Lith1* and *Lith2* genes reported by Wang et al. [186].

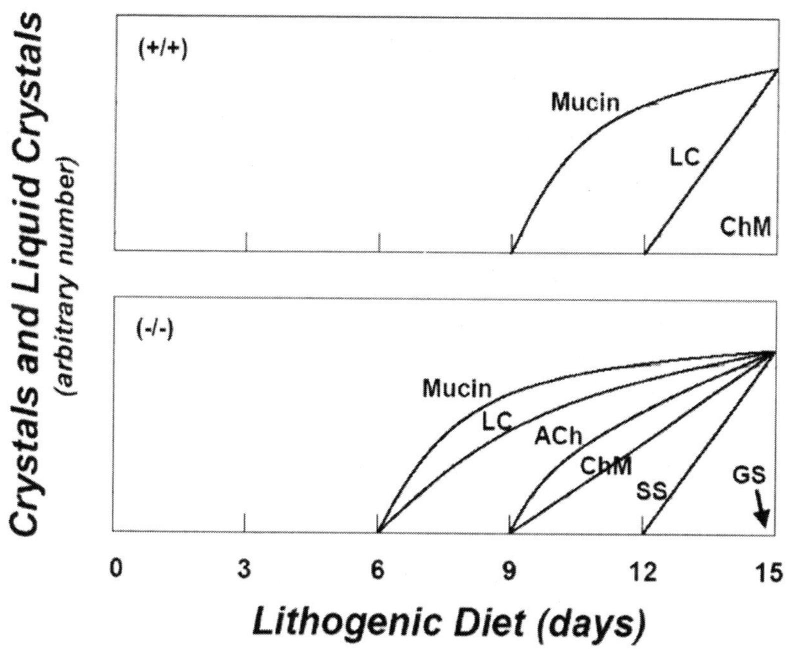

Figure 1.4.2. Schematic presentation of the crystal habits in the cholesterol crystallization sequence from fresh mouse gallbladder bile as functions of days on the lithogenic diet. The vertical axes represent arbitrary numbers of crystals and liquid crystals per high power microscopic field, all normalized to the same maximum. The panels show the time sequences as means for each group of CCK W (top panel) and KO mice (bottom panel). The arrow indicates the first appearance of true gallstones. Abbreviations: ACh, anhydrous cholesterol crystals, including arc-like and transitional tubular crystals; ChM, classic plate-like cholesterol monohydrate crystals; LC, liquid crystals, including small, aggregated and fused (multilamellar) varieties; SS, sandy stones; GS, true gallstones. See text for further description. Wang et al. Page 20 *Biochim Biophys.*

Further, Wang et al. found that besides the well-known liquid crystal to classic plate-like cholesterol monohydrate crystal pathway by Mazer and Halpern et al. [205-207] the anhydrous cholesterol crystal to solid cholesterol monohydrate crystal pathway by Wang [186, 187, 208] played a critical role in the early stage of cholesterol gallstone formation in mice with gallbladder stasis. Therefore, there were two cholesterol crystallization pathways in gallbladder biles of mice in response to the lithogenic diet, which are identical to those found in model biles for physiological lipid composition and in native human and mouse biles by Wang and Konikoff et al. [186, 187, 208, 209] Of special note is that the sequences of cholesterol crystallization and gallstone formation were more rapid in CCK KO mice than in other mouse models of gallstones on the same lithogenic diet by Marks and Borris, [177] which highlights the importance of gallbladder stasis. Why did CCK KO mice display rapid cholesterol crystallization and gallstone formation? Wang et al. found in their preliminary study that the lack of endogenous CCK induced a significant retardation of small intestinal transit times, which resulted in increased intestinal cholesterol absorption in mice with ablation of the *Cck* gene. These changes, in part, explained why the CSI values elevated earlier and gallbladder bile became supersaturated with cholesterol more rapidly in CCK KO mice than WT mice. Due to the absence of CCK-induced contraction, the resulting gallbladder stasis provided an environment for the longer stay of excess cholesterol in the lumen. Consequently, the elevation in bile cholesterol, coupled with longer contact time of saturated mixed micelles with cholesterol transporters on the apical membrane of gallbladder epithelial cells, facilitated cholesterol absorption by the gallbladder reported by Ginanni and Neidedhiser et al. [75, 210] Increased cholesterol concentrations in the gallbladder wall could further impair gallbladder emptying function as well as enhanced mucin production and triggered mucin hypersecretion and accumulation in the lumen. The gel-forming mucins secreted by specialized gallbladder mucin-producing cells, were able to form a gel phase in higher concentrations because they could form disulfide-stabilized oligo- or polymers, a phenomenon that accounted for their viscoelastic properties. Further, hydrophobic domains in the mucin molecule (on the nonglycosylated regions of the polypeptide core) allowed binding of lipids such as cholesterol, phospholipids, and bilirubin. The resulting water-insoluble complex of mucous glycoproteins and calcium bilirubin ate could provide a surface for nucleation of cholesterol monohydrate crystals and a framework of matrix for the growth of stones by Lee et al. [180, 181] On the study of the evolutionary sequences of gallstone formation, Fang et al. found very tiny cholesterol monohydrate crystals, for their first appearance, often within the mucin gel. Accumulated evidence has suggested that gallbladder mucins play an important role in the early stage of cholesterol gallstone formation, and are a strong pro-nucleating/crystallizing agent for accelerating cholesterol crystallization in native and model biles reported by Levy and Afdhal et al. [211, 212] The results from human and animal studies also support the concept that the hypersecretion of gallbladder mucins is a prerequisite for gallstone formation Wang, Lee and Mazer et al. [186, 203, 213] Further, mucins have been found within cholesterol gallstones where they could act as a matrix for cholesterol crystal and stone growth reported by Pensingh and Womack et al. [214, 215] Although in the past years, cholesterol crystal growth habits have been extensively studied principally in model bile systems by Pearson and Toor et al., [191, 216] little is known whether these pathophysiologically relevant phenomena take place in native gallbladder biles of humans and mice as well. Wang et al., for the first time, found that in mouse lithogenic biles, there were three modes of cholesterol crystal growth habits in the early stage of cholesterol gallstone formation, all of which enlarged solid cholesterol crystals in size. These observations were consistent with the results found in model bile systems by Toor and colleagues. [191] They observed that when the CSI values in bile are higher, the spiral dislocation growth and the twin crystal growth patterns are two predominant crystal growth habits by Toor et al. [191] Moreover, when the CSI values in bile are lower, there is the third mode of crystal growth habits: proportional enlargement patterns. Because it is not easy to determine lipid compositions of individual mouse gallbladder biles due to very small amounts of bile, Wang et al. could not establish a direct relationship between the CSI values and cholesterol crystal growth habits in Wang et al.'s study. Nevertheless, they found that defects in gallbladder contractility are associated with larger sizes of cholesterol monohydrate crystals mostly due to more rapid crystal growth by means of these three crystal growth patterns in CCK KO mice compared to WT mice.

In summary, the absence of endogenous CCK impairs gallbladder motility function due to deletion of the *Cck* gene, which enlarges gallbladder size and presumably provides longer residence time of excess cholesterol in the gallbladder lumen for cholesterol crystallization. These results reported herein are consistent with the lithogenic effects of gallbladder stasis observed in other species, including the human. These changes promote cholesterol crystallization and gallstone formation. It has been found that in humans, frequent gallbladder emptying through supra-physiological doses of i.v. administered CCK-8 could restore gallbladder contractility and prevent gallstones in subjects undergoing total parenteral nutrition by Portincassa et al. [217]. Thus, Wang et al.'s findings may provide an efficacious novel strategy for the prevention of cholesterol gallstones by promoting gallbladder emptying with a gallbladder-specific, CCK-1 receptor-selective agonist, particularly for pregnant women and subjects with gallbladder contractile dysfunction, as well as patients undergoing total parenteral nutrition.

References

[1] Huang, S.M., Yao, C.C., Pan, H., Hsiao, K.M., Yu, J.K., Lai, T.J., and Huang, S.D. 2010. Pathophysiological significance of gallbladder volume changes in gallstone diseases. *World J Gastroenterol* 16:4341-4347.

[2] Cervantes, J. 2000. Common bile duct stones revisited after the first operation 110 years ago. *World J Surg* 24:1278-1281.

[3] Maingot, R. 1980. *Types of cholecystitis: the management of acute cholecystitis and chronic calculous cholecystitisx*. East Sussex, England: Appleton-Century-Crofts. 12 pp.

[4] Masclee, A.A., Jansen, J.B., Driessen, W.M., Geuskens, L.M., and Lamers, C.B. 1989. Plasma cholecystokinin and gallbladder responses to intraduodenal fat in gallstone patients. *Dig Dis Sci* 34:353-359.

[5] Stolk, M.F., van Erpecum, K.J., Renooij, W., Portincasa, P., van de Heijning, B.J., and vanBerge-Henegouwen, G.P. 1995. Gallbladder emptying in vivo, bile composition, and nucleation of cholesterol crystals in patients with cholesterol gallstones. *Gastroenterology* 108:1882-1888.

[6] van Erpecum, K.J., van Berge Henegouwen, G.P., Stolk, M.F., Hopman, W.P., Jansen, J.B., and Lamers, C.B. 1992. Fasting gallbladder volume, postprandial emptying and cholecystokinin release in gallstone patients and normal subjects. *J Hepatol* 14:194-202.

[7] Portincasa, P., Di Ciaula, A., Vendemiale, G., Palmieri, V., Moschetta, A., Vanberge-Henegouwen, G.P., and Palasciano, G. 2000. Gallbladder motility and cholesterol crystallization in bile from patients with pigment and cholesterol gallstones. *Eur J Clin Invest* 30:317-324.

[8] Etgen, S. 2004. *Calculus II*. 9 pp.

[9] Portincasa, P., Di Ciaula, A., Wang, H.H., Palasciano, G., van Erpecum, K.J., Moschetta, A., and Wang, D.Q. 2008. Coordinate regulation of gallbladder motor function in the gut-liver axis. *Hepatology* 47:2112-2126.

[10] Braverman, D.Z., Johnson, M.L., and Kern, F., Jr. 1980. Effects of pregnancy and contraceptive steroids on gallbladder function. *N Engl J Med* 302:362-364.

[11] Carey, M.C., and Cahalane, M.J. 1988. Whither biliary sludge? *Gastroenterology* 95:508-523.

[12] Sherlock, S., Dooley, J., and . 2002. *Diseases of the liver and biliary system.* Oxford: Blackwell Science.

[13] Miura, F., Takada, T., Kawarada, Y., Nimura, Y., Wada, K., Hirota, M., Nagino, M., Tsuyuguchi, T., Mayumi, T., Yoshida, M., et al. 2007. Flowcharts for the diagnosis and treatment of acute cholangitis and cholecystitis: Tokyo Guidelines. *J Hepatobiliary Pancreat Surg* 14:27-34.

[14] Everhart, J.E., Yeh, F., Lee, E.T., Hill, M.C., Fabsitz, R., Howard, B.V., and Welty, T.K. 2002. Prevalence of gallbladder disease in American Indian populations: findings from the Strong Heart Study. *Hepatology* 35:1507-1512.

[15] Huang, S., Su, C., Wu, L., Chang, T., Wu, C., Lee, C., and Lui, W. 1989. Polarizing microscopy versus infrared absorption spectrcscopy in gallstone analysis. *Asian J Surg* 12:6.

[16] Zhu, J., Han, T.Q., Chen, S., Jiang, Y., and Zhang, S.D. 2005. Gallbladder motor function, plasma cholecystokinin and cholecystokinin receptor of gallbladder in cholesterol stone patients. *World J Gastroenterol* 11:1685-1689.

[17] Choi, M., Moschetta, A., Bookout, A.L., Peng, L., Umetani, M., Holmstrom, S.R., Suino-Powell, K., Xu, H.E., Richardson, J.A., Gerard, R.D., et al. 2006. Identification of a hormonal basis for gallbladder filling. *Nat Med* 12:1253-1255.

[18] Portincasa, P., Moschetta, A., and Palasciano, G. 2006. Cholesterol gallstone disease. *Lancet* 368:230-239.

[19] Portincasa, P., Moschetta, A., Petruzzelli, M., Palasciano, G., Di Ciaula, A., and Pezzolla, A. 2006. Gallstone disease: Symptoms and diagnosis of gallbladder stones. *Best Pract Res Clin Gastroenterol* 20:1017-1029.

[20] Sandler, R.S., Everhart, J.E., Donowitz, M., Adams, E., Cronin, K., Goodman, C., Gemmen, E., Shah, S., Avdic, A., and Rubin, R. 2002. The burden of selected digestive diseases in the United States. *Gastroenterology* 122:1500-1511.

[21] Shaffer, E.A. 2006. Gallstone disease: Epidemiology of gallbladder stone disease. *Best Pract Res Clin Gastroenterol* 20:981-996.

[22] Haslam, D.W., and James, W.P. 2005. Obesity. *Lancet* 366:1197-1209.

[23] Grundy, S.M. 2004. Cholesterol gallstones: a fellow traveler with metabolic syndrome? *Am J Clin Nutr* 80:1-2.

[24] Attili, A.F., Carulli, N., Roda, E., Barbara, B., Capocaccia, L., Menotti, A., Okoliksanyi, L., Ricci, G., Capocaccia, R., Festi, D., et al. 1995. Epidemiology of gallstone disease in Italy: prevalence data of the Multicenter Italian Study on Cholelithiasis (M.I.COL.). *Am J Epidemiol* 141:158-165.

[25] Afdhal, N. 2000. *Epidemiology, risk factors, and pathogenesis of gallstones.* New York: In: , editor. Basel: Marcel Dekker, Inc. 18 pp.

[26] Wittenburg, H., and Lammert, F. 2007. Genetic predisposition to gallbladder stones. *Semin Liver Dis* 27:109-121.

[27] van Erpecum, K.J., Venneman, N.G., Portincasa, P., and Vanberge-Henegouwen, G.P. 2000. Review article: agents affecting gall-bladder motility--role in treatment and prevention of gallstones. *Aliment Pharmacol Ther* 14 Suppl 2:66-70.

[28] Stolk, M.F., Van Erpecum, K.J., Peeters, T.L., Samsom, M., Smout, A.J., Akkermans, L.M., and Vanberge-Henegouwen, G.P. 2001. Interdigestive gallbladder emptying, antroduodenal motility, and motilin release patterns are altered in cholesterol gallstone patients. *Dig Dis Sci* 46:1328-1334.

[29] Portincasa, P., Di Ciaula, A., Baldassarre, G., Palmieri, V., Gentile, A., Cimmino, A., and Palasciano, G. 1994. Gallbladder motor function in gallstone patients: sonographic and in vitro studies on the role of gallstones, smooth muscle function and gallbladder wall inflammation. *J Hepatol* 21:430-440.

[30] Niebergall-Roth, E., Teyssen, S., and Singer, M. 1997. Neurohormonal control of gallbladder motility. *Scand J Gastroenterol* 32:14.

[31] Greaves, R., and O'Donnell, L. 2000. *Gallbladder motility and gallstones*. New York, NY: Marcel Dekker Inc. 21 pp.

[32] Pauletzki, J., Cicala, M., Holl, J., Sauerbruch, T., Schafmayer, A., and Paumgartner, G. 1993. Correlation between gall bladder fasting volume and postprandial emptying in patients with gall stones and healthy controls. *Gut* 34:1443-1447.

[33] Otsuki, M. 2000. Pathophysiological role of cholecystokinin in humans. *J Gastroenterol Hepatol* 15 Suppl:D71-83.

[34] Beglinger, C., Hildebrand, P., Adler, G., Werth, B., Luo, H., Delco, F., and Gyr, K. 1992. Postprandial control of gallbladder contraction and exocrine pancreatic secretion in man. *Eur J Clin Invest* 22:827-834.

[35] Maselli, M.A., Piepoli, A.L., Pezzolla, F., Guerra, V., Caruso, M.L., Mennuni, L., Lorusso, D., and Makovec, F. 2001. Effect of three nonpeptide cholecystokinin antagonists on human isolated gallbladder. *Dig Dis Sci* 46:2773-2778.

[36] Portincasa, P., and vanBerge-Henegouwen, G. 2000. *Gallbladder smooth muscle function and its dysfunction in cholesterol gallstone disease*. New York, NY: Marcel Dekker Inc. 25 pp.

[37] Portincasa, P., Di Ciaula, A., and vanBerge-Henegouwen, G.P. 2004. Smooth muscle function and dysfunction in gallbladder disease. *Curr Gastroenterol Rep* 6:151-162.

[38] Schneider, H., Sanger, P., and Hanisch, E. 1997. In vitro effects of cholecystokinin fragments on human gallbladders. Evidence for an altered CCK-receptor structure in a subgroup of patients with gallstones. *J Hepatol* 26:1063-1068.

[39] Upp, J.R., Jr., Nealon, W.H., Singh, P., Fagan, C.J., Jonas, A.S., Greeley, G.H., Jr., and Thompson, J.C. 1987. Correlation of cholecystokinin receptors with gallbladder contractility in patients with gallstones. *Ann Surg* 205:641-648.

[40] Wang, D.Q., Schmitz, F., Kopin, A.S., and Carey, M.C. 2004. Targeted disruption of the murine cholecystokinin-1 receptor promotes intestinal cholesterol absorption and susceptibility to cholesterol cholelithiasis. *J Clin Invest* 114:521-528.

[41] Miyasaka, K., Takata, Y., and Funakoshi, A. 2002. Association of cholecystokinin A receptor gene polymorphism with cholelithiasis and the molecular mechanisms of this polymorphism. *J Gastroenterol* 37 Suppl 14:102-106.

[42] Ding, X., Lu, C.Y., Mei, Y., Liu, C.A., and Shi, Y.J. 2005. Correlation between gene expression of CCK-A receptor and emptying dysfunction of the gallbladder in patients with gallstones and diabetes mellitus. *Hepatobiliary Pancreat Dis Int* 4:295-298.

[43] Inagaki, T., Choi, M., Moschetta, A., Peng, L., Cummins, C.L., McDonald, J.G., Luo, G., Jones, S.A., Goodwin, B., Richardson, J.A., et al. 2005. Fibroblast growth factor 15 functions as an enterohepatic signal to regulate bile acid homeostasis. *Cell Metab* 2:217-225.

[44] Modica, S., Murzilli, S., Salvatore, L., Schmidt, D.R., and Moschetta, A. 2008. Nuclear bile acid receptor FXR protects against intestinal tumorigenesis. *Cancer Res* 68:9589-9594.

[45] Goodwin, B., Jones, S.A., Price, R.R., Watson, M.A., McKee, D.D., Moore, L.B., Galardi, C., Wilson, J.G., Lewis, M.C., Roth, M.E., et al. 2000. A regulatory cascade of the nuclear receptors FXR, SHP-1, and LRH-1 represses bile acid biosynthesis. *Mol Cell* 6:517-526.

[46] Lu, T.T., Makishima, M., Repa, J.J., Schoonjans, K., Kerr, T.A., Auwerx, J., and Mangelsdorf, D.J. 2000. Molecular basis for feedback regulation of bile acid synthesis by nuclear receptors. *Mol Cell* 6:507-515.

[47] Sutherland, S.D. 1967. The neurons of the gall bladder and gut. *J Anat* 101:701-709.

[48] Mawe, G.M., Talmage, E.K., Cornbrooks, E.B., Gokin, A.P., Zhang, L., and Jennings, L.J. 1997. Innervation of the gallbladder: structure, neurochemical coding, and physiological properties of guinea pig gallbladder ganglia. *Microsc Res Tech* 39:1-13.

[49] Stengel, P.W., and Cohen, M.L. 2002. Muscarinic receptor knockout mice: role of muscarinic acetylcholine receptors M(2), M(3), and M(4) in carbamylcholine-induced gallbladder contractility. *J Pharmacol Exp Ther* 301:643-650.

[50] Yegen, B., Biren, T., Onat, F., Tankurt, E., Gurmen, N., Oktay, S., Chey, W.Y., and Ulusoy, N.B. 1995. Modulation of gallbladder contraction by pirenzepine in humans. *Am J Gastroenterol* 90:1489-1494.

[51] Parkman, H.P., Garbarino, R., and Ryan, J.P. 2001. Myosin light chain phosphorylation correlates with contractile force in guinea pig gallbladder muscle. *Dig Dis Sci* 46:176-181.

[52] Stone, B.G., Gavaler, J.S., Belle, S.H., Shreiner, D.P., Peleman, R.R., Sarva, R.P., Yingvorapant, N., and Van Thiel, D.H. 1988. Impairment of gallbladder emptying in diabetes mellitus. *Gastroenterology* 95:170-176.

[53] Shaw, S.J., Hajnal, F., Lebovitz, Y., Ralls, P., Bauer, M., Valenzuela, J., and Zeidler, A. 1993. Gallbladder dysfunction in diabetes mellitus. *Dig Dis Sci* 38:490-496.

[54] Raman, P.G., Patel, A., and Mathew, V. 2002. Gallbladder disorders and type 2 diabetes mellitus--a clinic-based study. *J Assoc Physicians India* 50:887-890.

[55] Palasciano, G., Portincasa, P., Belfiore, A., Baldassarre, G., Cignarelli, M., Paternostro, A., Albano, O., and Giorgino, R. 1992. Gallbladder volume and emptying in diabetics: the role of neuropathy and obesity. *J Intern Med* 231:123-127.

[56] Fiorucci, S., Scionti, L., Bosso, R., Desando, A., Bottini, P., Marino, C., and Morelli, A. 1992. Effect of erythromycin on gallbladder emptying in diabetic patients with and without autonomic neuropathy and high levels of motilin. *Dig Dis Sci* 37:1671-1677.

[57] Fiorucci, S., Bosso, R., Scionti, L., DiSanto, S., Annibale, B., Delle Fave, G., and Morelli, A. 1990. Neurohumoral control of gallbladder motility in healthy subjects and diabetic patients with or without autonomic neuropathy. *Dig Dis Sci* 35:1089-1097.

[58] Catnach, S.M., Ballinger, A.B., Stevens, M., Fairclough, P.D., Trembath, R.C., Drury, P.L., and Watkins, P.J. 1993. Erythromycin induces supranormal gall bladder contraction in diabetic autonomic neuropathy. *Gut* 34:1123-1127.

[59] Burgstaller, M., Barthel, S., and Kasper, H. 1992. Diabetic gastroparesis and gallbladder disease. Ultrasound diagnosis after multiple-component meals. *Dtsch Med Wochensch* 117:6.

[60] Altomare, D., Pilot, M.A., Scott, M., Williams, N., Rubino, M., Ilincic, L., and Waldron, D. 1992. Detection of subclinical autonomic neuropathy in constipated patients using a sweat test. *Gut* 33:1539-1543.

[61] Altomare, D.F., Portincasa, P., Rinaldi, M., Di Ciaula, A., Martinelli, E., Amoruso, A., Palasciano, G., and Memeo, V. 1999. Slow-transit constipation: solitary symptom of a systemic gastrointestinal disease. *Dis Colon Rectum* 42:231-240.

[62] Wedmann, B., Pfaffenbach, B., and Wegener, M. 1996. [Does chronic alcohol drinking modify digestive gastrobiliary motility?]. *Leber Magen Darm* 26:98-102.

[63] Chaudhry, V., Corse, A.M., O'Brian, R., Cornblath, D.R., Klein, A.S., and Thuluvath, P.J. 1999. Autonomic and peripheral (sensorimotor) neuropathy in chronic liver disease: a clinical and electrophysiologic study. *Hepatology* 29:1698-1703.

[64] Oliver, M.I., Miralles, R., Rubies-Prat, J., Navarro, X., Espadaler, J.M., Sola, R., and Andreu, M. 1997. Autonomic dysfunction in patients with non-alcoholic chronic liver disease. *J Hepatol* 26:1242-1248.

[65] Chawla, A., Puthumana, L., and Thuluvath, P.J. 2001. Autonomic dysfunction and cholelithiasis in patients with cirrhosis. *Dig Dis Sci* 46:495-498.

[66] Portincasa, P., Moschetta, A., Berardino, M., Di-Ciaula, A., Vacca, M., Baldassarre, G., Pietrapertosa, A., Cammarota, R., Tannoia, N., and Palasciano, G. 2004. Impaired gallbladder motility and delayed orocecal transit contribute to pigment gallstone and biliary sludge formation in beta-thalassemia major adults. *World J Gastroenterol* 10:2383-2390.

[67] Carey, M.C. 1993. Pathogenesis of gallstones. *Am J Surg* 165:410-419.

[68] Trotman, B.W., Ostrow, J.D., and Soloway, R.D. 1974. Pigment vs cholesterol cholelithiasis: comparison of stone and bile composition. *Am J Dig Dis* 19:585-590.

[69] Everson, G.T., Nemeth, A., Kourourian, S., Zogg, D., Leff, N.B., Dixon, D., Githens, J.H., and Pretorius, D. 1989. Gallbladder function is altered in sickle hemoglobinopathy. *Gastroenterology* 96:1307-1316.

[70] Attili, A., Casale, R., Di Lauro, G., Festuccia, V., Natali, L., and Pasqualetti, P. 1992. Assessment of gallbladder motility in patients with alcoholic hepatic cirrhosis after a fatty meal. A real-time ultrasonography study. *Minerva Gastroenterol Dietol* 38:4.

[71] Li, C.P., Hwang, S.J., Lee, F.Y., Chang, F.Y., Lin, H.C., Lu, R.H., Chu, C.J., and Lee, S.D. 2000. Evaluation of gallbladder motility in patients with liver cirrhosis: relationship to gallstone formation. *Dig Dis Sci* 45:1109-1114.

[72] Pompili, M., Rapaccini, G.L., Caturelli, E., Curro, D., Montuschi, P., D'Amato, M., Aliotta, A., Grattagliano, A., Cedrone, A., Anti, M., et al. 1995. Gallbladder emptying, plasma levels of estradiol and progesterone, and cholecystokinin secretion in liver cirrhosis. *Dig Dis Sci* 40:428-434.

[73] Moschetta, A., Stolk, M.F., Rehfeld, J.F., Portincasa, P., Slee, P.H., Koppeschaar, H.P., Van Erpecum, K.J., and Vanberge-Henegouwen, G.P. 2001. Severe impairment of postprandial cholecystokinin release and gall-bladder emptying and high risk of gallstone formation in acromegalic patients during Sandostatin LAR. *Aliment Pharmacol Ther* 15:181-185.

[74] Pereira, S.P., Hussaini, S.H., Murphy, G.M., Wass, J.A., and Dowling, R.H. 2001. Octreotide increases the proportions of arachidonic acid-rich phospholipids in gall-bladder bile. *Aliment Pharmacol Ther* 15:1435-1443.

[75] Ginanni Corradini, S., Ripani, C., Della Guardia, P., Giovannelli, L., Elisei, W., Cantafora, A., Codacci Pisanelli, M., Tebala, G.D., Nuzzo, G., Corsi, A., et al. 1998. The human gallbladder increases cholesterol solubility in bile by differential lipid absorption: a study using a new in vitro model of isolated intra-arterially perfused gallbladder. *Hepatology* 28:314-322.

[76] Behar, J., Lee, K.Y., Thompson, W.R., and Biancani, P. 1989. Gallbladder contraction in patients with pigment and cholesterol stones. *Gastroenterology* 97:1479-1484.

[77] Chen, Q., Amaral, J., Biancani, P., and Behar, J. 1999. Excess membrane cholesterol alters human gallbladder muscle contractility and membrane fluidity. *Gastroenterology* 116:678-685.

[78] Corradini, S.G., Elisei, W., Giovannelli, L., Ripani, C., Della Guardia, P., Corsi, A., Cantafora, A., Capocaccia, L., Ziparo, V., Stipa, V., et al. 2000. Impaired human gallbladder lipid absorption in cholesterol gallstone disease and its effect on cholesterol solubility in bile. *Gastroenterology* 118:912-920.

[79] Lee, J., Shirk, A., Oram, J.F., Lee, S.P., and Kuver, R. 2002. Polarized cholesterol and phospholipid efflux in cultured gall-bladder epithelial cells: evidence for an ABCA1-mediated pathway. *Biochem J* 364:475-484.

[80] Hauser, H., Dyer, J.H., Nandy, A., Vega, M.A., Werder, M., Bieliauskaite, E., Weber, F.E., Compassi, S., Gemperli, A., Boffelli, D., et al. 1998. Identification of a receptor mediating absorption of dietary cholesterol in the intestine. *Biochemistry* 37:17843-17850.

[81] Calvo, D., and Vega, M.A. 1993. Identification, primary structure, and distribution of CLA-1, a novel member of the CD36/LIMPII gene family. *J Biol Chem* 268:18929-18935.

[82] Acton, S., Rigotti, A., Landschulz, K.T., Xu, S., Hobbs, H.H., and Krieger, M. 1996. Identification of scavenger receptor SR-BI as a high density lipoprotein receptor. *Science* 271:518-520.

[83] Labonte, E.D., Howles, P.N., Granholm, N.A., Rojas, J.C., Davies, J.P., Ioannou, Y.A., and Hui, D.Y. 2007. Class B type I scavenger receptor is responsible for the high affinity cholesterol binding activity of intestinal brush border membrane vesicles. *Biochim Biophys Acta* 1771:1132-1139.

[84] Mardones, P., Quinones, V., Amigo, L., Moreno, M., Miquel, J.F., Schwarz, M., Miettinen, H.E., Trigatti, B., Krieger, M., VanPatten, S., et al. 2001. Hepatic cholesterol and bile acid metabolism and intestinal cholesterol absorption in scavenger receptor class B type I-deficient mice. *J Lipid Res* 42:170-180.

[85] Bietrix, F., Yan, D., Nauze, M., Rolland, C., Bertrand-Michel, J., Comera, C., Schaak, S., Barbaras, R., Groen, A.K., Perret, B., et al. 2006. Accelerated lipid absorption in mice overexpressing intestinal SR-BI. *J Biol Chem* 281:7214-7219.

[86] Johnson, M.S., Svensson, P.A., Boren, J., Billig, H., Carlsson, L.M., and Carlsson, B. 2002. Expression of scavenger receptor class B type I in gallbladder columnar epithelium. *J Gastroenterol Hepatol* 17:713-720.

[87] Miquel, J.F., Moreno, M., Amigo, L., Molina, H., Mardones, P., Wistuba, II, and Rigotti, A. 2003. Expression and regulation of scavenger receptor class B type I (SR-BI) in gall bladder epithelium. *Gut* 52:1017-1024.

[88] Davies, J.P., Levy, B., and Ioannou, Y.A. 2000. Evidence for a Niemann-pick C (NPC) gene family: identification and characterization of NPC1L1. *Genomics* 65:137-145.

[89] Altmann, S.W., Davis, H.R., Jr., Zhu, L.J., Yao, X., Hoos, L.M., Tetzloff, G., Iyer, S.P., Maguire, M., Golovko, A., Zeng, M., et al. 2004. Niemann-Pick C1 Like 1 protein is critical for intestinal cholesterol absorption. *Science* 303:1201-1204.

[90] Temel, R.E., Tang, W., Ma, Y., Rudel, L.L., Willingham, M.C., Ioannou, Y.A., Davies, J.P., Nilsson, L.M., and Yu, L. 2007. Hepatic Niemann-Pick C1-like 1 regulates biliary cholesterol concentration and is a target of ezetimibe. *J Clin Invest* 117:1968-1978.

[91] Spener, F. 2007. Ezetimibe in search of receptor(s)--still a never-ending challenge in cholesterol absorption and transport. *Biochim Biophys Acta* 1771:1113-1116.

[92] Yu, L., Hammer, R.E., Li-Hawkins, J., Von Bergmann, K., Lutjohann, D., Cohen, J.C., and Hobbs, H.H. 2002. Disruption of Abcg5 and Abcg8 in mice reveals their crucial role in biliary cholesterol secretion. *Proc Natl Acad Sci U S A* 99:16237-16242.

[93] Yu, L., Li-Hawkins, J., Hammer, R.E., Berge, K.E., Horton, J.D., Cohen, J.C., and Hobbs, H.H. 2002. Overexpression of ABCG5 and ABCG8 promotes biliary cholesterol secretion and reduces fractional absorption of dietary cholesterol. *J Clin Invest* 110:671-680.

[94] Berge, K.E., Tian, H., Graf, G.A., Yu, L., Grishin, N.V., Schultz, J., Kwiterovich, P., Shan, B., Barnes, R., and Hobbs, H.H. 2000. Accumulation of dietary cholesterol in sitosterolemia caused by mutations in adjacent ABC transporters. *Science* 290:1771-1775.

[95] Tauscher, A., and Kuver, R. 2003. ABCG5 and ABCG8 are expressed in gallbladder epithelial cells. *Biochem Biophys Res Commun* 307:1021-1028.

[96] Repa, J.J., Berge, K.E., Pomajzl, C., Richardson, J.A., Hobbs, H., and Mangelsdorf, D.J. 2002. Regulation of ATP-binding cassette sterol transporters ABCG5 and ABCG8 by the liver X receptors alpha and beta. *J Biol Chem* 277:18793-18800.

[97] Lawn, R.M., Wade, D.P., Garvin, M.R., Wang, X., Schwartz, K., Porter, J.G., Seilhamer, J.J., Vaughan, A.M., and Oram, J.F. 1999. The Tangier disease gene product ABC1 controls the cellular apolipoprotein-mediated lipid removal pathway. *J Clin Invest* 104:R25-31.

[98] Bodzioch, M., Orso, E., Klucken, J., Langmann, T., Bottcher, A., Diederich, W., Drobnik, W., Barlage, S., Buchler, C., Porsch-Ozcurumez, M., et al. 1999. The gene encoding ATP-binding cassette transporter 1 is mutated in Tangier disease. *Nat Genet* 22:347-351.

[99] Brooks-Wilson, A., Marcil, M., Clee, S.M., Zhang, L.H., Roomp, K., van Dam, M., Yu, L., Brewer, C., Collins, J.A., Molhuizen, H.O., et al. 1999. Mutations in ABC1 in Tangier disease and familial high-density lipoprotein deficiency. *Nat Genet* 22:336-345.

[100] Rust, S., Rosier, M., Funke, H., Real, J., Amoura, Z., Piette, J.C., Deleuze, J.F., Brewer, H.B., Duverger, N., Denefle, P., et al. 1999. Tangier disease is caused by mutations in the gene encoding ATP-binding cassette transporter 1. *Nat Genet* 22:352-355.

[101] Erranz, B., Miquel, J.F., Argraves, W.S., Barth, J.L., Pimentel, F., and Marzolo, M.P. 2004. Megalin and cubilin expression in gallbladder epithelium and regulation by bile acids. *J Lipid Res* 45:2185-2198.

[102] Hofmann, A.F. 2007. Biliary secretion and excretion in health and disease: current concepts. *Ann Hepatol* 6:15-27.

[103] Chignard, N., Mergey, M., Veissiere, D., Parc, R., Capeau, J., Poupon, R., Paul, A., and Housset, C. 2001. Bile acid transport and regulating functions in the human biliary epithelium. *Hepatology* 33:496-503.

[104] Dray-Charier, N., Paul, A., Veissiere, D., Mergey, M., Scoazec, J.Y., Capeau, J., Brahimi-Horn, C., and Housset, C. 1995. Expression of cystic fibrosis transmembrane conductance regulator in human gallbladder epithelial cells. *Lab Invest* 73:828-836.

[105] Scoazec, J.Y., Bringuier, A.F., Medina, J.F., Martinez-Anso, E., Veissiere, D., Feldmann, G., and Housset, C. 1997. The plasma membrane polarity of human biliary epithelial cells: in situ immunohistochemical analysis and functional implications. *J Hepatol* 26:543-553.

[106] Guarino, M.P., Cong, P., Cicala, M., Alloni, R., Carotti, S., and Behar, J. 2007. Ursodeoxycholic acid improves muscle contractility and inflammation in symptomatic gallbladders with cholesterol gallstones. *Gut* 56:815-820.

[107] Xu, Q.W., and Shaffer, E.A. 1996. The potential site of impaired gallbladder contractility in an animal model of cholesterol gallstone disease. *Gastroenterology* 110:251-257.

[108] Amaral, J., Xiao, Z.L., Chen, Q., Yu, P., Biancani, P., and Behar, J. 2001. Gallbladder muscle dysfunction in patients with chronic acalculous disease. *Gastroenterology* 120:506-511.

[109] Chen, Q., Amaral, J., Oh, S., Biancani, P., and Behar, J. 1997. Gallbladder relaxation in patients with pigment and cholesterol stones. *Gastroenterology* 113:930-937.

[110] DeCarvalho, S. 1985. Atherosclerosis. I. A leiomyoproliferative disease of the arteries resulting from breakdown of the endothelial barrier to potent blood growth factors. II. Perspectives in atheroprophylaxis. *Angiology* 36:697-710.

[111] Behar, J., Rhim, B.Y., Thompson, W., and Biancani, P. 1993. Inositol trisphosphate restores impaired human gallbladder motility associated with cholesterol stones. *Gastroenterology* 104:563-568.

[112] Chen, Q., Yu, P., de Petris, G., Biancani, P., and Behar, J. 1995. Distinct muscarinic receptors and signal transduction pathways in gallbladder muscle. *J Pharmacol Exp Ther* 273:650-655.

[113] Chen, Q., De Petris, G., Yu, P., Amaral, J., Biancani, P., and Behar, J. 1997. Different pathways mediate cholecystokinin actions in cholelithiasis. *Am J Physiol* 272:G838-844.

[114] Yu, P., Chen, Q., Xiao, Z., Harnett, K., Biancani, P., and Behar, J. 1998. Signal transduction pathways mediating CCK-induced gallbladder muscle contraction. *Am J Physiol* 275:G203-211.

[115] Jennings, L.J., Xu, Q.W., Firth, T.A., Nelson, M.T., and Mawe, G.M. 1999. Cholesterol inhibits spontaneous action potentials and calcium currents in guinea pig gallbladder smooth muscle. *Am J Physiol* 277:G1017-1026.

[116] Stolk, M.F., Van de Heijning, B.J., Van Erpecum, K.J., Verheem, A., Akkermans, L.M., and Van Berge-Henegouwen, G.P. 1996. Effect of bile salts on in vitro gallbladder motility: preliminary study. *Ital J Gastroenterol* 28:105-110.

[117] Xu, Q.W., Freedman, S.M., and Shaffer, E.A. 1997. Inhibitory effect of bile salts on gallbladder smooth muscle contractility in the guinea pig in vitro. *Gastroenterology* 112:1699-1706.

[118] Xiao, Z.L., Rho, A.K., Biancani, P., and Behar, J. 2002. Effects of bile acids on the muscle functions of guinea pig gallbladder. *Am J Physiol Gastrointest Liver Physiol* 283:G87-94.

[119] van de Heijning, B.J., van de Meeberg, P.C., Portincasa, P., Doornewaard, H., Hoebers, F.J., van Erpecum, K.J., and Vanberge-Henegouwen, G.P. 1999. Effects of ursodeoxycholic acid therapy on in vitro gallbladder contractility in patients with cholesterol gallstones. *Dig Dis Sci* 44:190-196.

[120] Dopico, A.M., Walsh, J.V., Jr., and Singer, J.J. 2002. Natural bile acids and synthetic analogues modulate large conductance Ca2+-activated K+ (BKCa) channel activity in smooth muscle cells. *J Gen Physiol* 119:251-273.

[121] Wang, H.H., Afdhal, N.H., Gendler, S.J., and Wang, D.Q. 2006. Evidence that gallbladder epithelial mucin enhances cholesterol cholelithogenesis in MUC1 transgenic mice. *Gastroenterology* 131:210-222.

[122] Wilhelmi, M., Jungst, C., Mock, M., Meyer, G., Zundt, B., Del Pozo, R., and Jungst, D. 2004. Effect of gallbladder mucin on the crystallization of cholesterol in bile. *Eur J Gastroenterol Hepatol* 16:1301-1307.

[123] Gustafsson, U., Benthin, L., Granstrom, L., Groen, A.K., Sahlin, S., and Einarsson, C. 2005. Changes in gallbladder bile composition and crystal detection time in morbidly obese subjects after bariatric surgery. *Hepatology* 41:1322-1328.

[124] Brotschi, E.A., Lamorte, W.W., and Williams, L.F., Jr. 1984. Effect of dietary cholesterol and indomethacin on cholelithiasis and gallbladder motility in guinea pig. *Dig Dis Sci* 29:1050-1056.

[125] Hemming, J.M., Guarraci, F.A., Firth, T.A., Jennings, L.J., Nelson, M.T., and Mawe, G.M. 2000. Actions of histamine on muscle and ganglia of the guinea pig gallbladder. *Am J Physiol Gastrointest Liver Physiol* 279:G622-630.

[126] Jennings, L.J., Salido, G.M., Pozo, M.J., Davison, J.S., Sharkey, K.A., Lea, R.W., and Singh, J. 1995. The source and action of histamine in the isolated guinea-pig gallbladder. *Inflamm Res* 44:447-453.

[127] Martinez-Cuesta, M.A., Moreno, L., Morillas, J., Ponce, J., and Esplugues, J.V. 2003. Influence of cholecystitis state on pharmacological response to cholecystokinin of isolated human gallbladder with gallstones. *Dig Dis Sci* 48:898-905.

[128] O'Riordan, A.M., Quinn, T., and Baird, A.W. 2001. Role of prostaglandin E(2) and Ca(2+) in bradykinin induced contractions of guinea-pig gallbladder in vitro. *Eur J Pharmacol* 431:245-252.

[129] Trevisani, M., Amadesi, S., Schmidlin, F., Poblete, M.T., Bardella, E., Maggiore, B., Harrison, S., Figueroa, C.D., Tognetto, M., Navarra, G., et al. 2003. Bradykinin B2 receptors mediate contraction in the normal and inflamed human gallbladder in vitro. *Gastroenterology* 125:126-135.

[130] Kano, M., Shoda, J., Satoh, S., Kobayashi, M., Matsuzaki, Y., Abei, M., and Tanaka, N. 2002. Increased expression of gallbladder cholecystokinin: a receptor in prairie dogs fed a high-cholesterol diet and its dissociation with decreased contractility in response to cholecystokinin. *J Lab Clin Med* 139:285-294.

[131] van Erpecum, K.J., Wang, D.Q., Moschetta, A., Ferri, D., Svelto, M., Portincasa, P., Hendrickx, J.J., Schipper, M., and Calamita, G. 2006. Gallbladder histopathology during murine gallstone formation: relation to motility and concentrating function. *J Lipid Res* 47:32-41.

[132] Moschetta, A., Bookout, A.L., and Mangelsdorf, D.J. 2004. Prevention of cholesterol gallstone disease by FXR agonists in a mouse model. *Nat Med* 10:1352-1358.

[133] Greaves, R.R., O'Donnell, L.J., and Farthing, M.J. 2000. Differential effect of prostaglandins on gallstone-free and gallstone-containing human gallbladder. *Dig Dis Sci* 45:2376-2381.

[134] Xiao, Z.L., Andrada, M.J., Biancani, P., and Behar, J. 2002. Reactive oxygen species (H(2)O(2)): effects on the gallbladder muscle of guinea pigs. *Am J Physiol Gastrointest Liver Physiol* 282:G300-306.

[135] Xiao, Z.L., Biancani, P., Carey, M.C., and Behar, J. 2003. Hydrophilic but not hydrophobic bile acids prevent gallbladder muscle dysfunction in acute cholecystitis. *Hepatology* 37:1442-1450.

[136] Kano, M., Shoda, J., Irimura, T., Ueda, T., Iwasaki, R., Urasaki, T., Kawauchi, Y., Asano, T., Matsuzaki, Y., and Tanaka, N. 1998. Effects of long-term ursodeoxycholate administration on expression levels of secretory low-molecular-weight phospholipases A2 and mucin genes in gallbladders and biliary composition in patients with multiple cholesterol stones. *Hepatology* 28:302-313.

[137] Al-Jiffry, B.O., Chen, J.W., Toouli, J., and Saccone, G.T. 2002. Endothelins induce gallbladder contraction independent of elevated blood pressure in vivo in the Australian possum. *J Gastrointest Surg* 6:699-705.

[138] Alcon, S., Morales, S., Camello, P.J., Hemming, J.M., Jennings, L., Mawe, G.M., and Pozo, M.J. 2001. A redox-based mechanism for the contractile and relaxing effects of NO in the guinea-pig gall bladder. *J Physiol* 532:793-810.

[139] Bird, N.C., Ahmed, R., Chess-Williams, R., and Johnson, A.G. 2002. Active relaxation of human gallbladder muscle is mediated by ATP-sensitive potassium channels. *Digestion* 65:220-226.

[140] Cullen, J.J., Maes, E.B., Aggrawal, S., Conklin, J.L., Ephgrave, K.S., and Mitros, F.A. 2000. Effect of endotoxin on opossum gallbladder motility: a model of acalculous cholecystitis. *Ann Surg* 232:202-207.

[141] Greaves, R.R., O'Donnell, L.J., Battistini, B., Forget, M.A., and Farthing, M.J. 2000. The differential effect of VIP and PACAP on guinea pig gallbladder in vitro. *Eur J Gastroenterol Hepatol* 12:1181-1184.

[142] Huang, S.C., Lee, M.C., Wei, C.K., and Huang, S.M. 2001. Endothelin receptors in human and guinea-pig gallbladder muscle. *Regul Pept* 98:145-153.

[143] Kline, L.W., Benishin, C.G., and Pang, P.K. 2000. Parathyroid hormone (PTH) and parathyroid hormone-related protein (PTHrP) relax cholecystokinin-induced tension in guinea pig gallbladder strips. *Regul Pept* 91:83-88.

[144] Lindaman, B.A., Hinkhouse, M.M., Conklin, J.L., and Cullen, J.J. 2002. The effect of phosphodiesterase inhibition on gallbladder motility in vitro. *J Surg Res* 105:102-108.

[145] Merg, A.R., Kalinowski, S.E., Hinkhouse, M.M., Mitros, F.A., Ephgrave, K.S., and Cullen, J.J. 2002. Mechanisms of impaired gallbladder contractile response in chronic acalculous cholecystitis. *J Gastrointest Surg* 6:432-437.

[146] Nissan, A., Freund, H.R., and Hanani, M. 2002. Direct inhibitory effect of erythromycin on human alimentary tract smooth muscle. *Am J Surg* 183:413-418.

[147] Parkman, H.P., James, A.N., Thomas, R.M., Bartula, L.L., Ryan, J.P., and Myers, S.I. 2001. Effect of indomethacin on gallbladder inflammation and contractility during acute cholecystitis. *J Surg Res* 96:135-142.

[148] Pozo, M.J., Perez, G.J., Nelson, M.T., and Mawe, G.M. 2002. Ca(2+) sparks and BK currents in gallbladder myocytes: role in CCK-induced response. *Am J Physiol Gastrointest Liver Physiol* 282:G165-174.

[149] Xiao, Z.L., Chen, Q., Biancani, P., and Behar, J. 2001. Abnormalities of gallbladder muscle associated with acute inflammation in guinea pigs. *Am J Physiol Gastrointest Liver Physiol* 281:G490-497.

[150] McKirdy, M.L., Johnson, C.D., and McKirdy, H.C. 1994. Inflammation impairs neurally mediated responses to electrical field stimulation in isolated strips of human gallbladder muscle. *Dig Dis Sci* 39:2229-2234.

[151] Jazrawi, R.P., Pazzi, P., Petroni, M.L., Prandini, N., Paul, C., Adam, J.A., Gullini, S., and Northfield, T.C. 1995. Postprandial gallbladder motor function: refilling and turnover of bile in health and in cholelithiasis. *Gastroenterology* 109:582-591.

[152] Portincasa, P., Colecchia, A., Di Ciaula, A., Larocca, A., Muraca, M., Palasciano, G., Roda, E., and Festi, D. 2000. Standards for diagnosis of gastrointestinal motility disorders. Section: ultrasonography. A position statement from the Gruppo Italiano di Studio Motilita Apparato Digerente. *Dig Liver Dis* 32:160-172.

[153] Everson, G.T., Braverman, D.Z., Johnson, M.L., and Kern, F., Jr. 1980. A critical evaluation of real-time ultrasonography for the study of gallbladder volume and contraction. *Gastroenterology* 79:40-46.

[154] Festi, D., Frabboni, R., Bazzoli, F., Sangermano, A., Ronchi, M., Rossi, L., Parini, P., Orsini, M., Primerano, A.M., Mazzella, G., et al. 1990. Gallbladder motility in cholesterol gallstone disease. Effect of ursodeoxycholic acid administration and gallstone dissolution. *Gastroenterology* 99:1779-1785.

[155] Pomeranz, I.S., and Shaffer, E.A. 1985. Abnormal gallbladder emptying in a subgroup of patients with gallstones. *Gastroenterology* 88:787-791.

[156] Palasciano, G., Portincasa, P., Belfiore, A., Baldassarre, G., and Albano, O. 1992. Opposite effects of cholestyramine and loxiglumide on gallbladder dynamics in humans. *Gastroenterology* 102:633-639.

[157] Portincasa, P., Peeters, T.L., van Berge-Henegouwen, G.P., van Solinge, W.W., Palasciano, G., and van Erpecum, K.J. 2000. Acute intraduodenal bile salt depletion leads to strong gallbladder contraction, altered antroduodenal motility and high plasma motilin levels in humans. *Neurogastroenterol Motil* 12:421-430.

[158] Colecchia, A., Sandri, L., Bacchi-Reggiani, M.L., Portincasa, P., Palasciano, G., Mazzella, G., Roda, E., and Festi, D. 2006. Is it possible to predict the clinical course of gallstone disease? Usefulness of gallbladder motility evaluation in a clinical setting. *Am J Gastroenterol* 101:2576-2581; quiz 2672.

[159] Forgacs, I.C., Maisey, M.N., Murphy, G.M., and Dowling, R.H. 1984. Influence of gallstones and ursodeoxycholic acid therapy on gallbladder emptying. *Gastroenterology* 87:299-307.

[160] Venneman, N.G., Besselink, M.G., Keulemans, Y.C., Vanberge-Henegouwen, G.P., Boermeester, M.A., Broeders, I.A., Go, P.M., and van Erpecum, K.J. 2006.

Ursodeoxycholic acid exerts no beneficial effect in patients with symptomatic gallstones awaiting cholecystectomy. *Hepatology* 43:1276-1283.

[161] Pozo, M.J., Camello, P.J., and Mawe, G.M. 2004. Chemical mediators of gallbladder dysmotility. *Curr Med Chem* 11:1801-1812.

[162] Shaffer, E.A. 2000. Review article: control of gall-bladder motor function. *Aliment Pharmacol Ther* 14 Suppl 2:2-8.

[163] Li, J., Pircher, P.C., Schulman, I.G., and Westin, S.K. 2005. Regulation of complement C3 expression by the bile acid receptor FXR. *J Biol Chem* 280:7427-7434.

[164] Ornitz, D.M. 2000. FGFs, heparan sulfate and FGFRs: complex interactions essential for development. *Bioessays* 22:108-112.

[165] Zhang, X., Ibrahimi, O.A., Olsen, S.K., Umemori, H., Mohammadi, M., and Ornitz, D.M. 2006. Receptor specificity of the fibroblast growth factor family. The complete mammalian FGF family. *J Biol Chem* 281:15694-15700.

[166] Kline, L.W., Zhang, M.L., and Pang, P.K. 1997. Cyclic AMP induces a relaxation response in the bullfrog Rana catesbeiana, but nitric oxide does not. *J Exp Biol* 200:2669-2674.

[167] Gomez, G., Upp, J.R., Jr., Lluis, F., Alexander, R.W., Poston, G.J., Greeley, G.H., Jr., and Thompson, J.C. 1988. Regulation of the release of cholecystokinin by bile salts in dogs and humans. *Gastroenterology* 94:1036-1046.

[168] Malagelada, J.R., Go, V.L., DiMagno, E.P., and Summerskill, W.H. 1973. Interactions between intraluminal bile acids and digestive products on pancreatic and gallbladder function. *J Clin Invest* 52:2160-2165.

[169] LaMorte, W.W., Matolo, N.M., Birkett, D.H., and Williams, L.F., Jr. 1981. Pathogenesis of cholesterol gallstones. *Surg Clin North Am* 61:765-774.

[170] Pauletzki, J., and Paumgartner, G. 2000. Review article: defects in gall-bladder motor function--role in gallstone formation and recurrence. *Aliment Pharmacol Ther* 14 Suppl 2:32-34.

[171] Wang, H.H., Portincasa, P., Liu, M., Tso, P., Samuelson, L.C., and Wang, D.Q. 2010. Effect of gallbladder hypomotility on cholesterol crystallization and growth in CCK-deficient mice. *Biochim Biophys Acta* 1801:138-146.

[172] Wang, D.Q., Cohen, D.E., and Carey, M.C. 2009. Biliary lipids and cholesterol gallstone disease. *J Lipid Res* 50 Suppl:S406-411.

[173] Carey, M.C., and Small, D.M. 1978. The physical chemistry of cholesterol solubility in bile. Relationship to gallstone formation and dissolution in man. *J Clin Invest* 61:998-1026.

[174] Holzbach, R.T., Marsh, M., Olszewski, M., and Holan, K. 1973. Cholesterol solubility in bile. Evidence that supersaturated bile is frequent in healthy man. *J Clin Invest* 52:1467-1479.

[175] Holan, K.R., Holzbach, R.T., Hermann, R.E., Cooperman, A.M., and Claffey, W.J. 1979. Nucleation time: a key factor in the pathogenesis of cholesterol gallstone disease. *Gastroenterology* 77:611-617.

[176] Sedaghat, A., and Grundy, S.M. 1980. Cholesterol crystals and the formation of cholesterol gallstones. *N Engl J Med* 302:1274-1277.

[177] Marks, J.W., and Bonorris, G. 1984. Intermittency of cholesterol crystals in duodenal bile from gallstone patients. *Gastroenterology* 87:622-627.

[178] Susann, P.W., Sheppard, F., and Baloga, A.J. 1985. Detection of occult gallbladder disease by duodenal drainage collected endoscopically. A clinical and pathologic correlation. *Am Surg* 51:162-165.

[179] Neoptolemos, J.P., Davidson, B.R., Winder, A.F., and Vallance, D. 1988. Role of duodenal bile crystal analysis in the investigation of 'idiopathic' pancreatitis. *Br J Surg* 75:450-453.

[180] Lee, S.P., and Nicholls, J.F. 1986. Nature and composition of biliary sludge. *Gastroenterology* 90:677-686.

[181] Lee, S.P., Maher, K., and Nicholls, J.F. 1988. Origin and fate of biliary sludge. *Gastroenterology* 94:170-176.

[182] Ko, C.W., Schulte, S.J., and Lee, S.P. 2005. Biliary sludge is formed by modification of hepatic bile by the gallbladder mucosa. *Clin Gastroenterol Hepatol* 3:672-678.

[183] Ivy, A., and Oldberg, E. 1928. A hormone mechanism for gallbladder contraction and evacuation. *Am J of Physiol* 86:15.

[184] Schjoldager, B.T. 1994. Role of CCK in gallbladder function. *Ann N Y Acad Sci* 713:207-218.

[185] Lacourse, K.A., Swanberg, L.J., Gillespie, P.J., Rehfeld, J.F., Saunders, T.L., and Samuelson, L.C. 1999. Pancreatic function in CCK-deficient mice: adaptation to dietary protein does not require CCK. *Am J Physiol* 276:G1302-1309.

[186] Wang, D.Q., Paigen, B., and Carey, M.C. 1997. Phenotypic characterization of Lith genes that determine susceptibility to cholesterol cholelithiasis in inbred mice: physical-chemistry of gallbladder bile. *J Lipid Res* 38:1395-1411.

[187] Wang, D.Q., and Carey, M.C. 1996. Complete mapping of crystallization pathways during cholesterol precipitation from model bile: influence of physical-chemical variables of pathophysiologic relevance and identification of a stable liquid crystalline state in cold, dilute and hydrophilic bile salt-containing systems. *J Lipid Res* 37:606-630.

[188] Bartlett, G.R. 1959. Phosphorus assay in column chromatography. *J Biol Chem* 234:466-468.

[189] Turley, S.D., and Dietschy, J.M. 1978. Re-evaluation of the 3 alpha-hydroxysteroid dehydrogenase assay for total bile acids in bile. *J Lipid Res* 19:924-928.

[190] Carey, M.C. 1978. Critical tables for calculating the cholesterol saturation of native bile. *J Lipid Res* 19:945-955.

[191] Toor, E.W., Evans, D.F., and Cussler, E.L. 1978. Cholesterol monohydrate growth in model bile solutions. *Proc Natl Acad Sci U S A* 75:6230-6234.

[192] Wang, H., Portincasa, P., and Wang, D. 2008. Molecular pathophysiology and physical chemistry of cholesterol gallstones. *Front Biosci* 13:23.

[193] Roslyn, J.J., Pitt, H.A., Mann, L.L., Ament, M.E., and DenBesten, L. 1983. Gallbladder disease in patients on long-term parenteral nutrition. *Gastroenterology* 84:148-154.

[194] Pitt, H.A., King, W., 3rd, Mann, L.L., Roslyn, J.J., Berquist, W.E., Ament, M.E., and DenBesten, L. 1983. Increased risk of cholelithiasis with prolonged total parenteral nutrition. *Am J Surg* 145:106-112.

[195] Haber, G.B., and Heaton, K.W. 1979. Lipid composition of bile in diabetics and obesity-matched controls. *Gut* 20:518-522.

[196] Vezina, W.C., Paradis, R.L., Grace, D.M., Zimmer, R.A., Lamont, D.D., Rycroft, K.M., King, M.E., Hutton, L.C., and Chey, W.Y. 1990. Increased volume and decreased

emptying of the gallbladder in large (morbidly obese, tall normal, and muscular normal) people. *Gastroenterology* 98:1000-1007.

[197] Kodama, H., Kono, S., Todoroki, I., Honjo, S., Sakurai, Y., Wakabayashi, K., Nishiwaki, M., Hamada, H., Nishikawa, H., Koga, H., et al. 1999. Gallstone disease risk in relation to body mass index and waist-to-hip ratio in Japanese men. *Int J Obes Relat Metab Disord* 23:211-216.

[198] Stampfer, M.J., Maclure, K.M., Colditz, G.A., Manson, J.E., and Willett, W.C. 1992. Risk of symptomatic gallstones in women with severe obesity. *Am J Clin Nutr* 55:652-658.

[199] Ko, C.W., Beresford, S.A., Schulte, S.J., Matsumoto, A.M., and Lee, S.P. 2005. Incidence, natural history, and risk factors for biliary sludge and stones during pregnancy. *Hepatology* 41:359-365.

[200] Marks, J.W., Bonorris, G.G., Albers, G., and Schoenfield, L.J. 1992. The sequence of biliary events preceding the formation of gallstones in humans. *Gastroenterology* 103:566-570.

[201] Shiffman, M.L., Sugerman, H.J., Kellum, J.M., Brewer, W.H., and Moore, E.W. 1991. Gallstone formation after rapid weight loss: a prospective study in patients undergoing gastric bypass surgery for treatment of morbid obesity. *Am J Gastroenterol* 86:1000-1005.

[202] Broomfield, P.H., Chopra, R., Sheinbaum, R.C., Bonorris, G.G., Silverman, A., Schoenfield, L.J., and Marks, J.W. 1988. Effects of ursodeoxycholic acid and aspirin on the formation of lithogenic bile and gallstones during loss of weight. *N Engl J Med* 319:1567-1572.

[203] Lee, S.P., LaMont, J.T., and Carey, M.C. 1981. Role of gallbladder mucus hypersecretion in the evolution of cholesterol gallstones. *J Clin Invest* 67:1712-1723.

[204] Holzbach, R.T., Corbusier, C., Marsh, M., and Naito, H.K. 1976. The process of cholesterol cholelithiasis induced by diet in the prairie dog: a physicochemical characterization. *J Lab Clin Med* 87:987-998.

[205] Mazer, N.A., and Carey, M.C. 1983. Quasi-elastic light-scattering studies of aqueous biliary lipid systems. Cholesterol solubilization and precipitation in model bile solutions. *Biochemistry* 22:426-442.

[206] Halpern, Z., Dudley, M.A., Lynn, M.P., Nader, J.M., Breuer, A.C., and Holzbach, R.T. 1986. Vesicle aggregation in model systems of supersaturated bile: relation to crystal nucleation and lipid composition of the vesicular phase. *J Lipid Res* 27:295-306.

[207] Halpern, Z., Dudley, M.A., Kibe, A., Lynn, M.P., Breuer, A.C., and Holzbach, R.T. 1986. Rapid vesicle formation and aggregation in abnormal human biles. A time-lapse video-enhanced contrast microscopy study. *Gastroenterology* 90:875-885.

[208] Konikoff, F.M., Chung, D.S., Donovan, J.M., Small, D.M., and Carey, M.C. 1992. Filamentous, helical, and tubular microstructures during cholesterol crystallization from bile. Evidence that cholesterol does not nucleate classic monohydrate plates. *J Clin Invest* 90:1155 1160.

[209] Wang, D.Q., and Carey, M.C. 1996. Characterization of crystallization pathways during cholesterol precipitation from human gallbladder biles: identical pathways to corresponding model biles with three predominating sequences. *J Lipid Res* 37:2539-2549.

[210] Neiderhiser, D.H., Harmon, C.K., and Roth, H.P. 1976. Absorption of cholesterol by the gallbladder. *J Lipid Res* 17:117-124.

[211] Levy, P.F., Smith, B.F., and LaMont, J.T. 1984. Human gallbladder mucin accelerates nucleation of cholesterol in artificial bile. *Gastroenterology* 87:270-275.

[212] Afdhal, N.H., Niu, N., Gantz, D., Small, D.M., and Smith, B.F. 1993. Bovine gallbladder mucin accelerates cholesterol monohydrate crystal growth in model bile. *Gastroenterology* 104:1515-1523.

[213] Pemsingh, R.S., MacPherson, B.R., and Scott, G.W. 1987. Mucus hypersecretion in the gallbladder epithelium of ground squirrels fed a lithogenic diet for the induction of cholesterol gallstones. *Hepatology* 7:1267-1271.

[214] Womack, N.A. 1971. The development of gallstones. *Surg Gynecol Obstet* 133:937-945.

[215] Pearson, J.P., and Foster, S.N. 1987. Mucus glycoprotein content of human cholesterol gallstones. *Digestion* 36:132-140.

[216] Portincasa, P., Venneman, N.G., Moschetta, A., van den Berg, A., Palasciano, G., vanBerge-Henegouwen, G.P., and van Erpecum, K.J. 2002. Quantitation of cholesterol crystallization from supersaturated model bile. *J Lipid Res* 43:604-610.

[217] Sitzmann, J.V., Pitt, H.A., Steinborn, P.A., Pasha, Z.R., and Sanders, R.C. 1990. Cholecystokinin prevents parenteral nutrition induced biliary sludge in humans. *Surg Gynecol Obstet* 170:25-31.

Chapter II

Etiology and Pathogenesis of Cholesterol Gallstones

I. Introduction

Cholesterol gallstone disease results from a complex interaction of genetic and environmental risk factors. Discoveries linking gene transcription, protein function, lipid metabolism, and regulation of biliary lipid secretion in the formation of cholesterol gallstones provide the impetus to review our understanding of the Disease as put forth by Portincassa et al. [1]

II. Pathobiology

Precipitation of excess cholesterol in bile as solid crystals is a prerequisite for cholesterol gallstone formation proposed by Hoffman and Lamont et al. [2, 3] Gallstones are abnormal masses of a solid mixture of cholesterol crystals, mucin, calcium bilirubinate, and proteins that have affected people for centuries advocated by Thudichum. [4]: multiple gallstones were found in a mummified Egyptian priestess discovered by Gordon-Taylor, [5] but the disease was first described in 1507 by a Florentine pathologist, Antonio Benivenius. [6] The Swiss medic Paracelsus viewed gallstones as a consequence of "tartaric" disease [7].

Patients present with single or multiple gallstones of different sizes, shapes (spherical or oval), and surfaces (smooth or morular). Both anhydrous Shieh and Konikoff et al. [8, 9] or monohydrate by Craven et al. [10] cholesterol crystals occur in human bile from cholesterol gallstone patients advocated by Portincassa et al. [11]

Cholesterol is only slightly soluble in aqueous media, but is made soluble in bile through mixed micelles by bile salts and phospholipids, mainly phosphatidylcholine, whose concentrations determine the degree of cholesterol saturation suggested by Carey. [12] The description of the ternary phase diagram by Admirand and Small (Figure 2.2.1) and later by Wang and Carey [13, 14] has clarified the importance of the relative amounts of bile salts and phospholipids needed to solubilize biliary cholesterol.

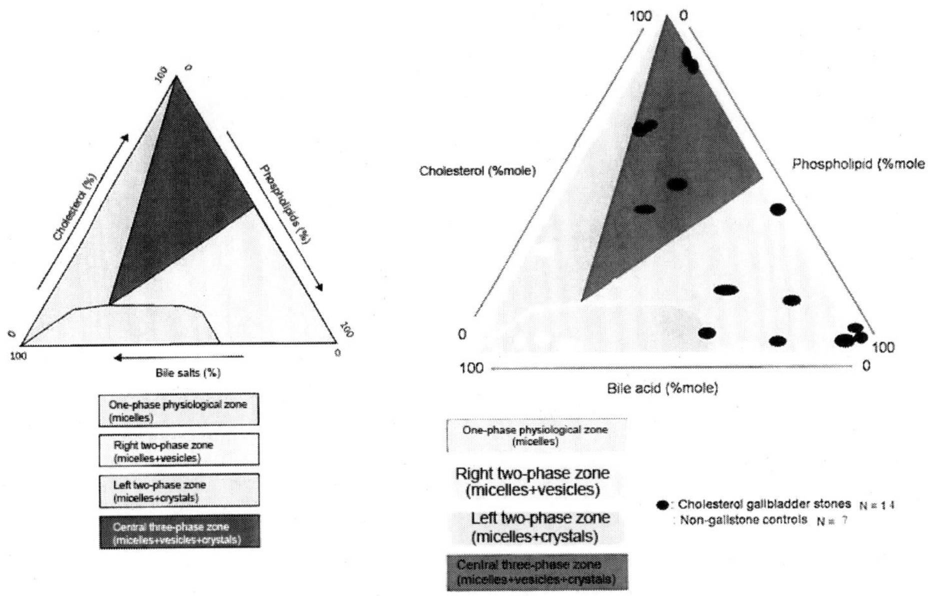

Figure 2.2.1.

Figure 2.2.1 demonstrates (a) schematic representation of the ternary bile salt-cholesterol-phospholipid phase diagram that describes the different pathways of cholesterol solubilization or precipitation, or both, in bile. The three axes of the triangle represent the concentrations of the three lipids. The triangle has been adapted from refs [15-18] for a putative bile of total lipid concentration 72 g/L, pH 7, and temperature 37°C. Cholesterol precipitates quickly with excess bile salts; at increasing amounts of phospholipids, cholesterol can reside in vesicles with phospholipids and crystal formation is slower or absent. Depicted are the one-phase zone in green (only micelles), and three zones with cholesterol supersaturation: a left two-phase zone (containing micelles, vesicles, and cholesterol crystals), and a right two-phase zone (containing micelles and vesicles). Bile from cholesterol gallstone patients plots within the orange and red zones. If the hydrophilic bile salt ursodeoxycholate is present, the yellow zone expands to the left at the expense of the crystals containing orange and red zones. Thus, a cholesterol-supersaturated bile of pathophysiological importance might lie in the three-phase zone (with crystals) if enriched with hydrophobic bile salts (i.e., deoxycholate), but in the right two-phase zone (without crystals) if enriched with hydrophilic bile salts (i.e., ursodeoxycholate) reported by Konikoff et al. [19] This partly explains why ursodeoxycholate prevents cholesterol crystallization and gallstone formation and is effective for oral litholysis in a subgroup of cholesterol gallstone patients. Figure 2.1b shows GB biliary lipids distribution in Taiwanese population. Ternary bile salt – cholesterol – phospholipid phase diagram demonstrating GB biliary lipids in Taiwanese gallstone patients and non-gallstone subjects as modified from Portincasa. [1] (b) In Taiwanese population, the GB biliary lipid distribution of gallbladder stone patients falls within the expected central three–phase zone and the unexpected right two–phase zone, whereas the GB biliary lipid distribution of non-gallstone subjects falls within the expected one–phase physiological zone and right two–phase zone as compared to the Western population. *Modified from courtesy of Lancet,* Elsevier Inc.

In supersaturated bile, phospholipids solubilize cholesterol into vesicles. Monohydrate crystals can precipitate from these cholesterol-enriched vesicles as suggested by Ko et al.,[20] become entrapped in gallbladder mucin gel together with bilirubinate (biliary sludge) reported by Holzbach et al., [21] and ultimately agglomerate into a macroscopic gallstone as reported by Apstein et al. [22] Nevertheless, supersaturated gallbladder bile with cholesterol crystals occurs frequently in healthy individuals as reported by Jirsa et al., [23] suggesting that microcrystals can be flushed into the duodenum during normal postprandial gallbladder contraction. In patients who form gallstones, pro-nucleating factors such as biliary glycoproteins and mucin as suggested by Portincassa et al., [24] as well as impaired gallbladder motility Portincassa et al. [25] allow these microcrystals to be retained and to eventually grow over months or years into macroscopic gallstones.

Role of the Liver and Biliary Lipid Secretion

Russell and Setchell find bile is composed mainly of water (>90%) [26] and is the primary excretory route for organic compounds such as cholesterol, lipid hormones, and drugs with low water solubility. The hepatocyte is the major site for cholesterol synthesis and peripheral uptake, and Crawford et al. find excess cholesterol is directly secreted into bile or converted into bile salts. [27]

Hofmann finds cholesterol and phosphatidylcholine are mainly secreted in bile as small unilamellar vesicles (40–200 nm in diameter) that form on the external hemi leaflet of the canalicular membrane. [28] Because of their detergent properties, Gerloff et al. find bile salts secreted from hepatocytes within the canalicular lumen directly convert vesicles into smaller (40–100 Å in diameter) structures called micelles. [29] Thus, "mixed" micelles containing bile salts and phospholipids and unilamellar vesicles are the physiological carriers of cholesterol in bile. Biliary lipid secretion is regulated by an elaborate network of ATP-binding cassette (ABC) transporters on the hepatocyte canalicular membrane. The ABC transporter (ABCB11), known as the bile salt export pump (BSEP), serves as the major canalicular bile salt export pump in mammalian liver as found by Gerloff et al. [30] The human multidrug resistant 3 p-glycoprotein, also known as ABCB4 (corresponding to the murine Mdr2 p-glycoprotein), functions as a "flippase", translocating phosphatidylcholine molecules from the inner to the outer leaflet of the canalicular membrane as found by Smit et al. [31] Finally, the ABC transporters ABCG5 and ABCG8 pump cholesterol into bile as found by Yu et al. [32] (Figure 2.1.). Two nuclear receptors in hepatocytes, the bile acid receptor or farnesoid X receptors suggested by Wang and Makishima et al. [33-35] (FXR) and the oxysterol receptors or liver X receptors as disclosed by Janowski and Zhang et al. [36, 37] (LXRs) play important roles in transcriptional regulation of the genes encoding these proteins. The expression of *ABCB11* reported by Ananthanarayanan et al. [3]) and ABCB4 Huang et al. [39] is under FXR control, while *ABCG5* and *ABCG8* are target genes of LXRs disclosed by Repa et al. [40]

The relevance of these transcriptional activations for cholesterol gallstone disease has been highlighted in a mouse model. After one week on a lithogenic diet, cholesterol gallstones formed in the gallbladder of FXR null mice, due to decreased biliary bile salt and phospholipid concentrations, associated with reduced expression of *ABCB11* and *ABCB4.* Treatment of gallstone-susceptible (C57L) mice with synthetic FXR ligands prevented cholesterol precipitation and gallstone formation due to the FXR-induced expression of *ABCB11* and *ABCB4,* which was associated with higher biliary concentrations of bile salts and phospholipids, and a subsequent lowering of the cholesterol saturation in bile compared to untreated animals demonstrated by Morschetta et al. [41] By contrast, activation of LXR by synthetic ligands rendered gallstone-resistant (AKR) mice prone to gallstone formation because of LXR-induced expression of *ABCG5* and *ABCG8*, which increased biliary cholesterol secretion and saturation.

Microsomal triglyceride transfer protein (MTTP) is critical for the production of very-low-density lipoproteins (VLDL).Amigo et al. [42] used mice in which *Mttp* had been inactivated in the liver (*Mttp* Δ/Δ mice). They measured several parameters of cholesterol metabolism, fatty acid synthesis, and biliary lipid levels in mice fed a normal or a lithogenic diet. They also assessed the incidence of diet-associated gallstones. They found hepatic *Mttp* inactivation markedly decreased plasma triglyceride and cholesterol levels and increased biliary cholesterol and bile acid output. Hepatic cholesterogenesis and fatty acid synthesis were significantly decreased in *Mttp* Δ/Δ mice compared with control mice. The incidence of gallstones decreased from 90% in control mice to 33% in *Mttp* Δ/Δ mice after 8 weeks of a lithogenic diet ($P < .0001$). The mechanism of the protective effect appears to be increased biliary phospholipid output in *Mttp* Δ/Δ mice, leading to significant unsaturation of gallbladder bile. These results indicate that modulation of *Mttp* expression in the liver affects hepatic lipid synthesis and storage as well as biliary lipid secretion. Inhibition of hepatic MTTP activity decreases the risk of experimental cholelithiasis by favoring phospholipid output into the bile.

The Gpbar1 [G-protein-coupled BA (bile acid) receptor 1] is a recently identified cell-surface receptor that can bind and is activated by BAs, but its physiological role is unclear. Using targeted deletion of the Gpbar1 gene in mice, Vassileva et al. [43] showed that the gene plays a critical role in the maintenance of bile lipid homoeostasis. Mice lacking Gpbar1 expression were viable, developed normally and did not show significant difference in the levels of cholesterol, BAs or any other bile constituents. However, they did not form cholesterol gallstones when fed a cholic acid-containing high-fat diet, and liver-specific gene expression indicated that Gpbar1- deficient mice have altered feedback regulation of BA synthesis. These results suggest that Gpbar1 plays a critical role in the formation of gallstones, possibly via a regulatory mechanism involving the cholesterol 7α-hydroxylase pathway.

The G2A receptor is a member of the ovarian cancer G protein– coupled receptor 1 family of stress-inducible G protein– coupled receptors. Laura et al. [44] examined the hepatobiliary effects of loss of function of G2A in mice fed either a chow or lithogenic diet. G2A-deficient (G2A$^{-/-}$) mice fed chow had a 25% reduction in biliary phosphatidylcholine content, reduced hepatic gene expression of the phosphatidylcholine transporter adenosine triphosphate–binding cassette B4, and an 8-fold increase in expression of the nuclear receptor liver X receptor (LXR). Despite the increased expression of LXR, transcription of several LXR target genes was reduced. G2A$^{-/-}$mice fed a lithogenic diet had rapid gallstone formation, an increased cholesterol saturation index, a 2.5-fold increase in farnesoid X receptor expression, a 5-fold increase in LXR expression, and a 90% reduction in cholesterol 7_-hydroxylase expression in comparison with wild-type mice. There were no changes in gallbladder volume. These data demonstrate that the G2A receptor is important for hepatobiliary bile salt, cholesterol, and phospholipid homeostasis and for the pathogenesis of cholesterol gallstone formation.

The relevance of these intriguing observations in mice to human gallstone disease is not yet clear. Through the quantitative trait loci approach, Paigen has identified genetic defects and described several *lith* genes in mice that are susceptible to cholesterol gallstones as reported by Paigen, khanula, Wang and Hillebrandt et al. [45-48] Description of candidate *lith* genes in the mouse by Wang et al. [48] will eventually help in the identification of the human *LITH* genes. Several family and twin studies, including haplotype analysis, have indicated the role of a few genes (*ABCG5*, *ABCG8*, *FXR*, *LDLR*, *CYP7A1*, *Apolipoprotein B-100*, *APOE*, *CCKAR*), as common genetic determinants for cholesterol gallstone diseases in humans as reported by Lammert et al. [49, 50] The precise understanding of the ultimate role of such genes as well as their functions is an active research field.

Role of Gallbladder Dysfunction in Gallstone Disease

Hepatic bile is concentrated in the gallbladder during fasting and emptied into the duodenum in response to feeding (Figure 2.1.2). Gallbladder-induced bile flow into the intestine facilitates digestion and absorption of lipids and lipid-soluble vitamins, and protects against intestinal bacterial overgrowth reported by Hofmann et al. [29] Meal-induced release of cholecystokinin (CCK) from the duodenum is the principal factor driving gallbladder smooth muscle contraction, accounting for 70–80% of the decrease of fasting gallbladder volume. A subgroup of cholesterol gallstone patients ("bad contractors") have severely decreased or even absent postprandial gallbladder emptying, whereas patients whose gallbladders empty ("good contractors") mostly have increased fasting and residual gallbladder volumes compared with controls reported by Portincassa and van Erpecum et al. [25, 51] Whether gallbladder dysmotility is a primary factor in cholesterol gallstone disease or secondary to inflammation reported by Xiao et al. [52] and excess cholesterol accumulation in gallbladder smooth muscle is debatable proposed by Portincassa et al. [53] Nevertheless, gallbladder motility is often impaired in many high-risk situations for gallstone formation, such as pregnancy, obesity and rapid weight loss in obese patients, diabetes mellitus, and total parenteral nutrition by van Erpecum et al. [54] Also, impaired gallbladder motility is an independent risk factor for gallstone recurrence after successful extracorporeal shockwave lithotripsy reported by Moschetta and Wang et al. [55, 56] Further, acromegalics are at high risk for gallstone formation during treatment with the somatostatin analogue octreotide, which suppresses postprandial CCK release and gallbladder contractility by Moschetta et al. [57]

Genetic deletion of the CCK-1 receptors in the mouse induces gallbladder stasis, increasing the risk of gallstone formation proposed by Wang et al. [58] A primary role for gallbladder motility in gallstone formation is also indirectly supported by the observation that daily CCK injection during total parenteral nutrition by Sitzmann et al. [59] or inclusion of dietary fat to enhance CCK release during rapid weight loss restores gallbladder contractility and can prevent gallstone formation by Gerhard et al. [60]

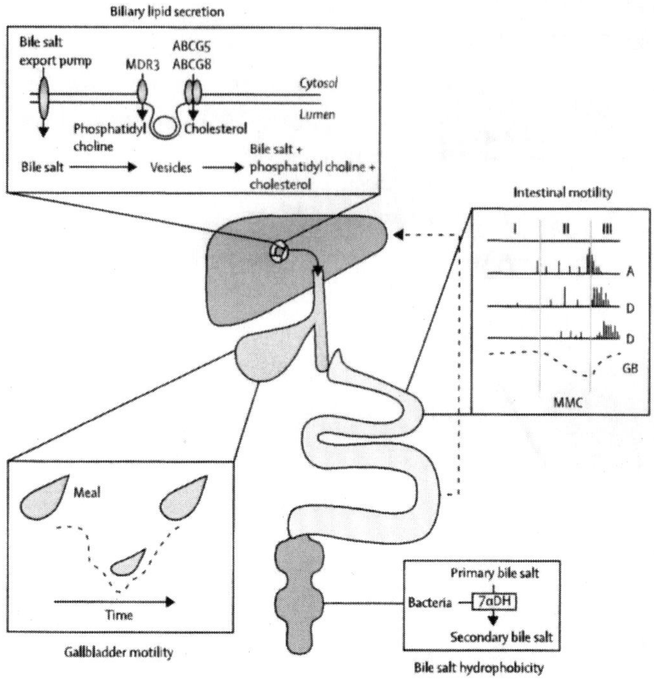

Figure 2.2.2. Role of the liver, gallbladder, intestine, and the enterohepatic circulation in cholesterol gallstone disease. The four boxes represent key physiological events in cholesterol gallstone prevention. Box A shows the pathways of biliary lipid secretion and nascent bile formation in the liver; Box B shows a schematic of normal time-dependent changes in gallbladder volumes before and after a meal; C shows the rhythmic cycles of gastric and small intestinal motility synchronized with periodic. fluctuations of fasting gallbladder volume (20–30% decrease of maximal fasting gallbladder volume occurs during end-phase II of the migrating motor complex, MMC). D represents hydrophobic secondary bile salts (deoxycholate and lithocholate), produced in the colon by bacterial 7α-dehydroxylation of the primary bile salts (cholate and chenodeoxycholate, respectively). The broken line represents the enterohepatic circulation of bile salts: after their secretion in bile and appearance in the duodenum, bile salts are reabsorbed in the ileum into the portal vein circulation and re-uptaken by the liver. 7αDH=7α-dehydroxylation. *Courtesy of Lancet, Elsevier Inc.*

Bile salts secreted into the duodenum are reabsorbed in the distal ileum and transported back to the liver where they are secreted into bile—the so-called enterohepatic circulation by Hofmann et al. [29] (figure 2.2.2). The circulating bile salt pool comprises primary and secondary bile salts. Primary bile salts (cholate and chenodeoxycholate) are synthesized de novo from cholesterol and secondary, more hydrophobic, bile salts (deoxycholate and lithocholate) are produced in the colon by bacterial 7α-dehydroxylation of primary bile salts as reported by Russell et al. [27] Slow intestinal transit can increase the rates of deoxycholic acid formation; indeed, impaired intestinal motility as well as increased biliary deoxycholate levels are found in some patients with cholesterol gallstone disease Carey and Lammert et al. [11, 61]

Evidence for a causal relation between impaired intestinal motility, deoxycholate formation and bile lithogenicity comes from studies in humans Shoda et al. [62] and mice by Heaton et al. [63] First, patients with cholesterol gallstones have increased amounts of Gram-positive anaerobic bacteria and increased 7α-dehydroxylating activity in their caecum, with subsequent higher levels of biliary deoxycholate compared with controls reported by van

Erpecum et al. [64] Second, treatment with octreotide (a known risk factor for cholesterol gallstone disease) prolongs colonic transit, biliary deoxycholate concentration, and biliary cholesterol precipitation reported by Thomas et al. [65] Further, antibiotic treatment decreases faecal 7α-dehydroxylation activity, and lowers biliary deoxycholate and cholesterol concentration reported by Thomas et al. [66] Animals susceptible to cholesterol gallstone formation have high levels of biliary deoxycholate, associated with cholesterol supersaturation and gallstone formation by Berr et al. [67] Altered gallbladder and intestinal motility can have a role in gallstone formation. Normally, a 20–30% fall in fasting gallbladder volume occurs in the fasting state, just before phase III (i.e., intense, regular coordinated contractions) of the intestinal migrating motor complex (MMC, see figure 2.1.2), associated with a rise in plasma motilin concentrations as reported by van Erpecum and DiMagno et al0. [68, 69] Gallstone patients have less frequent MMC cycles, absent fasting gallbladder emptying, and abnormal pattern of motilin release compared with controls as reported by Stolk et al. [70] In fact, more frequent food consumption and avoidance of long fasting periods seems to protect against gallstones suggested by Attili et al. [71] Intestinal absorption of dietary cholesterol can also contribute to stone formation. Animal studies indicate that high cholesterol absorption efficiency and subsequent rapid biliary secretion of cholesterol promote cholesterol gallstone disease by Wang et al. [72] Also, delayed or impaired small intestinal transit time has been associated with enhanced intestinal cholesterol absorption, biliary cholesterol secretion and gallstone prevalence advocated by Berr et al. [66] Nonetheless, conflicting data exist from research in human beings, with some studies showing that high dietary cholesterol either increases by Denbesten, Lee and Nervi et al. [73-75] or has no effect on cholesterol saturation of bile by Andersen and Hellstrom. [76]

III. Risk Factors

Several risk factors are involved in gallstone formation, such as having given birth, estrogen replacement therapy, oral-contraceptive use, and rapid weight loss reported by Grepco, Benion and Liddle et al. [77-80] Similar to atherosclerosis, the risk of cholesterol gallstone disease increases with age, obesity, type 2 diabetes, dyslipidaemia (hypertriglyceridaemia and low HDL [high density lipoprotein] serum cholesterol), hyperinsulinaemia, and sedentary lifestyle reported by Shaffer and Cuevas et al. [81, 82] All these conditions are risk factors for the metabolic syndrome, of which cholesterol gallstone disease is deemed as just another complication suggested by Eckel and Grundy. [83, 84] The consumption of the high calorie diet that is more common in the West is clearly a key factor in cholesterol gallstone disease. In fact, gallstone composition has changed over the past decades in East Asian countries, with a prominent increase in the prevalence of cholesterol gallstones, possibly because dietary habits have become more unhealthy insinuated by Honda and Tsunoda et al. [85, 86] Nevertheless, there is still little agreement about the risk of specific dietary components for gallstones suggested by Johnston and Kaplan. [87] The difficulty in estimating the ingestion of specific dietary constituents by individuals could account for the large variability in data for humans as in Cuevas et al.'s report. [82] Studies on the association between total fat intake and risk of cholesterol gallstone disease have reported either positive by Caroll-Bosc et al. [88] or non-significant by Maclure et al. [89] A high intake of cis-unsaturated fats was associated with a lower risk for gallstone disease in men suggested by Tsai et al. [90] Additional dietary factors associated with gallstone disease are cholesterol, highly refined carbohydrates, alcohol, and dietary fiber reported by Newbridge, Denbesten Cuevas et al. [73-76, 82, 91]

Risk Factors for Gallstone Formation

Gallstone formation is multifactorial, including constitutional and environmental factors. Some factors, such as diet, activity, rapid weight loss, and obesity, are modifiable, whereas others (eg, age, female gender, genetics, and ethnicity) cannot change. Several case-control studies, which compare those with gallstones versus those without, have identified important associations for harboring gallstone suggested by Shaffer [92].

Age

Gallstone disease is rare in neonates and young children. Once thought only related to pigment stones developing in the setting of hemolysis, cholesterol stones are becoming increasingly more common in children reported by Palasciano and Kaechele et al. [93, 94] Risk factors for gallstone disease in children include female gender, obesity, and Mexican American origin. The frequency of gallstones increases with age, rising noticeably after age 40 to become 4 to 10 times more likely in older individuals proposed by Thudichum. [4] Although age correlates positively with increased cholesterol secretion and saturation, the stone type found in advanced age tends to be pigment. Although gallstones are inclined to be clinically silent, symptoms and severe complications increase with age, leading to cholecystectomy in more than 40% of those above age 40 in a report from Germany by Volzke et al. [95] High prevalence rates of gallstones can occur in such older women (70 to 79 years old): 57% have a history of cholecystectomy or current sonographic evidence for gallstones.

Gender and Female Sex Hormones

Female gender is one of the most powerful influences on gallstone disease, with women almost twice as likely as men to form stones reported by Shaffer. [92] This is especially true for women in their fertile years, with the gap narrowing into the postmenopausal period when men catch up. Women are also more likely to undergo cholecystectomy. The basis for this finding seems related to the female sex hormones, because parity, oral contraceptive use, and estrogen replacement therapy are risk factors for gallstone disease reported by Cirillo et al. [96] During pregnancy, biliary sludge can appear in 5% to 30% of women; gallstones develop in 2% to 5% reported by Maringhini et al. [97] In the puerperium, sludge disappears in two-thirds whereas small gallstones (<1 cm) resolve in one-third. Additional risk factors include obesity (pregnancy weight), reduced levels of high-density lipoprotein (HDL) cholesterol, parity, and insulin resistance (the metabolic syndrome). Female sex hormones adversely influence hepatic bile secretion and gallbladder function. Estrogens increase cholesterol secretion and diminish bile salt secretion. Progestins act by reducing bile salt secretion and impairing gallbladder emptying leading to stasis as suggested by Portincassa et al. [1]

Obesity

Obesity connotes excess body fat, an entity that cannot be directly measured. Hence, it is best defined as a body mass index (BMI), which is used to express weight adjusted for height, as kilograms divided by height in meters squared (kg/m^2). The normal range of BMI is 20 to 25. Overweight is a BMI of 25 to 30. Obesity (>30) may be further divided into severe (>35–39) or extreme (morbid) when BMI is greater than 35 and accompanied by comorbid conditions, such as diabetes or cardiovascular disease, or when the BMI is greater than 40. Overweight for children and adolescents is a BMI for age at or above the 95th percentile of a specified reference population of 30 or greater suggested by Ogden et al. [98] The prevalence of obesity has risen drastically over the past several decades, acquiring the status of an epidemic not only in developed counties, such as the United States, but also in developing nations, such as China. Obesity is a major, well-established risk factor for gallstone disease, particularly abdominal/centripetal obesity (e.g., as measured by waist-to-hip ratio). The risk is especially high in women and rises linearly with increasing obesity reported by Maclure et al. [89] Women with extreme obesity have a 7-fold elevation in the development of gallstones compared with nonobese controls; their annual incidence of developing gallstones is 2%. Obesity earlier in life (late teens) carries the greatest risk, whereas slimness protects against cholelithiasis as reported by Thudichum and Admirand. [4, 15] Obesity is associated with increased cholesterol synthesis and secretion into bile. Obesity dramatically increases the risk of gallstone formation, especially in females reported by Attili, Everhart, Nakeeb and Heaton et al. [80, 99-102] In a large population study, Heaton et al. [103] have shown that a high waist-hip ratio predicts gallstones in men, whereas a high BMI and high weight gain after age 20 do not. In the Framingham study, the clinical risk increased two-fold in those women 20% above the median weight. [104] In the large ultrasonographically surveyed Copenhagen cohort (n = 5581), Jorgensen [3] found that gallstone prevalence correlated positively with body mass index in women but not in men, a feature also seen in the GREPCO [77] study of Roman civil servants and in West Britain reported by Heaton et al. [103] In the Sirmione study, [105] gallstone prevalence was significantly higher in obese subjects of younger age, and incidence rates over 5 years of follow-up were three times higher in obese than in nonobese subjects. In Texas, most Mexican-American teenagers with cholesterol stones were found to be markedly obese reported by Hanis et al. [106] In the large MICOL study of 29,584 individuals carried out on 14 cohorts between 1984 and 1987 in Italy reported by Attili et al.,[80] obesity proved to be one of the most consistent associations with gallstones in both males and females. A well-established pathophysiologic link between obesity and gallstone formation is cholesterol-supersaturated bile by Shaffer and Amaral. [107, 108] Obese people hypersecrete biliary cholesterol, bile salts, and phospholipids, but the rate of cholesterol secretion supersedes that of the other biliary lipids, leading to cholesterol-supersaturated bile reported by Carey and Small. [109] Weight reduction aggravates this phenomenon, as hepatic stores of cholesterol are mobilized, bile salt synthesis is decreased, and normal gallbladder emptying is interrupted, leading to further supersaturation of bile and rapid gallstone formation reported by Shiffman et al. [110, 111] In theory, increased flux of cholesterol from the bile into gallbladder muscle cells stiffens the sarcolemmal membranes, decouples signal transduction, and inhibits gallbladder muscle function suggested by Yu and Behar et al. [112, 113] Nevertheless, ultrasound data on gallbladder volume and emptying in obese humans are conflicting between Everhart and Vezina et al.'s reports. [99, 114]. While most studies suggest increased resting gallbladder volume in obese subjects, some reports demonstrate that these large gallbladders empty normally. [99, 114]

Dyslipidemia, Diabetes Mellitus, and the Metabolic Syndrome

Given that cholesterol gallstone disease is a metabolic problem, it should correlate with lipid abnormalities, diabetes mellitus, and adiposity. Although most gallstones in the Western world consist of cholesterol, there is no definite association with hypercholesterolemia as suggested by Shaffer. [92] Rather, a low HDL cholesterol carries an increased risk of developing stones, as does hypertriglyceridemia. The association between diabetes mellitus and gallstones is confounded by age, obesity, and a family history of gallstones also by Shaffer. [92] The link between diabetes, obesity, and gallstones most likely comes through the metabolic syndrome. The metabolic syndrome characterizes a specific body phenotype (abdominal obesity), insulin resistance (type 2 diabetes mellitus), and dyslipidemia (hypertriglyceridemia), all risks for cardiovascular disease. Insulin resistance predisposes to cholesterol gallstone disease as reported by Ruhl and Nervi et al., [115, 116] suggesting that hepatic insulin resistance must somehow affect cholesterol and bile salt metabolism.

Rapid Weight Loss

At least 25% of morbidly obese individuals have evidence of gallstone disease even before undergoing weight reduction surgery reported by Li et al. [117] Low calorie diets and rapid weight loss (particularly after bariatric surgery), ironically, are then associated with the development of gallstones in 30% to 71% of these obese individuals losing weight reported by Everhart, Broomfield and Shaffer et al. [92, 118, 119] Weight loss exceeding 1.5 kg/week after bariatric surgery particularly increases the risk for stone formation reported by Weinster et al. [120] Further, stones are most likely to become apparent during the first 6 weeks after surgery when weight loss is most profound observed by Al-Jiffry et al. [121]

Diet

Although nutrition, intuitively, should represent a key factor contributing to gallstone formation, findings are often conflicting and difficult to examine as reported by Reshetnyak. [122] Other than energy intake as calories leading to obesity, the importance of dietary content is unclear. Diets high in cholesterol, fatty acids, carbohydrates, or legumes seem to increase the risk of cholelithiasis. In contrast, unsaturated fats, coffee, fiber, ascorbic acid (vitamin C), calcium, and moderate consumption of alcohol reduce the risk suggested by Shaffer. [92] The shift to a more Western diet, high in refined carbohydrates and fat (triglycerides) and low in fiber, best explains the profound increase in cholesterol gallstones in American Indians (unmasking their presumed genetic burden) and in post–World War II European countries; this also may underline the shift from pigment to cholesterol stones in Asian countries. Genetic variations, especially in those genes controlling cholesterol metabolism, presumably underscore why some respond to dietary change by developing cholesterol gallstones reported by Sun et al. [123].

Total Parental Nutrition

Total parental nutrition (TPN) is a well-known risk factor for developing microlithiasis (biliary sludge) and gallstone disease, along with acalculous cholecystitis in critically ill patients suggested by Marschall and Einarsson. [124] In an intensive care setting, biliary sludge appears after 5 to 10 days of fasting. After 4 weeks of TPN, half of those on TPN develop gallbladder sludge; after 6 weeks all show evidence of sludge. Most are asymptomatic. Fortunately, sludge resolves within 4 weeks of discontinuing TPN and resuming an oral intake, a pattern similar to sludge appearing during pregnancy and rapid weight loss: sludge disappearing after the inciting event resolves reported by Carey. [125] A possible explanation for this relates to loss of the enteric stimulation of the gallbladder in the absence of eating, leading to gallbladder stasis suggested by Marschall and Einarsson. [124] Additionally, ileal disorders, such as Crohn's disease or ileal resection, in which TPN is frequently required, can affect the enterohepatic cycling of bile acids and thus augment bilirubin absorption and excessive pigment secretion reported by He et al. [126]

Lifestyle Factors and Socioeconomic Status

It is controversial if an association between gallbladder disease and socioeconomic status exists suggested by Sun et al. [127] Any inverse relation likely reflects socioeconomic status as an indirect marker for other risk factors, such as obesity and dietary issues. Physical activity helps prevent cholelithiasis, independent of its role in weight loss reported by Dikkers and Tiege. [128] Reduced activity heightens the risk. The role of smoking in cholelithiasis is unclear.

Family History and Genetics

Familial and epidemiologic studies demonstrate that genetic susceptibility is important in the formation of gallstones suggested by Claudel et al. [129] Occurrence within families can be a product of genetic and shared environmental factors. Familial studies reveal an increased frequency in family clusters (about 5 times more common in families of affected persons) and relatives of gallstone patients, but more convincingly in monozygotic (12%) as opposed to dizygotic twins (6%) suggested by Sarin et al. [130] Genetic effects account for 25%, shared environmental effects for 13%, while unique environmental effects for 62% of the phenotypic variance reported by Katsika et al. [131] The extraordinary susceptibility of American Indians might relate to thrifty genes that conferred a survival advantage when Paleo-Indians migrated across the land bridge from Asia to the Americas during the last great ice age (50,000–10,000 years ago). This might also explain their proclivity to acquire the metabolic syndrome and its sequelae reported by Shaffer. [92] The search for gene variants has implicated polymorphisms of apolipoprotein E4 being associated with biliary cholesterol supersaturation and cholesterol stones reported by Bertomeu et al. [132] other studies, however, failed to find such a correlation by Mella et al. [133] The frequency of reputed lithogenic genetic variants may coincide with the gallstone prevalence in certain populations reported by Grünhage et al.

[134] but none has reached common recognition in population studies. The search for single gene mutation, lithogenic alleles associated with cholesterol gallstones has focused on the adenosine triphosphate–binding cassette (ABC) transporters located in the hepatocyte canalicular membrane. Specific mutations have been identified for cholesterol gallstone formation in animal models and seem to be a susceptibility factor for human gallstone formation. The ABCB4 gene mutation (impairing lecithin secretion) represents a risk factor causing the low phospholipid-associated cholelithiasis (LPAC) syndrome: symptomatic and recurring cholelithiasis in young patients (<40 years) reported by Rosmorduc et al. [135] This monogenetic defect however is an uncommon cause of cholelithiasis in young adults, evident in less than 2% of cases indicated by Nakken et al. [136] More promising is the genome analysis that identified ABCG8 19H and ABCB4 variants (for cholesterol secretion) as susceptibility factors for human gallstones reported by Mella and Buch et al. [134, 137] This confers odds ratios of 2 to 3 and 7 or heterozygous and homozygous carriers, respectively, but accounts for only 11% of their total gallstone risk. Furthermore, a genome-wide search has uncovered 2 susceptibility loci, at least for symptomatic gallbladder disease located on chromosome 1p of Mexican Americans reported by Puppala et al. [138] Cholelithiasis seems to be a polygenetic disorder. The association between gallbladder disease and family history has been hypothesized since the mid 1900s. Jackson and Gay [139] investigated the family members of 100 consecutive white patients undergoing gallbladder surgery utilizing oral cholecystography and cholecystectomy. For 72% of the families, definite or suggestive evidence of gallbladder disease was obtained in a sibling, parent, or offspring. Because of an observed 3:1 female-to-male ratio in the study, they suggested that gallstone disease may be inherited as a sex-linked dominant trait. In a cross-sectional ultrasonographic study of a large cohort in Copenhagen (n = 4,581), Jorgensen [140] found a 2:1 positive association between gallstone disease in first degree relatives of subjects with gallstones, irrespective of the symptom status of the patients. In a 430 pair subset of the Sirmione study by Saama, Barbara and Progeto et al. [105, 141, 142] the relative risk of gallstones was 3.3-fold higher in sons and daughters of parents with gallstones when controlled for age and other confounding variables. Nürnberg et al. [143] examined by ultrasonography 1,616 symptom-free patients, mostly female, aged 12 to 93 years with gallstones in Northern Germany. They found a threefold increased family prevalence of gallstones in the younger age groups, compared with stone-free controls. Recently, a similar familial frequency of gallstones was found by Kratzer et al. among 1,116 young-to-middle-aged healthy blood donors who were mostly men. In the Italian MICOL study reported by Attili et al. [80] subjects with a history of gallstones in either parent had an increased risk of having gallstones; the risk was significantly higher when both parents had gallstone disease. The present analysis is consistent with these earlier studies in that a 2.5:1 incidence of symptomatic gallstones was found in both the association and family studies. Willem van der Linden in Northern Sweden did very useful work on the familial occurrence of gallstones during the 1960s and 70s. He attempted to sort out diagnostic and ascertainment bias with respect to control groups, as well as verifying the presence of stones by oral cholecystography or cholecystectomy. Van der Linden and Lindelof [144] restricted their investigation to proven gallstone patients who were married and who had siblings of the opposite sex. If the patient was a man, the occurrence of gallstones in his wife was compared with that of his sister nearest in age to his wife. If the patient was a woman, her husband was compared with her brother nearest in age to her husband. Employing this approach, 263 individuals (87 males, 176 females— mean ages 49

and 51 years, respectively) were evaluated rigorously for gallstones. The data showed a clear 2:1 ratio in favor of a familial occurrence for gallstone disease. Because familial occurrence does not necessarily reflect genetic factors, van der Linden and Westlin [145] then studied the occurrence of gallstone disease in spouses who had lived together continuously and presumably shared the same environment, especially diet, during adult life. They used similar methodology and found that women married to patients with gallstone disease do not suffer more often from the disease than do other women. The impact of heredity has been corroborated in three large, carefully controlled prevalence studies (by cholecystography/surgery/ultrasonography) from Sweden reported by van der Linden et al., [146] Israel reported by Gilat et al. [147] and North India reported by Sarin et al. [130] In each case, the data showed significantly higher, (≥2:1) prevalence rates of gallstones in the first-degree relatives of the probands compared with controls. Hanis et al. [106] also established in Mexican-Americans that the probability of an individual with gallbladder disease having a first degree relative similarly affected was 1.8 times the random probability. Several anecdotal reports of concordance of cholesterol gallstones in small numbers of monozygous twins have been published. In a large Danish study, 900 unselected twin pairs born between 1870 and 1910 were sent a questionnaire, which requested that they describe "any and all admissions to hospital, where, when and for what condition." Diagnosis of gallstones was obtained from the chart descriptions of the hospitalized cases. In the entire cohort, the crude incidence of cholelithiasis was 2.6%. Of a total of 101 twin pairs with a hospital diagnosis of cholelithiasis, concordance for the disease was found among 14/25 monozygotic pairs compared with 6/40 (same sex) and 0/36 (different sex) dizygotic pairs. Zero concordance among white twins of different sex most likely reflects the different frequencies of symptomatic cholelithiasis between men and women. Furthermore, if silent gallstone cases were ascertained, the actual frequency and concordance of gallstones might have been much more impressive. Kesaniemi et al. [148] randomly selected male twins (17 monozygotic and 18 dizygotic pairs) from the Finnish Twin Cohort. The males were living apart but residing in the Helsinki area. Their ages ranged from 43 to 58 years (mean 50) and mean body weight was 78 kg. Employing oral cholecystography and history of cholecystectomy, gallstones were ascertained in seven monozygotic and three dizygotic subjects, with two monozygotic and none of the dizygotic twin pairs being concordant for gallstones giving 40% pairwise concordance for the former and 0% for the latter.

These studies, albeit imperfect, constitute the best information on familial occurrence and monozygotic twin concordance for gallstones. While epidemiologic studies and the increased risk of a positive family history of gallbladder disease in a first degree relative suggest a role of genetic factors for gallbladder disease, direct evidence for the genetic determination of gallbladder disease is limited. In a recent study by Duggirala et al. [149] of 579 individuals from 32 Mexican-American families, questionnaire data on prior cholecystectomy was used to determine gallbladder disease status.

Using a maximum likelihood-based variance decomposition approach the heritability of symptomatic gallbladder disease was estimated to be 44% - 18%. This heritability is similar to the 29% - 14% we have reported in family study of Midwestern white families. Similarly, age and gender were also found to be significant covariates in this Mexican– American study.

Underlying Chronic Diseases

Liver Disease

Cirrhosis is a well-established risk factor for gallstones particularly in the more advanced stages reported by Acalovschi and Conte et al. [150, 151]. The overall prevalence is much higher than the general population at 25% to 30% reported by Conte et al. [152] Increasing Child-Pugh score and obesity are more likely associated with gallstones. Most stones in cirrhosis are of the black pigment type reported by Alvaro et al. [153] The biologic mechanism likely relates to altered pigment secretion, abnormal gallbladder motility, or increased estrogen levels reported by Shaffer. [92] The threat of these stones becoming symptomatic seems higher in women, those more advanced in age, and patients with viral hepatitis compared with alcohol-related cirrhosis suggested by Acalovschi et al. [154] Gallstone disease is also associated with hepatitis C virus (even when not yet cirrhotic) reported by Acalovschi et al. [155] and non-alcoholic fatty liver disease, the connection being the metabolic syndrome and obesity reported by Loria et al. [156]

Crohn's Disease

Crohn's disease, when associated with extensive ileal disease or loss, conveys a 2 to 3 fold increased risk of developing gallstones reported by Whorwell et al. [157] Although once believed due to bile acid malabsorption and depletion leading to cholesterol gallstones, recent studies have found an increased frequency of pigment stones. Unabsorbed bile acids that escape into the colon function as a biologic detergent to solubilize bilirubin and thus increase its absorption and enterohepatic cycling. The resultant increased pigment in bile then promotes stone formation reported by Vitek and Carey. [158].

Cystic Fibrosis

The gallstone prevalence in cystic fibrosis is increased: 10% to 30% versus less than 5% in age-matched controls reported by Vitek and Carey. [158] Like ileal Crohn's disease, cystic fibrosis is associated with bile acid malabsorption; in this instance, the bile salts bind to undigested dietary nutrients. Such bile salt depletion could lead to cholesterol stone formation or the escape of bile salts into the colon might enhance bilirubin absorption, resulting in pigment stones suggested by Portincassa et al. [1]

Other Diseases

In the irritable bowel syndrome (IBS), cholecystectomy is a more common operation because of diagnostic confusion leading to inappropriate surgery reported by Kennedy and Jones [159] or because the IBS symptoms are a consequence of the surgery.

Drugs

Octreotide

More than 50% of patients receiving octreotide (eg, acromegalic and cancer patients) or those with a somatostatinoma develop cholelithiasis; the majority are asymptomatic reported by Trenddle et al. [160] Somatostatin abrogates the postprandial release of cholecystokinin, presumably leading to gallbladder stasis.

Ceftriaxone

The third-generation cephalosporin antibiotic, ceftriaxone, is secreted unmetabolized into bile reaching high concentrations and producing biliary sludge reported by Bickford et al. [161] Usually, patients remain asymptomatic; sludge resolves once the medication is discontinued.

Statins

Drugs that inhibit hydroxymethylglutaryl–coenzyme A (HMG-coA) reductase not only diminish cholesterol synthesis in the liver but also decrease its secretion into bile, seeming to prevent cholesterol gallstone disease reported by Tsai et al. [162]

IV. Gallstone Pathogenesis

Gallstones are formed by the concentration or accretion of normal or abnormal bile constituents. There are three main types: cholesterol gallstones, mixed gallstones and pigment gallstones. Cholesterol and mixed gallstones account for 80% of the total, and pigment stones comprise the remaining 20%. Cholesterol gallstones and mixed gallstones both usually contain more than 50% cholesterol monohydrate plus a mixture of calcium salts, bile pigments, proteins and fatty acids.

Mixed gallstones contain cholesterol and a calcium bilirubinate component. Cholesterol is essentially water insoluble and requires aqueous dispersion into either micelles or vesicles, both of which require the presence of a second lipid to 'liquefy' the cholesterol. If there is an excess of cholesterol in relation to phospholipids and bile acids, unstable, cholesterol-rich vesicles remain, which aggregate into larger multilamellar vesicles, from which cholesterol crystals precipitate.

The final stage in the formation of cholesterol and mixed gallstones is the transformation of cholesterol crystals into stones by aggregation and compaction of cholesterol and aggregation of calcium bilirubinate, respectively. Cholesterol gallstones occur because of the following metabolic malfunctions: bile supersaturation with cholesterol; nucleation of cholesterol monohydrate with subsequent crystal retention and stone growth; and abnormal gallbladder motor function with delayed emptying and stasis. Bile cholesterol saturation is caused by two metabolic defects in biliary lipid secretion: cholesterol hypersecretion and bile acid hyposecretion.

Excessive cholesterol secretion is related to increased cholesterol synthesis in the liver and this is associated with obesity, ageing, pregnancy, hyperlipidaemia, oral contraceptive use and hypolipodaemic agents. The individual risk for developing cholesterol gallstones in response to specific environmental factors is believed to be determined by complex genetics, involving numerous unknown 'lithogenic' genes reviewed by Reshetnyak. [163]

Pathogenesis of Cholesterol Stones

The pathogenesis of GD is suggested to be multifactorial and probably develops from complex interactions between many genetic and environmental factors as pointed out by Sun and Marschall et al. [127, 164] Unphysiological biliary supersaturation from hypersecretion of cholesterol, gallbladder hypomotility and the accumulation of mucin gel contribute to the formation of cholesterol GS, while black pigment stones derive from the precipitation of calcium hydrogen bilirubinate where pigment supersaturation and deposition of inorganic salts, phosphate and calcium bicarbonate accelerate the nucleation. Pigment supersaturation is common in hemolytic disorders, enterohepatic cycling of unconjugated bilirubin and ileal disorders and/or surgery reported by Carey. [165] Cholesterol GD results from a biochemical imbalance of lipids and bile salts in the gallbladder bile as pointed out by He et al. [166]

Cholesterol stones are formed in the gallbladder due to impaired relationships between the major bile components, cholesterol, phospholipids and bile acids pointed out by Dikkers and Tietge. [167]. The pathophysiology of GS formation involves three steps: saturation, crystallization and growth. Bile cholesterol supersaturation is an obligatory, but not the only, factor that contributes to GS formation. An important role in this is played by the state of pronucleating and antinucleating factors and the functional state of the gallbladder.

The biochemical composition and physicochemical properties of bile are modified when it is located in the gallbladder. Diminished evacuatory function of the gallbladder with its preserved concentrating capacity may give rise to biliary sludge and GS. In excess cholesterol or deficiency of phospholipids and/or bile acids (a high cholesterol saturation index), bile cholesterol is transported, not only in the form of mixed micelles, but also as phospholipid vesicles. Cholesterol-supersaturated unilamellar and then multilamellar vesicles that are less stable are formed. Nuclear receptors (NRs) play a key role in the transcriptional control of critical steps of hepatobiliary transport and phase I/II metabolism of endo- and xenobiotics such as bile acids and drugs. Apart from these metabolic roles, NRs may also play a key role in the control of hepatic inflammation. Hereditary and acquired alterations of NRs contribute to our understanding of the pathogenesis of cholestasis and GD. Further, NRs may represent attractive drug targets for these disorders suggested by Claudel et al. [168] Cholesterol nucleation is known to be an initial stage in the formation of cholesterol GS suggested by Small. [169] The present-day interpretation of the mechanisms responsible for cholesterol transport and formation of cholesterol monohydrate crystal in the bile suggests that cholesterol molecules nucleate from the liquid-crystalline phase (a mesophase) after the aggregation and possible fusion of cholesterol-rich unilamellar vesicles (Figure 2.4.1) suggested by Carey, Cohen and Loginov et al. [170-172] Under certain conditions, cholesterol can aggregate and precipitate in them as cholesterol monohydrate crystals to give rise to the core of a GS. The important factor in such mesophasic nucleation is associated with further interaction between the monohydrate crystals and the molecules of protein and unconjugated bilirubin. All these organic substances are precursors in the lithogenic bile and structural components of most human GS elucidated by Been et al. [173]

Polarizing light microscopy is the main technique for visualization of cholesterol crystal formation processes in normal and lithogenic bile as observed by Chijiiwa and Holan et al. [174, 175] This technique has revealed that cholesterol crystallizes from bile *via* metastable intermediates by Konikoff et al. [176] Loginov et al. [172] have shown that mixed (single and multiple) stones are composed of alternating concentric, cholesterol-rich and bilirubin-rich layers.

The reason for this alternation and the periodic emergence of layers of various compositions remain unclear. By taking into account the data on the zonal stratification of bile on its drying and the relationship of the formation of cholesterol and bilirubin the deposits to the dehydration or watering of a solution, it can be presumed that the layering of stones depends on bile concentrations in a period of lithogenesis Loginov et al. [177] Cholesterol can crystallize even when the concentration of a bile solution is outside or slightly below the normal range. Bilirubin precipitation increases as lithogenic bile concentrates progressively. Therefore, the concentrating or watering of a bile solution may be of great importance in the formation of cholesterol- and bilirubin-containing layers in the GS. Bile proteins and bilirubin, in addition to cholesterol crystals, can be a matrix in stone formation. Mucin-glycoprotein gel is one of the most important and identified pronucleators. It should be noted the mucus of the gallbladder in normalcy constantly secretes the mucin; however, its secretion increases due to inflammation observed by Jungst et al. [178].

Bacterial infection is of great significance in the development of inflammation in GD. In health, bile is sterile as it has bactericidal activity put forth by Hofmann [179]. When there are changes in bile composition or cholestasis in the gallbladder, bacteria can rise into the gallbladder through the bile duct and promote lithogenesis. Cystic bile destabilized by chronic inflammation of gallbladder wall contains high arachidonyl-lecithin levels (Figure 2.4.3). The observed increase in the activity of the phospholipase A2 secreted by bacteria leads to the hydrolysis of phospholipids and the accumulation of free fatty acids, including arachidonic acid reported by Uchyiyama et al. [180] The latter activates the generation of prostaglandins, thromboxanes and leukotrienes to cause mucin glycoproteins to be hypersecreted by the gallbladder mucosa. In infection, cholic acid is converted to lithocholic acid. The higher production of lithocholic acid in the cystic bile promotes aggregation of cholesterol monohydrate crystals.

In parallel with this, there are morphological changes in the gallbladder mucosa. The surface epithelium passes into goblet, mucus cells that secret much mucus, the columnar epithelium flattens and microvilli are lost. This results in impaired water and electrolyte absorption processes. Mucin and mucus hypersecretion gives rise to a parietal colloid solution that is turned to viscoelastic glycoprotein-mucin gel. The latter promotes the aggregation of phospholipid vesicles and the nucleation and precipitation of cholesterol monohydrate crystals and/or bilirubin. Cholesterol monohydrate crystals, mucus glycoprotein mucin bands and calcium bilirubinate granules form the basis for biliary sludge and a pigmented matrix of the core of most cholesterol gallstone reported by Reshetnyak. [163]

Hypersecretion is induced by the increased expression of one of the genes encoding the synthesis of mucin (*MUC5AC*) and by the decreased expression of the epidermal growth factor receptor gene involved in the regulation of mucin synthesis, which are observed in all patients with GD suggested by Kim et al. [181] The elevated levels of glycosaminoglycans mainly due to a sulfated fraction are characteristic.

In addition to mucin, the proteins that accelerate cholesterol precipitation include N-aminopeptidase, immunoglobulins and phospholipases C. The antinucleators include apolipoproteins A1 and A2, which slow cholesterol precipitation, aspirin and other nonsteroidal anti-inflammatory drugs suggested by Reshetnyak. [163].

Long-term corticosteroid therapy is well known to cause dyslipoproteinemia, characterized by elevated plasma total cholesterol, triglycerides and low-density lipoprotein cholesterol. The major catabolic pathway for cholesterol is its transformation into bile acids, involving P450 cytochrome and subsequent bile excretion from the body. The elevated level of total cholesterol may change a bile acid/cholesterol ratio and lead to the formation of GS in patients with SLE or in patients who use oral contraceptives.

Long-term therapy with each of these agents enhances cholesterol excretion into bile and results in its supersaturation with cholesterol through competitive inhibition of bile acid synthesis from cholesterol on cytochrome P_{45} (Figure 2.4.1)

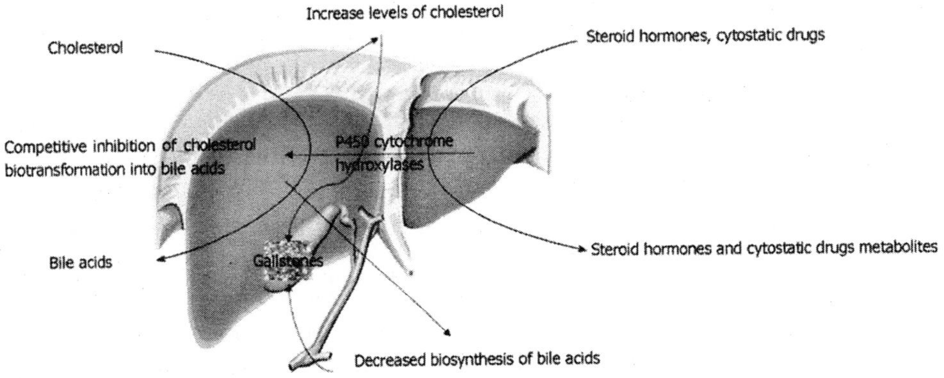

Figure 2.4.1. Diagram of steroid hormones-induced inhibition of cholesterol catabolism. *Courtesy of World J Hepatology, Baishideng Publishing Group.*

Cholesterol nucleation is known to be an initial stage in the formation of cholesterol GS. The present-day interpretation of the mechanisms responsible for cholesterol transport and formation of cholesterol monohydrate crystal in the bile suggests that cholesterol molecules nucleate from the liquid-crystalline phase (a mesophase) after the aggregation and possible fusion of cholesterol-rich unilamellar vesicles (Figure 2.4.2). [163]. Under certain conditions, cholesterol can aggregate and precipitate in them as cholesterol monohydrate crystals to give rise to the core of a GS.

The bulk of intrahepatic stones are formed due to biliary tract infection reported by Wu et al. [182]. The neck of the gallbladder hosts the biggest bacterial load in comparison with the body and the fundus. This difference might be attributed to the presence of Rokitansky-Aschoff sinuses, the main histological characteristic of the region[reported by Manolis et al. [183] This is frequently the opportunistic flora (Escherichia coli, streptococcus, staphylococcus and typhoid bacillus) that, by setting in motion its capsular O-antigen, can persist in the GS for decades reported by Crawford et al. [184] Intrahepatic stones contain abundant free fatty acids and free bile acids due to the deconjugation with bacterial enzymes.

Bacterial infection is of great significance in the development of inflammation in GD. In health, bile is sterile as it has bactericidal activity. When there are changes in bile composition or cholestasis in the gallbladder, bacteria can rise into the gallbladder through the bile duct and promote lithogenesis. Cystic bile destabilized by chronic inflammation of gallbladder wall contains high arachidonyl-lecithin levels (Figure 2.4.3). [163]

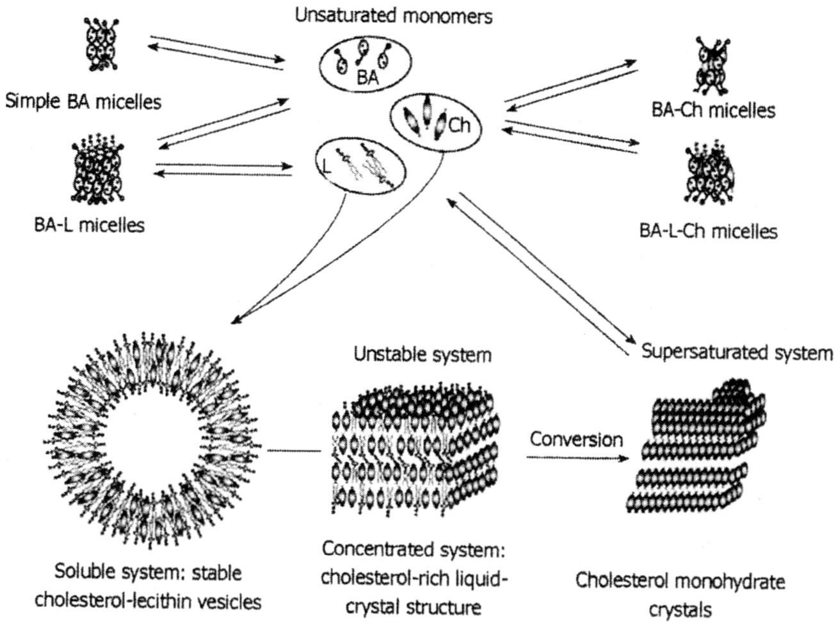

Figure 2.4.2. Formation of molecular structures in the system containing bile acids, lecithin and cholesterol. Cholesterol-supersaturated vesicles can stick together and agglomerate to form multilayer (liposomal) liquid-crystal structures. When gallbladder contractility is decreased, liposomes may be converted to solid cholesterol monocrystals. *Courtesy of World J Hepatology, Baishideng Publishing Group.*

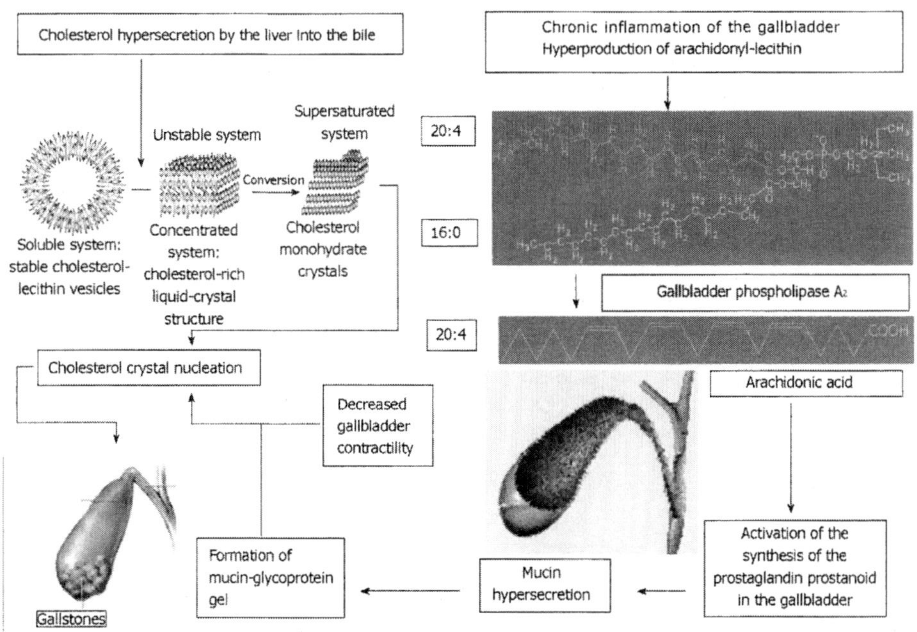

Figure 2.4.3. It shows a diagram of gallstone formation by taking into account the above impaired bile production and excretion process. *Courtesy of World J Hepatology, Baishideng Publishing Group.*

Bacteria are readily cultured from cholesterol stones with pigment centers, allowing for analysis of their virulence factors. Bacteria sequestered in cholesterol stones cause infectious manifestations but less than bacteria in pigment stones. Possibly, because of their isolation, cholesterol stone bacteria are less often present in bile and blood, induce less immunoglobulin G, are less often killed by a patient's serum and demonstrate fewer infectious manifestations than pigment stone bacteria reported by Stewart et al. [185]. The O-antigen capsule genes are bile induced and the capsule produced by the enzymes of this operon is specifically required for biofilm formation on cholesterol GS. Salmonella enterica serovar Typhi can establish a chronic, asymptomatic infection of the human gallbladder, suggesting that this bacterium utilizes novel mechanisms to mediate enhanced colonization and persistence in a bile-rich environment. GS are one of the most important risk factors for developing carriage and authors have previously demonstrated that salmonellae form biofilms on human GS *in vitro* reported by Crawford et al. [184] Thus, the microorganisms induce increased mucin production and destroy both components that solubilize cholesterol in the micelles by inducing its crystallization. The performed investigations indicate that stones of various compositions are formed responsible for biliary tract inflammation. Thus, the bacteria that produce beta-glucuronidase and mucus or beta-glucuronidase only give rise to pigment or mixed stones while the microorganisms that produce only mucus or do not produce any of these factors are more common in the cores of cholesterol stones reported by Stewart et al. [186].

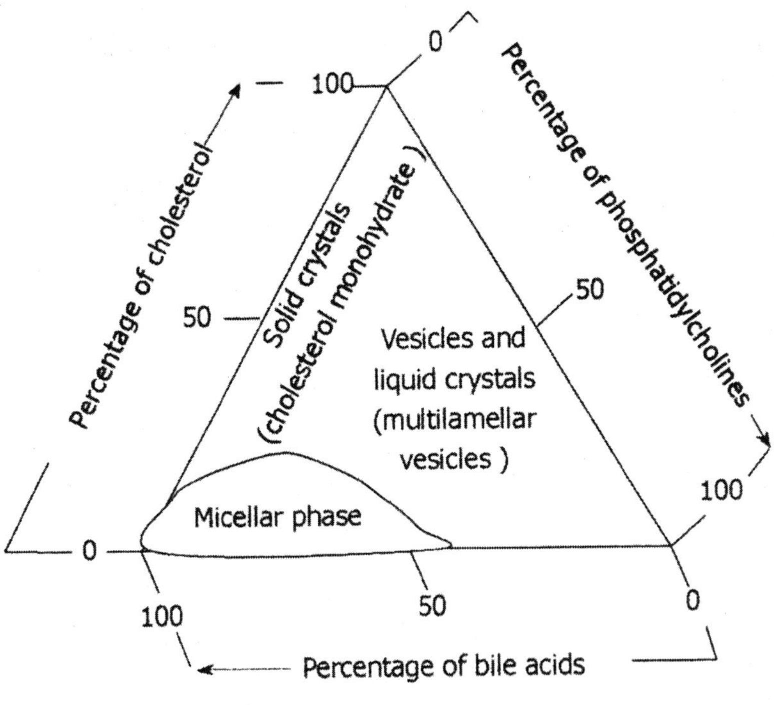

Figure 2.4.4.The phase state of the main bile components (cholesterol, phosphatidylcholines, and bile acids) in the triangular coordinate system. *Courtesy of World J Hepatology, Baishideng Publishing Group.*

The second half of the last century was marked by the emergence of new medical treatments for GD: litholytic therapy (stone dissolution) and lithotripsy (stone shattering). About 30% of patients with gallbladder stones may undergo litholytic therapy [22]. GS dissolution is based on the pathophysiology of cholepoiesis and choleresis in cholelithiasis and is carried out with bile acids. Scientists established experimentally that the ratio between the concentration of bile acids leads to a redistribution of phases in a triangular coordinate system [114] (Figure 2.4.4) [163].

Foreign bodies, such as suture materials, clips, swallowed metal or plastic fragments, or parasites, may become foci of nucleation. Surgical clips are the most common cause of iatrogenic cholelithiasis reported by Chong [187]. The stones' growth rate is 3-5 mm per year and in some cases it may be more reported by Chenko and Mayer. [188, 189].

V. The Physicochemical Basis of Cholesterol Gallstone Formation in Man [15]

The concentrations of bile, salt, lecithin, and cholesterol were determined on each of 66 samples of gall bladder bile from patients with cholesterol gallstones and 25 samples of normal gall bladder bile. When these three constituents were plotted simultaneously on triangular coordinates, a complete separation of the normal and "abnormal" bile was achieved. This separation was the result of an increase in the quantity of cholesterol relative to the amounts of bile salts and lecithin contained in the bile from patients with cholesterol gallstones. An in vitro model system was constructed (on triangular coordinates) that allows prediction of the maximum amount of cholesterol that can be solubilized in solutions containing varying proportions of bile salt and lecithin. When the bile data were compared with the solubility of cholesterol derived from the model system, normal biles were found to be less than saturated with cholesterol, whereas biles from patients with cholesterol gallstones were saturated and in some cases contained insoluble cholesterol in the form of microcrystals. It is suggested that the physical state of bile (i.e., the presence or absence of insoluble cholesterol) is determined by the relative concentrations of bile salt, lecithin, and cholesterol, and the other biliary constituents do not appear to significantly affect the solubility of cholesterol in bile.

The formation of cholesterol gallstones can be separated conceptually into two steps reported by Small [190]. In the first step, the capacity of bile to solubilize cholesterol is exceeded; therefore part of the cholesterol precipitates, presumably in the form of microcrystals. During the second step in gallstone formation microcrystals of cholesterol unite or grow to form macroscopic gallstones. These two steps probably proceed simultaneously. Admirand and Small consider the first step of cholesterol gallstone formation, namely the conditions that bring about the precipitation of cholesterol in bile.

Theory

Pure cholesterol is almost totally insoluble in water observed by Ekwall and Gourges et al., [191, 192] yet the cholesterol in normal human bile is completely soluble. It is assumed that cholesterol is solubilized in bile in the form of mixed micelles of bile salt and lecithin suggested by Small, Isaksson, Verschure, Furusawa, Tamesue and Juniper et al. [190, 193-197] In this case, the formation and persistence of insoluble cholesterol in bile could be the result of an increase in the quantity of cholesterol, a decrease in the quantity of bile salt or lecithin, or a combination of these factors. Previous studies have shown wide variations in the concentrations of bile salt, lecithin, and cholesterol in normal human gall bladder bile. Consistent differences between normal bile and bile from patients with cholesterol gallstones have been difficult to demonstrate pointed out by Isaksson, Polonovski, Tera, Mirvish, Dam et al. [198-206] Although some of this difficulty is due to differences in the analytical methods used, some confusion may have arisen from the way in which the data have been expressed. For example, when the quantities of bile salt, lecithin, and cholesterol per 100 ml of bile were compared, no significant differences were found in the concentration of any of these substances between the bile from normal subjects and from patients with cholesterol gallstones observed by Large et al. [202]. This method of expressing the quantity of bile constituents per unit volume of bile might be expected to produce a wide range of values since it is dependent upon the degree to which the bile has been concentrated at the time the sample is obtained. Furthermore, the quantity of any single constituent (e.g., cholesterol) has little meaning without its being compared to the quantities of both other major components. The use of binary ratios such as cholesterol: bile salt or cholesterol: lecithin failed to show consistent differences between normal bile and bile from patients with cholesterol gall stones observed by Dam et al. [206] Isaksson used an in vitro system to determine the maximum solubility of cholesterol in mixtures of bile salt and lecithin. [207] If the ratio of cholesterol to bile salt plus lecithin was above 1: 11, cholesterol precipitated out of solution. Applying the results of the in vitro system to the clinical situation, Isaksson found that in 70-95%o of the patients with cholesterol gallstones the ratio was above the 1: 11 critical level. This method of comparison was not entirely satisfactory since occasionally normal bile had high ratios, and some biles from patients with cholesterol gallstones had normal ratios. Isaksson's ratio does not distinguish between the individual effects of bile salt and lecithin. It has been demonstrated previously that the molecular function of bile salt and lecithin in relation to the micellar solubilization of cholesterol are distinctly different observed by Bourges et al. and Small [192, 208-210] and not strictly additive. Thus, the effects of each component must be judged separately. In Small et al.'s study they have expressed the relative quantity of bile salts, lecithin, and cholesterol in each bile sample as a percentage of the total quantity of all three components. To compare the composition of normal biles with that of biles from patients with cholesterol gallstones, each bile was plotted as a single point on triangular coordinates. This method permits simultaneous representation of the relative quantities of bile salts, lecithin, and cholesterol in any bile sample. When the data are expressed in this fashion, a clear-cut separation between normal and abnormal biles is achieved. Abnormal biles have more cholesterol relative to the quantities of bile salt and lecithin than do normal biles. To determine if the basis of this separation was related to the limits of cholesterol solubility in pure lecithin and bile salt solutions, the results obtained in human bile were compared to an in vitro model system. The model system was derived from previous studies by Small, Bourges, and Dervichian [192, 208-211] in which the physical state of all possible mixtures of four components (bile salt, lecithin, cholesterol, and water) was determined and the fine structure of the different phases (i.e. ,crystal, liquid crystal, and micellar) was defined. The techniques for representing this “quaternary system as a regular tetrahedron” have been described elsewhere by Bourges et al. [192] .In Small's paper, these techniques have been modified to show the effects of changes in composition of the three solid components (bile salt, lecithin, and cholesterol) at constant water concentrations similar to that found in gall bladder bile. This technique permits one to examine the individual effects of bile salts and lecithin on cholesterol solubilization. A comparison of the results obtained in human bile and from the in vitro system showed that the solubility of cholesterol in both was similar. Since the in vitro system contained only bile salt, lecithin, and cholesterol, it is suggested that only these three substances determine the solubility of cholesterol in bile.

In the **methods** section, a **clinical studies** was conducted in which bile specimens were obtained from 91 subjects by needle aspiration of the gall bladder during abdominal surgery. All gall bladders were aspirated as completely as possible to exclude the possibility of unrepresentative sampling due to stratification of bile observed by Tera et al. [212] The subjects were divided into two groups: (a) 25 subjects in whom there was no history of biliary tract disease, and in whom (after aspiration of the gall bladder) there were no palpable gallstones, and (b) 66 patients with cholesterol or mixed gallstones classified according to the scheme of Rains. [213]. The mean ages of both groups were similar, 52 years in normals and 57 in gallstone patients. 3 of the 25 normal subjects and 7 of the 66 patients with gallstones were female. The relatively small percentage of females in both groups was accounted for by the fact that all of the specimens were obtained at Veteran Administration Hospitals. The bile samples were sealed and refrigerated within minutes after collection and were warmed to room temperature before analysis. An aliquot of each bile was centrifuged, and the sediment was observed under a polarizing microscope for the presence of crystals. When crystals were found, their melting point was determined on a microscope heating stage. Flat parallelogram-shaped crystals, similar to those described by Juniper and Burson, [214] having melting points between 146 and 149^0C, were considered to be cholesterol crystals. When present in adequate amounts, these crystals were isolated and run on silica gel thin-layer chromatography as described by Hofmann. [215]. In all cases the crystals had the same Rf as the pure cholesterol standard. No crystals were observed in the 25 normal biles. All chemical determinations were performed in duplicate on aliquots of uncentrifuged bile. The per cent solids was calculated by dividing the dry weight by wet weight. All weighings were timed and extrapolated to time zero to correct for errors due to evaporation or hydration. Specimens that were obviously white bile or contained less than 4% total solids were not included in the study. The per cent solids varied between 5 and 25%o with an average of 10%. Total bile salts were enzymatically determined by a modification of the method of Talalay. [216] The reagents were similar with the exception that hydroxysteroid dehydrogenase 2 solution was made with 0.03 M tris buffer (pH=7.2) containing 0.001 moles of disodium ethylenediaminetetraacetate per liter. Methanolic bile solutions were prepared by diluting 0.1-0.5 ml of bile to a volume of 10 ml with methanol. The reaction mixture contained: 10 ml of pyrophosphate buffer; 0.5 ml of distilled water; 0.3 ml of β-diphosphopyridine nucleotide solution;. 1.0 ml of hydrazine hydrate solution; 0.1 ml of hydroxysteroid dehydrogenase solutions; and 0.1 cc methanolic bile solution. The OD of the reaction mixtures were measured at 340 mμ, and the quantity of bile salt determined from a standard curve (obtained with pure bile salts) which was run with each series of determinations. The accuracy of the method was ± 3%. Cholesterol was measured by the method of Abell, Levy, Brodie, and Kendall [217] and the method of Schoenheimer and Sperry, [218] and there was no significant differences between the values obtained with either technique. Phospholipid, which in bile is almost entirely lecithin reported by Polonovski and Isaksson et al., [198, 201] was determined by the method of Fiske and Subbarow. [219]

In Vitro Studies

To determine the limits of cholesterol solubility in pure bile salt-lecithin solutions in vitro, a large number of dry mixtures of bile salt, lecithin, and cholesterol were prepared as previously described by Isaksson and Bourges et al. [192, 209] The bile salt (a mixture of conjugated taurine and glycine dihydroxy and trihydroxy bile salts) and the purified egg lecithin used in this experiment were the same as described previously by Isaksson et al. [209] Water was added to each dry mixture so that the final solutions contained 20% solids by weight. The mixtures were allowed to equilibrate and then were examined grossly and microscopically for the presence of crystals and (or) liquid crystalline phases observed by Isaksson et al. [209] Similar mixtures were diluted with water so that their final concentrations were 5 and 10%o solids by weight. Those mixtures which contained both cholesterol crystals and an aqueous solution, or a mixture of cholesterol crystals, liquid crystals, and an aqueous solution were designated two- or three-phase systems, whereas those mixtures which contained only a single solution were considered one aqueous phase [micellar by Bourges and Isaksson et al. [192, 209].

In the **results** section concerning **clinical studies,** the mean values for all determinations on normal gall bladder biles and gall bladder biles from patients with cholesterol gallstones are compared. The millimolar concentrations of bile salt, lecithin, and cholesterol are shown and the sum of these three components and the per cents of total millimolar concentration contributed by each component are also shown.

The method of representing bile composition on triangular coordinates. The per cent of the total moles of bile salt, lecithin, and cholesterol constituted by each of these components are shown on the scales along the sides of the triangle. Since the sum of bile salt, lecithin, and cholesterol equals 100%, the composition of any bile containing these components can be represented as a single point within triangular coordinates [24]. Thus, a bile containing 80% bile salt, 15% lecithin, and 5% cholesterol is represented by a single point formed at the intersection of the dashed lines extended from the 80% level on the bile salt scale at the base of the triangle, the 15% level on the lecithin scale at the right of the triangle, and the 5% level on the cholesterol scale at the left of the triangle. in any one sample is equal to 100%o, each bile can be represented by a single point within triangular coordinates (see reference [117], p. 277). [220]. The position of this point within the triangle is dictated by the relative concentrations of each of the components. Thus, a bile containing 80% bile salt, 15% lecithin, and 5% cholesterol would be plotted. When the results from each of the 91 bile samples were plotted on one graph, there was a complete separation between the normal and abnormal biles. This separation appears to be the result of an increase in the quantity of cholesterol relative to the quantities of bile salt and lecithin present in gall bladder bile from the patients with cholesterol or mixed gallstones. Further, nearly all of the abnormal biles having relatively high cholesterols contained small cholesterol crystals0. These biles are two-phase systems containing liquid bile and microscopic cholesterol crystals. No liquid crystals were noted.

In Vitro Studies

The physical state of cholesterol in pure bile salt-lecithin systems containing 90% water and 10%o solids are the results were identical when the experiment was performed on a series of mixtures containing 5% solids or a series containing 20% solids. More dilute solutions (below 3%o solids) became unstable with time, whereas concentrated solutions with greater than 25% solids contained liquid crystalline phases which altered the solubility characteristics of both lecithin and cholesterol. Each of the mixtures listed has been plotted according to its composition on triangular coordinates. The physical state of each mixture is indicated: closed circles to represent a single liquid phase and open circles to indicate 2- or 3-phase systems (i.e., mixtures containing insoluble cholesterol). A line has been drawn by inspection separating the open and closed circles, and it thus represents the maximum solubility of cholesterol in varying proportions of lecithin and bile salt. Thus, any mixture beneath the line is less than saturated. Mixtures falling on the line are saturated, and any mixture above the line contains more cholesterol than can be maintained in solution. In the absence of lecithin, approximately 97 molecules of bile salt are necessary to solubilize three molecules of cholesterol. As the proportion of lecithin increases, progressively more cholesterol is solubilized to maximum of about 10 molecules per 60 of bile salt and 30 molecules of lecithin. This amount is similar to the maximum solubility of cholesterol determined by Isaksson [18]. Further increase in the proportion of lecithin results in decreased cholesterol solubilization in the micellar solution. At a molecular ratio of 40 molecules of bile salt to 60 of lecithin almost no cholesterol is solubilized in a micellar solution. Note that the state of insoluble cholesterol is crystalline at low lecithin concentrations but is liquid crystalline at higher lecithin concentrations.

The correlation of the findings in human bile with those of the model system is shown to be similar. It is significant that all normal biles have compositions within micellar zone, whereas biles from patients with cholesterol or mixed gallstones fall on, or above the line of maximum saturation with cholesterol. The biles of those patients that have cholesterol values clearly above the maximum saturation of cholesterol in the micellar solution nearly all contained microscopic crystals of cholesterol. These biles are two-phase systems: cholesterol crystals 3 and a micellar solution. Biles from gallstone patients falling very close to the line did not contain cholesterol crystals and are one-phase systems. Thus, they can be considered to be saturated with cholesterol. These facts suggest that the physical state of bile is determined by the relative concentrations of lecithin, bile salt, and cholesterol present in the bile and not by other components. The model system serves to predict the maximum amount of cholesterol that can be solubilized by any bile, and thus the degree of cholesterol saturation. In order to correlate Admirand and Small's findings with those of other laboratories, yhey have taken from the literature mean values for bile salt, lecithin, and cholesterol in normal biles and biles from patients with cholesterol or mixed gallstones. The methods of chemical analysis for each of the three components frequently differed, but Admirand and Small have taken the values as reported with the exception of one study in which only "cholate" was measured by Larrge et al. [202]

Admirand and Small have corrected this value by assuming that cholate represents 45%o of total bile salts by Laege and Wootton et al. [221, 222]. The correlation of the values with the model system are shown and it is noted that the composition of normal gall bladder bile is such that all the plotted values fall within the micellar zone. The biles from patients with cholesterol gallstones again contain more cholesterol than the maximum solubilization of cholesterol as determined from the model system.

In the **discussion** section, the model system defines the maximum quantity of cholesterol that can be solubilized in mixed micelles of bile salt and lecithin. The triangular diagram shown was constructed by determining the physical state of a large number of mixtures of bile salt, lecithin, and cholesterol in varying proportions. The total quantity of these three substances (i.e., total solids) was the same in all mixtures. Each mixture contained 10% solids and 90% water by weight. This concentration was selected because it approximated the mean concentration total solids in the 91 samples of gall bladder bile. It might be argued that the findings of the model system containing 10% solids are not applicable to the more dilute or concentrated bile samples.

This possibility can be excluded since the limits of the micellar zone at 10%o solids are the same at 5 or 20% solids. Therefore, in terms of water and total solids the model system is similar to the 91 samples of human gall bladder bile included in Admirand and Small's study. There are changes in cholesterol solubilization in the in vitro system when the total solids are less than 3%o. Thus, the limits of cholesterol solubilization are probably not applicable to very dilute biles. For this reason, dilute biles have been excluded from Admirand and Small's study. A mixture of taurine and glycine conjugated bile salts was used to construct the model system. Almost identical results have been obtained when the free bile salt sodium cholate was used at an alkaline pH simulated by Bourges et al. [192]. Alterations in pH do not affect the physical state of mixtures containing conjugated bile salts until the pH falls below about 4.5, at which point glycine conjugates tend to precipitate. In contrast, the solubilizing capacity of the systems using free sodium cholate is dependent upon the maintenance of an alkaline pH. At a pH above 9.5 sodium cholate is completely ionized.

Under this condition sodium cholate is as effective as conjugated bile salts in solubilizing lecithin and cholesterol. At somewhat lower pH levels, where a portion of free bile salt is in the form of protonated bile acid, solubilization is less efficient. Below pH 6 no solubilization occurs since cholic acid precipitates from solution. The model system contained only bile salts, lecithin, cholesterol, and water and thus was devoid of many of the normal biliary constituents such as bilirubin, inorganic ions, mucus, and protein.

Despite the absence of these substances the model system apparently predicts which bile samples will contain insoluble cholesterol crystals. It thus may be suggested that the solubility of cholesterol in bile is determined solely by the amount of cholesterol relative to the quantities of bile salts and lecithin present.

Admirand and Small emphasize that all of the findings discussed in the present study deal only with one step in the formation of cholesterol gallstones, namely the precipitation of cholesterol microcrystals. The process by which these microcrystals unite or grow to form macroscopic gallstones is unknown. Factors such as inflammation, stasis, mucus content, divalent cation concentration, bile pigment, pH etc., which do not appear to be significant in the precipitation of cholesterol microcrystals, may be important in the process by which these microcrystals form macroscopic cholesterol gallstones.

VI. Intestinal Absorption, Hepatic Synthesis, and Biliary Secretion of Cholesterol: Where Are We for Cholesterol Gallstone Formation? [223]

With a 10%-15% prevalence, gallstone disease is one of the most prevalent and costly digestive diseases in Western countries reported by Portincassa and Wang et al. [1, 224] About two-thirds of gallstones are cholesterol gallstones reported by Wang et al., [225] while the remaining are pigment stones that contain less than 30% cholesterol. The prevalence of gallstones increases with age and is associated with a number of major risk factors advocsated by Portincassa et al. [1, 131] Overall, cholesterol gallstone disease is deemed as the gallbladder/bile expression of the metabolic syndrome, as it is often associated with obesity, type 2 diabetes, dyslipidemia, and hyperinsulinemia. The combination of multiple disturbances affecting cholesterol homeostasis in bile is essential for cholesterol gallstone formation. The interactions of five primary defects result in rapid cholesterol nucleation and crystallization in bile, the key step for gallstone formation by Portincassa and Wang et al. [1, 226] (1) LITH genes and genetic defects; (2) unphysiological sustained supersaturation of bile with cholesterol due to hepatic hypersecretion; (3) enhanced intestinal cholesterol absorption; (4) accelerated phase transitions of cholesterol; and (5) prolonged gallbladder stasis due to disrupted gallbladder motility accompanied with immunomediated gallbladder inflammation, as well as hypersecretion of mucins and accumulation of mucin gel in the gallbladder lumen by Portincassa, Crawczyk and Wang et al. [1, 72, 227] Growth of solid, platelike cholesterol monohydrate crystals to form gallstones is a consequence of persistent hepatic hypersecretion of biliary cholesterol together with enhanced gallbladder mucin secretion and incomplete evacuation by the gallbladder due to its impaired motility function. Krawczyk et al. [228] report that patients with cholesterol-enriched stones displayed a high biliary cholesterol output and relatively low absorption efficiency of intestinal cholesterol. Apparently, this metabolic trait could precede gallstone formation, which may be a feature of those ethnic groups at (possibly genetic) high risk of gallstones. In their case-control studies, the authors examined four cohorts, each including gallstone patients and matched controls: one cohort of German subjects (112 patients and 152 controls), two cohorts of Chilean ethnic groups (100 Hispanic patients and 100 controls), and one cohort of Amerindian Mapuches (20 patients and 20 controls). Using chromatography/mass spectrometry, serum levels of surrogates were measure as markers of both intestinal cholesterol absorption (phytosterols: sitosterol and campesterol) and hepatic de novo synthesis (cholesterol precursors: lathosterol and desmosterol). In addition, serum sterol levels were employed as markers for evaluating increased risk of gallstones in an 8-year ultrasonographic follow-up study (Hispanics, 35 gallstone patients and 35 controls). Sterol levels were also measured in gallbladder bile from a subgroup of patients and controls (n = 17 each). Common variants of ABCG5/G8 were genotyped. Cholesterol gallstone patients had distinctive serum sterol profiles (i.e., low levels of phytosterols, high levels of cholesterol precursors, and low ratios of phytosterols: cholesterol precursors). Differences were more pronounced in women than in men and in Chilean Hispanics than in Germans. In bile, both phytosterols and cholesterol were increased and relative lipid compositions of gallbladder bile plotted above the micellar phase boundary.

In the follow-up study, individuals with incident stones had significantly lower serum phytosterol levels even before the appearance of gallstones. Based on the ratios of phytosterols: cholesterol precursors, the following sequences were established: Amerindians< Hispanics<Germans. The overall genotype distributions of the variants of ABCG5/G8 did not differ between cases with gallstones and stone-free controls, and therefore, these results could not fully explain the sterol metabolism. Cholesterol homeostasis in humans is the consequence of the fine regulatory mechanisms involving intestinal absorption and hepatic de novo synthesis, as well as biliary secretion and fecal excretion of cholesterol. In enterocytes, sterol uptake and secretion is mediated by two brush border transport proteins. The Niemann-Pick C1-like 1 protein (NPC1L1) acts as an intestinal sterol influx transporter that actively facilitates the uptake of cholesterol by Davis, Katsica and Wang et al. [229-231] Two ATP-binding cassette (ABC) transporters, ABCG5 and ABCG8, work as a heterodimeric efflux pump, for mediating cholesterol transport back to the intestinal lumen. Because in humans both NPC1L1 and ABCG5/G8 are also expressed in the hepatocyte at the canalicular membrane, both transporters contribute to the overall balance of cholesterol absorption/secretion at two different sites: intestine and liver by Davis et al. [32, 232] Where exactly excess biliary cholesterol comes from (i.e., intestinal absorption, hepatic de novo synthesis, reverse cholesterol transport by high-density lipoprotein [HDL]) is still an open issue and should be interpreted together with the function of these cholesterol transporters at different levels. Krawczyk et al. suggested that, at least in their particular setting, reduced cholesterol absorption, which is associated with increased cholesterol synthesis, may drive impaired cholesterol homeostasis in gallstone disease, with higher cholesterol clearance. The authors also speculated that the early events might be the biliary/intestinal cholesterol efflux (sterol clearance) followed by increased synthesis of cholesterol, since they did not occur simultaneously. Overall, however, such events should result in "sustained" rather than "fluctuating" supersaturation of bile with cholesterol. Genetic factors and LITH genes play a role in the pathogenesis of cholesterol gallstones by Wang et al. [230]. In principle, a gain-of-function of ABCG5/G8 in humans might recapitulate both steps, leading to decreased intestinal absorption versus increased biliary output of cholesterol. The ABCG8 p.D19H and p.T400K coding variants might play a role as putative susceptibility variants for gallstone formation in humans by Katsika et al. [134, 137, 233]. Despite much evidence in this respect, the authors could not confirm such an interesting hypothesis, possibly due to the small cohort size. The issue becomes even more intriguing when considering that high cholesterol content is typical of Westernized diets and that the small intestine is a unique organ providing dietary and reabsorbed biliary cholesterol to the body by de Bari et al. [229] Furthermore, high efficiency of intestinal cholesterol absorption may occur, as shown in several inbred strains of mice by Wang et al. [72, 234]. Slow/sluggish intestinal motility is a feature in gallstone disease and is an additional factor predisposing to increased cholesterol absorption, more hydrophobe absorption, and secondary bile salt synthesis by the intestinal anaerobic microbiota. Thus, high dietary cholesterol matched with increased intestinal cholesterol absorption both appear to be key and independent risk factors for the formation of cholesterol gallstones by Wang et al. [229]. This mechanism might be actively operating in subgroups of subjects who are at lower genetic risk of developing gallstones but are victims of environmental dietary factors. Indeed, the potent and selective inhibitor of NPC1L1 ezetimibe reduced biliary cholesterol secretion by suppressing intestinal cholesterol absorption and protected gallbladder motor function by desaturating bile, thus preventing the formation of

cholesterol gallstones in mice. [231, 235] The results are straightforward, since in mice NPC1L1 is expressed only in the intestine. In hamsters and humans, however, NPC1L1 is also detected at a significantly lower expression level in the liver compared with the intestine. Because NPC1L1 is a cholesterol transporter that is expressed on the canalicular membrane of hepatocytes, it could function to limit cholesterol excretion, presumably by reabsorbing cholesterol from bile.19 However, it was found that ezetimibe can significantly reduce hepatic secretion of biliary cholesterol in cholesterol-fed hamsters.20 Furthermore, in gallbladder biles of Mexican patients with gallstones, ezetimibe reduced biliary cholesterol saturation and retarded cholesterol crystallization by Wang et al. [231]. These results strongly suggest that the secretion efficiency of biliary cholesterol is most likely determined by the net effect between the efflux and influx of cholesterol molecules across the canalicular membrane of hepatocyte, which could be regulated by ABCG5/G8 and the NPC1L1 pathways.11 It is highly likely that because biliary cholesterol secretion is a unique path for excretion of cholesterol from the body in humans and hamsters, hepatic ABCG5/G8 may play a stronger role in the regulation of biliary cholesterol secretion than NPC1L1. In addition, in the gut-liver axis, the intestinal NPC1L1 plays a significant role in providing dietary and reabsorbed biliary cholesterol to the body, and the inhibition of its functions by ezetimibe significantly reduces cholesterol absorption. Consequently, the bio-availability of cholesterol from intestinal sources for biliary secretion is decreased significantly.9 Moreover, intestinal absorption of dietary cholesterol and reabsorption of biliary cholesterol could play a major role in a subgroup of patients with cholesterol gallstones. Such aspects need to be prospectively investigated .because of some gallstone patients with increased hepatic de novo cholesterol synthesis; the results of Krawczyk et al. suggested a potential therapeutic role for statins. Statins decrease hepatic cholesterol biosynthesis by inhibiting the rate-limiting 3-hydroxy-3-methyl-glutarylcoenzyme a reductase pathway and may therefore lower the risk of cholesterol gallstones by reducing the cholesterol concentration in bile. Although this was the case with pravastatin in a previous report [236] and in a recent large cohort study investigating the statin use and risk of gallstone disease followed by cholecystectomy by Bodmer et al, [237] evidence remains scarce and speculative. In general, the contribution of de novo synthesis on the formation of lithogenic bile and cholesterol gallstones appears to be modest by Turley et al. [238] In a small group of cholesterol gallstone patients, it was found that statins neither influenced biliary cholesterol secretion nor reduced cholesterol saturation index in gallbladder bile by Smit et al. [239] They did not influence cholesterol crystal detection time in these patients, either by Smit et al. [240] Lastly, simvastatin reduced plasma cholesterol concentrations, but could not prevent gallstone formation and biliary cholesterol crystallization in the prairie dog model of cholesterol gallstones by Davis et al. [241] The combination therapy of statins with the hydrophilic ursodeoxycholic acid yielded either limited by Tazuma et al. [242] or similar by Sackmann et al. [243] dissolution rates versus ursodeoxycholic acid alone in patients with radiolucent cholesterol gallstones. These issues also remain unsettled in the study of Krawczyk et al., since none of the patients were treated with statins. Krawczyk et al. showed that the ratio of phytosterol:- cholesterol precursors in serum was even more predictive than "orthodox" variables determining the typical metabolic syndrome. Also, the ratio was consistent with the gallstone prevalence in different geographical areas and populations: <20% in Germans (and similar in Italians by Attili et al. [244]), ~27% in Hispanics, and 35% in Mapuches. Whether serum phytosterol levels may become additional predictive biomarkers for increased gallstone risk even at a younger age (as is the case for other aspects of cholesterol metabolism) is still a matter of debate. Of note, nonalcoholic fatty liver disease (another ''fellow traveler'' with the metabolic syndrome) also showed similar cholesterol metabolic profiles compared with gallstone disease by Simonen et al. [245] The process referred to as reverse cholesterol transport (i.e., cholesterol from peripheral [extrahepatic] tissues returning to the liver) needs to be considered as well. HDL delivers cholesterol to the hepatocyte for selective uptake by scavenger receptor class B type I, an HDL receptor Acton et al. [246] that contributes to the hepatic cholesterol pool used for bile acid synthesis and excretion of cholesterol in the bile and feces. Thus, knowing the ultimate interaction between complex pathways involving cholesterol absorption, transport, synthesis, and secretion in subgroups of patients precipitating solid cholesterol crystals in bile and forming gallstones obviously requires further attention. In conclusion, Krawczyk et al. investigated subtle mechanisms governing cholesterol homeostasis in the body (intestine, liver, and bile) with respect to cholesterol gallstone disease. Whether intestinal cholesterol absorption is decreased in certain gallstone patients and associated with a gain-of-function of the cholesterol intestinal and biliary transporter ABCG5/G8 (as well as of a number of other LITH genes) is a matter of research. Serum phytosterol levels might become additional predictive biomarkers for evaluating increased risk of gallstones. A new strategy aiming at inhibiting both hepatic synthesis and intestinal absorption of cholesterol for reducing its biliary output might be envisioned for a genetically defined subgroup of individuals at a high risk for gallstones. Overall, data need to be integrated with those suggesting that the absorption of intestinal cholesterol indeed plays a role in the pathogenesis of gallstone disease, and that other groups of patients might benefit from drugs (such as ezetimibe) inhibiting this process. [231] Although the ultimate and major sources of biliary cholesterol remain to be established in different populations, a more and more intriguing story about cholesterol cholelithiasis is developing and linking with complex metabolic disturbances and genetics. This will require appropriate preventive and medicinal approaches in the future.

VII. Phytosterol and Cholesterol Precursor Levels Indicate Increased Cholesterol Excretion and Biosynthesis in Gallstone Disease [228]

In hepatocytes and enterocytes sterol uptake and secretion is mediated by Niemann-Pick C1- like 1 (NPC1L1) and ATP-binding cassette (ABC)G5/8 proteins, respectively. Whereas serum levels of phytosterols represent surrogate markers for intestinal cholesterol absorption, cholesterol precursors reflect cholesterol biosynthesis. Crawczyk et al. compare serum and biliary sterol levels in ethnically different populations of patients with gallstone disease (GSD) and stone-free controls to identify differences in cholesterol transport and synthesis between these groups. In this case-control study four cohorts were analyzed: 112 German patients with GSD and 152 controls; two distinct Chilean ethnic groups: Hispanics (100 GSD, 100 controls), and Amerindians (20 GSD, 20 controls); additionally an 8-year follow-up of 70 Hispanics was performed. Serum sterols were measured by gas chromatography / mass spectrometry. Gallbladder bile sterol levels were analyzed in cholesterol GSD and controls. Common ABCG5/8 variants were genotyped. Comparison of serum sterols showed lower levels of phytosterols and higher levels of cholesterol precursors in GSD patients than in controls. The ratios of phytosterols to cholesterol precursors were lower in GSD patients, whereas biliary phytosterol and cholesterol concentrations were elevated as compared with controls. In the follow-up study, serum phytosterol levels were significantly lower even before GSD was detectable by ultrasound. An ethnic gradient in the ratios of phytosterols to cholesterol precursors was apparent (Germans > Hispanics > Amerindians). ABCG5/8 variants did not fully explain the sterol metabolic trait of GSD in any of the cohorts.

Conclusion

Individuals predisposed to GSD display increased biliary output of cholesterol in the setting of relatively low intestinal cholesterol absorption, indicating enhanced whole-body sterol clearance. This metabolic trait precedes gallstone formation and is a feature of ethnic groups at higher risk of cholesterol GSD. In humans, cholesterol homeostasis is maintained by the precise interaction between intestinal uptake, de novo synthesis, hepatic output, and fecal disposal. Among these mechanisms, intestinal uptake and biosynthesis represent the sole sources of new cholesterol. At the intestinal level, two brush border proteins, NPC1L1 and ABCG5/8, determine cholesterol uptake. The Niemann-Pick C1-like 1 (NPC1L1) transporter, selectively blocked by ezetimibe, is critical for the absorption of intestinal cholesterol by Lammert and Altmann et al. [247, 248] Conversely, the two ATP-binding cassette (ABC) transporters ABCG5 and ABCG8 function as a heterodimeric efflux pump, mediating cholesterol transport back into the intestinal lumen by Berge and Lee et al. [249, 250] Additionally, NPC1L1 and ABCG5/8 are expressed at the canalicular membrane of hepatocytes as well by Lammert et al. [247] Both at the intestinal level and in the liver, NPC1L1 and ABCG5/8 transport not only cholesterol but also sterols that are synthesized exclusively by plants, namely phytosterols (e.g., sitosterol, campesterol). Hence, in Npc1l1 knockout mice serum levels of campesterol and sitosterol are hardly detectable by Davis et al. [232]. In parallel, Abcg5/8-deficient animals demonstrate reduced biliary cholesterol secretion, whereas phytosterol absorption is enhanced because of impaired hepatic and intestinal excretion. [32] As phytosterols are not synthesized in the human body, their serum levels provide direct insights into the transport function of hepatic and intestinal cholesterol transporters by Lammert et al. [251] Measurements of cholesterol precursors (e.g., lathosterol, desmosterol) in serum allow indirect estimation of de novo cholesterol synthesis by Miettinen et al. [252] The comparison of serum surrogate markers informs about the sources of cholesterol and its transport in a given individual by Kempen et al. [253] Genetic studies have shown that dysfunction of the ABCG5/8 transporters can lead not only to an improper flux of sterols, but also to cholesterol gallstone formation, one of the most common diseases in Westernized and developing countries by Berge et al. [254] Hepatic hypersecretion of biliary cholesterol, followed by cholesterol crystal formation, is presumably the primary defect in the formation of cholesterol gallstones. Although the precise source of cholesterol (i.e., exogenous or endogenous) present in gallstones has not been fully clarified, the ongoing working hypothesis is that the underlying molecular mechanism leading to cholesterol hypersecretion is a gain of sterol transport activity at the canalicular level by Crawczyk and Acalovischi et al. [255, 256] In fact, a recent genome- wide association study (GWAS) and the analysis of sib-pairs with gallstones have demonstrated that the common ABCG8 variant p.D19H is a major determinant of gallstone formation in humans, presumably by gain-of-function of the transporter by Grunhage and Buch et al. [134, 137] Furthermore, carriers of other rare loss-of-function mutations in ABCG5/8 suffer from phytosterolemia, a disease characterized by intestinal hyperabsorption and diminished biliary secretion of phytosterols and cholesterol. Of note, patients with this rare genetic disease appear to be resistant to gallstone formation [249, 250]. In order to gain further insights into the sterol metabolic trait leading to cholesterol gallstone formation, we performed case-control studies comparing serum levels of surrogates for cholesterol absorption (phytosterols) and de novo synthesis (cholesterol precursors) in two ethnically different populations at high risk of cholesterol gallstone disease (Germany and Chile). Additionally, in an 8-year follow-up study we assessed the predictive value of sterol serum levels as markers for increased risk of developing gallstones. Subsequently, we corroborated our results by comparing the biliary levels of sterols in an additional cohort of gallstone patients and in a group of stone-free controls.

Patients and Methods

Study Cohorts

The general description of the study cohorts is presented. Crawczyk et al. selected 35 stone-free subjects in Chile between 1992 and 1993 who subsequently developed GSD during an 8-year follow-up period, and paired them by age, gender, and body mass index (BMI) at the first survey with 35 subjects who remained free of gallstones during this follow-up period. In order to study biliary sterol contents in GSD and controls, gallbladder bile was obtained by needle aspiration from cholesterol gallstone patients (n = 17) during elective laparoscopic cholecystectomy. Gallbladder bile was also obtained from 17 patients without gallstones who underwent surgery because of hepatic focal lesions (cysts, focal liver metastases of colon cancer) or resectable gastrointestinal malignancies (gastric or colon cancer). Routine biochemical analyses, including liver function tests, were performed within one week before surgery. Only patients without major elevations of serum aminotransferase activities (≤1.5-fold normal levels) and without cholestasis (i.e., normal serum bilirubin, c-glutamyl transferase and alkaline phosphatase activities) were included. Immediately after collection, bile samples were investigated for the presence or absence of typical cholesterol crystals and the absence of blood contamination by polarizing light microscopy. Bile samples were stored at ~70°C for lipid and phytosterol measurements. In all individuals, fasting serum specimens, containing butylated hydroxytoluene, were collected at the time of the clinical survey and stored at ~70°C; blood samples with ethylenediaminetetraacetic acid were simultaneously obtained for DNA isolation.

Genotyping

All studied individuals were genotyped for the ABCG5 p.Q604E (rs6720173, c__29001998_10) and ABCG8 p.D19H (rs11887534, c__26135643_10), p.Y54C (rs4148211, c__29535502_10), p.T400K (rs4148217, c__375061_10), and p.A632V (rs6544718, c__25642779_10) variants. The ABCG8 p.D19H and p.T400K coding variants have been described previously as putative susceptibility variants for gallstone formation in humans by Grunhage, Katsica and Buch et al. [134, 137, 233] Measurement of Sterols and Clinical Chemical Parameters. Serum levels of cholesterol, phytosterols (sitosterol, campesterol) and cholesterol precursors (lathosterol, desmosterol) were measured in serum samples by gas chromatography / mass spectrometry (GC/MS) after alkaline hydrolysis, extraction, and derivatization, as described [257]. We excluded individuals with sterol levels suggesting familial hypercholesterolemia or hereditary sitosterolemia. Subsequently, ratios allowing the estimation of de novo cholesterol synthesis and intestinal cholesterol absorption were calculated as described. [258] In bile, besides sitosterol and campesterol, a panel of other phytosterols frequently present in food was also quantified by GC-MS, including avenasterol, brasicasterol, campestanol, sitostanol, and stigmasterol. [259] Because biliary compound concentrations in gallbladder bile varied substantially between patients, bile salt contents were also measured enzymatically [260] and used to normalize sterol contents in bile. Biliary phospholipids were measured enzymatically using phospholipase D and choline oxidase [261] Serum triglyceride levels, liver function tests as well as glucose, insulin and C-peptide levels were determined by standard clinical chemical assays. Values of concurrent fasting glucose and insulin were used to estimate insulin resistance by the homeostasis model assessment (IR-HOMA) index. IR-HOMA was calculated according to the following formula: insulin (lU/ mL) _ fasting plasma glucose (mmol/L)/22.5. Statistical Analysis. All data are given as means ± standard deviation (SD). The SAS 9.1 program (SAS Institute, Cary, NC) was used for all data processing. Demographic data and baseline characteristics were checked for normal distribution with Kolmogorov-Smirnov goodness-of-fit tests. Significant differences were evaluated in contingency tables using either Fisher's exact tests or v2-tests. Continuous variables were compared between groups using Student t tests or Mann- Whitney rank sum tests. Two-sided $P < 0.05$ was considered significant, unless previous studies indicated that lower or higher values were to be expected; then, one-sided tests were performed. Pearson's correlation coefficient was used to evaluate univariate associations between the sitosterol:lathosterol and campesterol: lathosterol ratios and different ethnic groups, age, BMI and gender. Analysis of covariance was performed to obtain estimates of sitosterol:lathosterol and campesterol: lathosterol ratios between ethnic groups adjusted for age, BMI and gender. The area under the receiver operating characteristic curve (AUC) was calculated foreach serum surrogate marker of cholesterol synthesis and absorption as well as the specified ratios; the P-values for the AUC indicate significance in comparison to 0.5. For ABCG5/8 genotypes, Hardy-Weinberg equilibrium was checked using exact tests (http://ihg.gsf.de/ cgi-bin/hw/hwa1.pl). [134] Potential associations between gene variants and cholelithiasis were tested in contingency tables (genotypes: Armitrage's trend tests; alleles: v2-tests).

In the **results** section, in Germans and Chilean Hispanics, cases and matched controls are similar in age, gender, and BMI distribution. Compared with the Chilean Hispanic cohort, the German patients are older, leaner, and include more men. The small Amerindian Chilean cohort (Mapuche) was composed only of women who were relatively younger than the Hispanics and Germans. Of note, serum total cholesterol and low-density lipoprotein (LDL) cholesterol concentrations were lower in Mapuches compared with Hispanics independently of gallstone status. Serum lipids are similar in cases and controls in the German cohort. In contrast, in the Chilean Hispanic cohort total and LDL cholesterol levels are significantly lower in cases compared with controls. In the Chilean Hispanic and Amerindian cohorts, fasting glucose and insulin levels were also determined, yielding comparable results between cases and controls. As shown in Table 1, the IR-HOMA indexes are high and in the range of insulin resistance for both cases and controls, but they do not differ between groups.

Patients with Gallstones Display Serum Sterol Levels Reflecting Lower Intestinal Cholesterol Absorption and Higher Hepatic Cholesterol Synthesis

The mean levels of the phytosterol sitosterol as well as the sitosterol to cholesterol ratios are significantly lower in both German and Chilean Hispanic patients with GSD, indicating that these patients display decreased intestinal sterol absorption as compared with stone-free individuals. In contrast, German gallstone patients show significantly higher mean lathosterol concentrations and lathosterol to cholesterol ratios, which reflect increased de novo cholesterol synthesis in comparison to controls. Of note, the same differences were observed for lathosterol levels in Chilean Hispanics with GSD, and similar trends were observed for desmosterol. Taken together, the sitosterol to lathosterol ratio is significantly decreased in patients with gallstones in comparison to controls. Further, the results are in line with markedly lower levels of another phytosterol, campesterol, and decreased campesterol to lathosterol ratios in individuals with gallstones. In the German cohort the differences were more pronounced in women than in men. Of note, the magnitude of the differences in cholesterol precursors and phytosterol levels between GSD and controls are more pronounced in Chilean Hispanics as compared with Germans. Based on the above associations between sterols and the gallstone phenotype, we calculated the AUC for sterol levels to assess their clinical value as predictive markers for gallstone formation. The analysis of Chilean cohort German females0 shows the two ratios of sitosterol: lathosterol and lathosterol:cholesterol, which have the best predictive values. Additionally, the AUC for campesterol:lathosterol is significant in female German gallstone patients (AUC = 0.602, 95% confidence interval [CI] 0.510-0.693, P = 0.033); nevertheless, this association could not be replicated in the Chilean cohort. Effect of the ABCG5/8 polymorphisms on serum sterol levels and gallstone susceptibility. Genotype frequencies do not deviate from respective frequencies deposited in the Entrez single nucleotide polymorphism (SNP) database. The p.Y53C variant in the Chilean cohort, the p.D19H variant in Chilean controls, and the p.A632V variant in German cases depart from Hardy-Weinberg equilibrium. This result might be attributed to the matching of individuals in the Chilean cohort (see Patients and Methods) and hints at a possible association with GSD in Germans. However, the overall genotype distributions of the variants do not differ between cases and stone-free controls. German carriers of the ABCG8 p.D19H gallstone risk allele [C] by Grunhage and Buch et al. [134, 137] are characterized by a trend to elevated serum lathosterol as well as lower phytosterol (sitosterol, campesterol) levels, indicating increased hepatic synthesis and lower intestinal absorption of cholesterol. In contrast, these trends are not evident in the Chilean cohort. Interestingly, the p.Y54C variant s associated with phytosterol levels in the Chilean but not the German cohort. Chilean carriers of genotype [AA] display significantly higher sitosterol and campesterol levels as compared with carriers of the [G] allele ($P < 0.01$ and $P < 0.05$, respectively). On the other hand, the other common polymorphisms of the hepatobiliary cholesterol transporter ABCG5/8 are not significantly associated with the serum levels of sterol precursors and phytosterol.

Follow-up Study

Serum Levels of Phytosterols Represent Predictive Markers for the Risk of Developing Gallstones. Table 3 presents the general characteristics of the sub cohort of the Chilean individuals who were followed up for 8 years from 1992/1993 to 2000/2001. Individuals who developed gallstones during the follow-up period had significantly lower cholesterol levels as compared with gallstone-free subjects. In contrast, there are no differences in terms of serum glucose, insulin, or lipid concentrations. Table 4 demonstrates remarkable differences in serum sterol levels: Individuals who developed gallstones during the follow-up period had significantly (P _ 0.001) decreased sitosterol and campesterol levels at inclusion. In line with this observation, the ratios of phytosterols to cholesterol in future gallstone patients were significantly ($P < 0.001$) lower as compared with patients who remained stone-free. The initially different serum sterol levels between cases and controls converged during follow- up. In contrast, the prevalence of variables determining the metabolic syndrome (MS) and MS per se did not differ between patients who developed stones during follow-up and individuals who did not (Table 3). In this respect, serum phytosterol levels might be regarded as predictive markers for increased gallstone risk. Serum Sterol Levels Differ Between Ethnicities.

The ratios of phytosterols to cholesterol precursors differ significantly ($P < 0.0001$) between the German and Chilean cohorts included in this study. Indeed, the ratio is highest in the German individuals and lowest in Mapuches. Of note, these results are in line with the prevalence rates of gallstones in these populations, which are the lowest in Germans (~20%), [95] but higher in Hispanics (27%) and highest in Mapuches (35%). [262, 263] Because in our cohorts age and BMI correlate significantly with phytosterol to cholesterol precursor levels (data not shown) and the ratio of males to females differs between the cohorts, analysis of covariance was used to compare noncholesterol sterol ratios adjusted for BMI, age, and gender. The differences between the German and Chilean cohorts remained significant (campesterol: lathosterol, $P = 0.005$; sitosterol:lathosterol, $P = 0.021$) after this adjustment.

Gallstone Patients Display Increased Concentrations of Phytosterols and Cholesterol in Bile

Finally, as an estimation of hepatic sterol clearance we studied the cholesterol and plant sterol contents in gallbladder bile from cholesterol gallstone and stone-free control patients. Both groups were similar in age (43 6 17 versus 45 6 19 years), gender distribution (72% females), and BMI (27 6 6 versus 25 6 3 kg/m2). Figure 3 demonstrates that individuals with GSD display significantly (P? 0.003) higher biliary concentrations of total phytosterols in comparison to controls (60-70% increase). Also, mean molar cholesterol concentrations show a trend to higher levels (6.2 6 1.6% versus 4.7 ± 1.4%). Mean molar bile salt concentrations in biles from cases and controls were 79.5 ± 4.2% and 82.4 ± 4.7%, respectively; the corresponding mean biliary phospholipid levels were 14.3 ± 3.7% and 12.9 ± 3.6%. Figure 4 plots the composition of gallbladder biles in cases and controls in the ternary equilibrium phase diagram, demonstrating that cases and controls plot above and below the micellar phase boundary, respectively. In addition, gallbladder biles from GSD patients are enriched in sitosterol, avenasterol, sitostanol, and stigmasterol as compared with biles from stone-free controls (data not shown). Discussion The regulation of cholesterol synthesis and transport, the latter mediated by the ABCG5/8 and NPC1L1 proteins, is substantial for whole-body cholesterol homeostasis. Hence, genetically underlined defects of proteins involved in these processes can distort the overall cholesterol balance, resulting in atherosclerosis, dyslipidemia, or gallstones. The precise sources of the excess free cholesterol secreted into the bile in GSD remain largely unknown. It has been suggested that cholesterol in gallstones is of exogenous origin (dietary), whereas the overall contribution of de novo synthesis to biliary cholesterol secretion is generally modest by Gurantz et al. [238, 264] Here we analyzed the association between GSD and surrogate markers of cholesterol absorption and synthesis as well as common genetic variants of the cholesterol transporter ABCG5/8. Figure 5 summarizes our hypothesis on cholesterol transport and synthesis in individuals at risk for gallstones. Overall, they display lower concentrations of phytosterols such as sitosterol— valid surrogate markers for intestinal cholesterol absorption— as compared with controls. In parallel, serum levels of the cholesterol precursor lathosterol are higher in these subjects, indicating that they synthesize more cholesterol. The decreased sitosterol to lathosterol ratios indicate reduced cholesterol absorption and in turn increased cholesterol synthesis. These results underpin a particular derangement of cholesterol homeostasis, i.e., increased whole sterol clearance, as a critical factor in GSD. The increasing prevalence of gallstones in Westernized countries26 and the correlation between intestinal cholesterol absorption rates and stone frequency in several strains of inbred mice27 point to dietary factors as drivers of stone susceptibility in general. Because our study indicates that patients at risk for gallstones present with increased cholesterol synthesis and relatively lower cholesterol absorption rates, 1,28 we hypothesize that higher cholesterol clearance is the specific metabolic trait triggering GSD in this setting. There are several conclusions that can be drawn from our results. First, this study suggests that serum sterol levels, in particular the sitosterol:lathosterol and lathosterol:cholesterol ratios, might have predictive value as ''biomarkers'' for an increased risk of gallbladder stone formation. Of note, the cohort that took part in the follow-up study was carefully matched in terms of the most common lithogenic factors (Table 3). Our analysis showed that at inclusion in the study individuals who were prone to develop gallstones later on displayed lower serum phytosterol levels. Hence, increased biliary/intestinal cholesterol efflux can be regarded as a trait that is not only characteristic for individuals with gallstones but is also present before the formation of stones. On the other hand, we did not detect increased concentrations of markers of cholesterol synthesis at this point. This suggests that higher clearance of sterols is the primary defect, which subsequently triggers an increased synthesis of cholesterol (Figure 5). As cholesterol homeostasis changes with time, the prolithogenic state is not a permanent metabolic trait, and it could be modulated, for example, by environmental factors. Indeed, the differences in sterol levels that were present at inclusion disappeared during follow-up, supporting that the prolithogenic metabolic trait does not persist during gallstone formation. Conceptually, the increased cholesterol output into bile and diminished cholesterol absorption in the intestine can be connected with a gain-of-function of the ABCG5/8 biliary hemitransporters for cholesterol. In fact, previous studies showed that an increased expression of these proteins enhances biliary cholesterol output and reduces intestinal absorption [265]. Our previous genetic studies in large cohorts have shown that the common lithogenic variant p.D19H of the ABCG8 transporter predisposes to GSD. [134, 266] However, the overall genetic association does not reach statistical significance in the present study, most likely due to the smaller cohort size. However, Krawczyk et al.'s findings in serum sterol levels are clearly consistent with an ABCG5/8 gain-of-function, increasing sterol output and subsequently synthesis. ABCG5/8 gain-of-function could also be explained by induction of transporter activity and/or increased transporter expression. Indeed, enhanced hepatic protein expression of ABCG5/8 has been described in some gallstone subjects,30 and functional studies have demonstrated that biliary cholesterol secretion correlates with hepatic expression of ABCG5/G8 in most mouse models. [267, 268]. The higher sterol contents in bile in GSD (Figures 3, 4) are also in line with the gain-of-function of hepatic sterol transport activity, and the preferential increment of biliary phytosterols relative to cholesterol is consistent with the higher transport affinity of ABCG5/8 for plant sterols as compared with cholesterol by Buch et al. [269] In this respect, a new strategy aiming both at decreasing biliary cholesterol output and inhibiting cholesterol synthesis might be envisioned for a genetically defined subgroup of individuals at high risk for stones. On the other hand, dysfunction of NPC1L1 at the hepatic and the intestinal level could also contribute to the GSD phenotype. Previously rare and common variants of NPC1L1 have been reported to influence sterol absorption by Kosters and Kamisako et al. [270, 271] Although NPC1L1 has never been regarded as a Lith gene, we cannot exclude the possibility that loss-of-function of this transport could contribute to GSD. Recently, several other LITH genes have also been detected 10. Although polymorphisms in these loci only moderately affect gallstone risk, we cannot exclude that they contribute to gallstone formation in the individuals included in our study. Interestingly, in the German cohort the association between cholesterol synthesis and transport with GSD was more pronounced in women than in m n. This observation might be related to a lower number of en in the German cohort, which decreases the power of this analysis. Also, the Chilean cohort was predominantly female. Our findings suggest that a distorted cholesterol homeostasis is more evident in women in whom GSD is in general more common. Cholesterol absorption and synthesis can also be affected by insulin sensitivity, which is, at least in part, determined genetically, but also associated with BMI and central obesity. Of note, both obesity and insulin resistance modulate cholesterol absorption and synthesis. 36 Indeed, lean subjects with lower insulin sensitivity show higher cholesterol synthesis and lower sterol absorption. In our Hispanic and Amerindian cohorts, GSD and controls are similar in terms of BMI and insulin resistance, thus the specific sterol metabolic trait associated with GSD is not confounded by these variables. Cases and controls included in the follow-up study were matched for these variables at inclusion, and members of both subgroups developed obesity, insulin resistance and metabolic syndrome to similar extents. Although these changes might suggest that the metabolic variables contributed to GSD, our refined analysis showed that only individuals with lower sterol absorption at study entry were susceptible to gallstone development. Notably, we showed previously that this increment in metabolic syndrome traits in Chile during the period from 1992 to 2001 is higher than expected and related to changes of socioeconomic status by Yu et al. [272] This study is notable because none of the subjects were under cholesterol reducing therapy with ezetimibe or statins. In fact, the cohorts were recruited before ezetimibe was introduced as a drug for hypercholesterolemia, and the use of statins was an exclusion criterion both in cases and controls. The results, therefore, provide novel and unique insights into cholesterol flux and its relation to gallstone formation. Previous studies on the effect of drugs lowering cholesterol synthesis (i.e., statins) and absorption (i.e., ezetimibe) are controversial. Analyses performed in large human cohorts have documented lower prevalence of clinical relevant gallstone disease (i.e., cholecystectomy) among individuals on long-term therapy with statins by Bodmer et al. [237] In other studies, statins neither influenced biliary cholesterol secretion nor reduced cholesterol saturation indices in general [239]. The data from our patients, which are given as means, indicate that subgroups of patients are at higher (genetic) risk of stone formation. In these cases, increased cholesterol synthesis could be a critical additional factor driving stone formation, and they could benefit from drugs lowering cholesterol synthesis, which has indeed been observed on an individual basis by Smit et al. [236] With respect to ezetimibe, studies in mouse models and a single study in humans by Wang and Zuniga et al. [231, 235] have shown that it can reduce biliary cholesterol secretion and cholesterol concentrations in gallbladder bile. In this respect, future prospective studies using surrogate markers of cholesterol synthesis and transport in large cohorts of patients under cholesterol-lowering therapy are warranted. Previously, it has been postulated that in selected patients ratios of serum campesterol and sitosterol to cholesterol reflect the biliary cholesterol secretion rates by Cohen et al. [273] Because in our study we used the surrogate markers for cholesterol transport and synthesis, which indicated a link between cholesterol homeostasis and GSD, we further strengthened our findings by analysis of biliary lipid compositions, demonstrating that gallstone patients display increased biliary levels of both phytosterols and cholesterol. These results are in line with data published by Miettinen et al.44 Their analysis of 150 individuals with cholesterol stones showed preferentially increased levels of plant sterols in bile from cholesterol gallstone patients. [274] The latest analysis of a cohort of pediatric patients with gallstones indicated that increased cholesterol synthesis and decreased cholesterol absorption are likely to underlie the formation of gallbladder stones in younger individuals by Cuevas et al. [275] Interestingly, the same profile is characteristic for another liver phenotype, fatty liver disease by Simonen et al. [245] As fatty liver is one of the risk factors for gallstone formation by Lindenthal et al. [276] distorted cholesterol homeostasis may represent a metabolic link between both entities. Moreover, we observed pronounced differences across the ethnic groups. These results, together with lower cholesterol levels in Chilean individuals as compared with Germans, point to a more pronounced prolithogenic phenotype in Chileans and at least partially explain the previously reported differences of gallstone prevalence rates among the ethnicities included in the current study Lammert and Empen et al. [95, 262, 263] In summary, serum sterol levels represent surrogate markers indicating that gallstone-susceptible patients display enhanced secretion of cholesterol and non-cholesterol sterols into bile, which is coupled with an increased synthesis of new cholesterol. Furthermore, increased cholesterol synthesis might be secondary to decreased intestinal cholesterol absorption resulting from gain-of-function of the ABCG5/8 transporter system. The latter link remains hypothetical; however, our results suggest a new possibility for preventing gallstones in patients carrying risk gene variants.

References

[1] Portincasa, P., Moschetta, A., and Palasciano, G. 2006. Cholesterol gallstone disease. *Lancet* 368:230-239.

[2] Hofmann, A.F., Amelsberg, A., and vanSonnenberg, E. 1993. Pathogenesis and treatment of gallstones. *N Engl J Med* 328:1854-1855.

[3] Lamont, J.T., and Carey, M.C. 1992. Cholesterol gallstone formation. 2. Pathobiology and pathomechanics. *Prog Liver Dis* 10:165-191.

[4] Thudichum, J. 1983. *A treatise on gallstones: their chemistry, pathology, and treatment.* London: John Churchill and Sons.

[5] Gordon-Taylor, G. 1937. On gallstones and their sufferers. *Br J Surg* 25:11.

[6] Shehadi, W.H. 1979. The biliary system through the ages. *Int Surg* 64:63-78.

[7] Theophrastus Bombastus, v.H. 1589. *Das Buch von den tartarischen Krankheiten nach dem alten Namen vom Stein/sand und Gries.* Basel: Conrad Waldkirk. 5 pp.

[8] Shieh, H.S., Hoard, L.G., and Nordman, C.E. 1977. Crystal structure of anhydrous cholesterol. *Nature* 267:287-289.

[9] Konikoff, F.M., Chung, D.S., Donovan, J.M., Small, D.M., and Carey, M.C. 1992. Filamentous, helical, and tubular microstructures during cholesterol crystallization from bile. Evidence that cholesterol does not nucleate classic monohydrate plates. *J Clin Invest* 90:1155-1160.

[10] Craven, B.M. 1976. Crystal structure of cholesterol monohydrate. *Nature* 260:727-729.

[11] Portincasa, P., van Erpecum, K.J., Jansen, A., Renooij, W., Gadellaa, M., and vanBerge-Henegouwen, G.P. 1996. Behavior of various cholesterol crystals in bile from patients with gallstones. *Hepatology* 23:738-748.

[12] Carey, M.C. 1978. Critical tables for calculating the cholesterol saturation of native bile. *J Lipid Res* 19:945-955.

[13] Wang, D.Q., and Carey, M.C. 1996. Characterization of crystallization pathways during cholesterol precipitation from human gallbladder biles: identical pathways to corresponding model biles with three predominating sequences. *J Lipid Res* 37:2539-2549.

[14] Wang, D.Q., and Carey, M.C. 1996. Complete mapping of crystallization pathways during cholesterol precipitation from model bile: influence of physical-chemical variables of pathophysiologic relevance and identification of a stable liquid crystalline state in cold, dilute and hydrophilic bile salt-containing systems. *J Lipid Res* 37:606-630.

[15] Admirand, W.H., and Small, D.M. 1968. The physicochemical basis of cholesterol gallstone formation in man. *J Clin Invest* 47:1043-1052.

[16] Danzinger, R.G., Hofmann, A.F., Schoenfield, L.J., and Thistle, J.L. 1972. Dissolution of cholesterol gallstones by chenodeoxycholic acid. *N Engl J Med* 286:1-8.

[17] Makino, I., Shinozaki, K., Yoshino, K., and Nakagawa, S. 1975. [Dissolution of cholesterol gallstones by long-term administration of ursodeoxycholic acid]. *Nihon Shokakibyo Gakkai Zasshi* 72:690-702.

[18] Sauerbruch, T., Delius, M., Paumgartner, G., Holl, J., Wess, O., Weber, W., Hepp, W., and Brendel, W. 1986. Fragmentation of gallstones by extracorporeal shock waves. *N Engl J Med* 314:818-822.

[19] Moschetta, A., vanBerge-Henegouwen, G.P., Portincasa, P., Palasciano, G., and van Erpecum, K.J. 2001. Cholesterol crystallization in model biles: effects of bile salt and phospholipid species composition. *J Lipid Res* 42:1273-1281.

[20] Konikoff, F.M., Danino, D., Weihs, D., Rubin, M., and Talmon, Y. 2000. Microstructural evolution of lipid aggregates in nucleating model and human biles visualized by cryogenic transmission electron microscopy. *Hepatology* 31:261-268.

[21] Ko, C.W., Sekijima, J.H., and Lee, S.P. 1999. Biliary sludge. *Ann Intern Med* 130:301-311.

[22] Apstein, M.D., and Carey, M.C. 1996. Pathogenesis of cholesterol gallstones: a parsimonious hypothesis. *Eur J Clin Invest* 26:343-352.

[23] Holzbach, R.T., Marsh, M., Olszewski, M., and Holan, K. 1973. Cholesterol solubility in bile. Evidence that supersaturated bile is frequent in healthy man. *J Clin Invest* 52:1467-1479.

[24] Jirsa, M., and Groen, A. 2001. Role of biliary proteins and non-protein factors in kinetics of cholesterol crystallisation and gallstone growth. *Front Biosci* 6:14.

[25] Portincasa, P., Di Ciaula, A., Baldassarre, G., Palmieri, V., Gentile, A., Cimmino, A., and Palasciano, G. 1994. Gallbladder motor function in gallstone patients: sonographic and in vitro studies on the role of gallstones, smooth muscle function and gallbladder wall inflammation. *J Hepatol* 21:430-440.

[26] Portincasa, P., Moschetta, A., Mazzone, A., Palasciano, G., Svelto, M., and Calamita, G. 2003. Water handling and aquaporins in bile formation: recent advances and research trends. *J Hepatol* 39:864-874.

[27] Russell, D.W., and Setchell, K.D. 1992. Bile acid biosynthesis. *Biochemistry* 31:4737-4749.

[28] Crawford, A.R., Smith, A.J., Hatch, V.C., Oude Elferink, R.P., Borst, P., and Crawford, J.M. 1997. Hepatic secretion of phospholipid vesicles in the mouse critically depends on mdr2 or MDR3 P-glycoprotein expression. Visualization by electron microscopy. *J Clin Invest* 100:2562-2567.

[29] Hofmann, A.F. 1999. The continuing importance of bile acids in liver and intestinal disease. *Arch Intern Med* 159:2647-2658.

[30] Gerloff, T., Stieger, B., Hagenbuch, B., Madon, J., Landmann, L., Roth, J., Hofmann, A.F., and Meier, P.J. 1998. The sister of P-glycoprotein represents the canalicular bile salt export pump of mammalian liver. *J Biol Chem* 273:10046-10050.

[31] Smit, J.J., Schinkel, A.H., Oude Elferink, R.P., Groen, A.K., Wagenaar, E., van Deemter, L., Mol, C.A., Ottenhoff, R., van der Lugt, N.M., van Roon, M.A., et al. 1993. Homozygous disruption of the murine mdr2 P-glycoprotein gene leads to a complete absence of phospholipid from bile and to liver disease. *Cell* 75:451-462.

[32] Yu, L., Hammer, R.E., Li-Hawkins, J., Von Bergmann, K., Lutjohann, D., Cohen, J.C., and Hobbs, H.H. 2002. Disruption of Abcg5 and Abcg8 in mice reveals their crucial role in biliary cholesterol secretion. *Proc Natl Acad Sci U S A* 99:16237-16242.

[33] Wang, H., Chen, J., Hollister, K., Sowers, L.C., and Forman, B.M. 1999. Endogenous bile acids are ligands for the nuclear receptor FXR/BAR. *Mol Cell* 3:543-553.

[34] Makishima, M., Okamoto, A.Y., Repa, J.J., Tu, H., Learned, R.M., Luk, A., Hull, M.V., Lustig, K.D., Mangelsdorf, D.J., and Shan, B. 1999. Identification of a nuclear receptor for bile acids. *Science* 284:1362-1365.

[35] Parks, D.J., Blanchard, S.G., Bledsoe, R.K., Chandra, G., Consler, T.G., Kliewer, S.A., Stimmel, J.B., Willson, T.M., Zavacki, A.M., Moore, D.D., et al. 1999. Bile acids: natural ligands for an orphan nuclear receptor. *Science* 284:1365-1368.

[36] Janowski, B.A., Willy, P.J., Devi, T.R., Falck, J.R., and Mangelsdorf, D.J. 1996. An oxysterol signalling pathway mediated by the nuclear receptor LXR alpha. *Nature* 383:728-731.

[37] Zhang, Z., Li, D., Blanchard, D.E., Lear, S.R., Erickson, S.K., and Spencer, T.A. 2001. Key regulatory oxysterols in liver: analysis as delta4-3-ketone derivatives by HPLC and response to physiological perturbations. *J Lipid Res* 42:649-658.

[38] Ananthanarayanan, M., Balasubramanian, N., Makishima, M., Mangelsdorf, D.J., and Suchy, F.J. 2001. Human bile salt export pump promoter is transactivated by the farnesoid X receptor/bile acid receptor. *J Biol Chem* 276:28857-28865.

[39] Huang, L., Zhao, A., Lew, J.L., Zhang, T., Hrywna, Y., Thompson, J.R., de Pedro, N., Royo, I., Blevins, R.A., Pelaez, F., et al. 2003. Farnesoid X receptor activates transcription of the phospholipid pump MDR3. *J Biol Chem* 278:51085-51090.

[40] Repa, J.J., Berge, K.E., Pomajzl, C., Richardson, J.A., Hobbs, H., and Mangelsdorf, D.J. 2002. Regulation of ATP-binding cassette sterol transporters ABCG5 and ABCG8 by the liver X receptors alpha and beta. *J Biol Chem* 277:18793-18800.

[41] Moschetta, A., Bookout, A.L., and Mangelsdorf, D.J. 2004. Prevention of cholesterol gallstone disease by FXR agonists in a mouse model. *Nat Med* 10:1352-1358.

[42] Amigo, L., Castro, J., Miquel, J.F., Zanlungo, S., Young, S., and Nervi, F. 2006. Inactivation of hepatic microsomal triglyceride transfer protein protects mice from diet-induced gallstones. *Gastroenterology* 131:1870-1878.

[43] Vassileva, G., Golovko, A., Markowitz, L., Abbondanzo, S.J., Zeng, M., Yang, S., Hoos, L., Tetzloff, G., Levitan, D., Murgolo, N.J., et al. 2006. Targeted deletion of Gpbar1 protects mice from cholesterol gallstone formation. *Biochem J* 398:423-430.

[44] Johnson, L.E., Elias, M.S., Bolick, D.T., Skaflen, M.D., Green, R.M., and Hedrick, C.C. 2008. The G protein-coupled receptor G2A: involvement in hepatic lipid metabolism and gallstone formation in mice. *Hepatology* 48:1138-1148.

[45] Khanuja, B., Cheah, Y.C., Hunt, M., Nishina, P.M., Wang, D.Q., Chen, H.W., Billheimer, J.T., Carey, M.C., and Paigen, B. 1995. Lith1, a major gene affecting cholesterol gallstone formation among inbred strains of mice. *Proc Natl Acad Sci U S A* 92:7729-7733.

[46] Paigen, B., Schork, N.J., Svenson, K.L., Cheah, Y.C., Mu, J.L., Lammert, F., Wang, D.Q., Bouchard, G., and Carey, M.C. 2000. Quantitative trait loci mapping for cholesterol gallstones in AKR/J and C57L/J strains of mice. *Physiol Genomics* 4:59-65.

[47] Hillebrandt, S., Matern, S., and Lammert, F. 2003. Mouse models for genetic dissection of polygenic gastrointestinal diseases. *Eur J Clin Invest* 33:155-160.

[48] Wang, D.Q., and Afdhal, N.H. 2004. Genetic analysis of cholesterol gallstone formation: searching for Lith (gallstone) genes. *Curr Gastroenterol Rep* 6:140-150.

[49] Lammert, F., and Matern, S. 2005. The genetic background of cholesterol gallstone formation: an inventory of human lithogenic genes. *Curr Drug Targets Immune Endocr Metabol Disord* 5:163-170.

[50] Lammert, F., and Sauerbruch, T. 2005. Mechanisms of disease: the genetic epidemiology of gallbladder stones. *Nat Clin Pract Gastroenterol Hepatol* 2:423-433.

[51] van Erpecum, K.J., van Berge Henegouwen, G.P., Stolk, M.F., Hopman, W.P., Jansen, J.B., and Lamers, C.B. 1992. Fasting gallbladder volume, postprandial emptying and cholecystokinin release in gallstone patients and normal subjects. *J Hepatol* 14:194-202.

[52] Xiao, Z.L., Amaral, J., Biancani, P., and Behar, J. 2005. Impaired cytoprotective function of muscle in human gallbladders with cholesterol stones. *Am J Physiol Gastrointest Liver Physiol* 288:G525-532.

[53] Portincasa, P., Di Ciaula, A., and vanBerge-Henegouwen, G.P. 2004. Smooth muscle function and dysfunction in gallbladder disease. *Curr Gastroenterol Rep* 6:151-162.

[54] van Erpecum, K.J., Venneman, N.G., Portincasa, P., and Vanberge-Henegouwen, G.P. 2000. Review article: agents affecting gall-bladder motility--role in treatment and prevention of gallstones. *Aliment Pharmacol Ther* 14 Suppl 2:66-70.

[55] Pauletzki, J., Althaus, R., Holl, J., Sackmann, M., and Paumgartner, G. 1996. Gallbladder emptying and gallstone formation: a prospective study on gallstone recurrence. *Gastroenterology* 111:765-771.

[56] Portincasa, P., van Erpecum, K.J., van De Meeberg, P.C., Dallinga-Thie, G.M., de Bruin, T.W., and van Berge-Henegouwen, G.P. 1996. Apolipoprotein E4 genotype and gallbladder motility influence speed of gallstone clearance and risk of recurrence after extracorporeal shock-wave lithotripsy. *Hepatology* 24:580-587.

[57] Moschetta, A., Stolk, M.F., Rehfeld, J.F., Portincasa, P., Slee, P.H., Koppeschaar, H.P., Van Erpecum, K.J., and Vanberge-Henegouwen, G.P. 2001. Severe impairment of postprandial cholecystokinin release and gall-bladder emptying and high risk of gallstone formation in acromegalic patients during Sandostatin LAR. *Aliment Pharmacol Ther* 15:181-185.

[58] Wang, D.Q., Schmitz, F., Kopin, A.S., and Carey, M.C. 2004. Targeted disruption of the murine cholecystokinin-1 receptor promotes intestinal cholesterol absorption and susceptibility to cholesterol cholelithiasis. *J Clin Invest* 114:521-528.

[59] Sitzmann, J.V., Pitt, H.A., Steinborn, P.A., Pasha, Z.R., and Sanders, R.C. 1990. Cholecystokinin prevents parenteral nutrition induced biliary sludge in humans. *Surg Gynecol Obstet* 170:25-31.

[60] Gebhard, R.L., Prigge, W.F., Ansel, H.J., Schlasner, L., Ketover, S.R., Sande, D., Holtmeier, K., and Peterson, F.J. 1996. The role of gallbladder emptying in gallstone formation during diet-induced rapid weight loss. *Hepatology* 24:544-548.

[61] Shoda, J., He, B.F., Tanaka, N., Matsuzaki, Y., Osuga, T., Yamamori, S., Miyazaki, H., and Sjovall, J. 1995. Increase of deoxycholate in supersaturated bile of patients with cholesterol gallstone disease and its correlation with de novo syntheses of cholesterol and bile acids in liver, gallbladder emptying, and small intestinal transit. *Hepatology* 21:1291-1302.

[62] Heaton, K.W., Emmett, P.M., Symes, C.L., and Braddon, F.E. 1993. An explanation for gallstones in normal-weight women: slow intestinal transit. *Lancet* 341:8-10.

[63] Van Erpecum, K.J., and Van Berge-Henegouwen, G.P. 1999. Gallstones: an intestinal disease? *Gut* 44:435-438.

[64] Thomas, L.A., Veysey, M.J., Bathgate, T., King, A., French, G., Smeeton, N.C., Murphy, G.M., and Dowling, R.H. 2000. Mechanism for the transit-induced increase in colonic deoxycholic acid formation in cholesterol cholelithiasis. *Gastroenterology* 119:806-815.

[65] Thomas, L.A., Veysey, M.J., Murphy, G.M., Russell-Jones, D., French, G.L., Wass, J.A., and Dowling, R.H. 2005. Octreotide induced prolongation of colonic transit increases faecal anaerobic bacteria, bile acid metabolising enzymes, and serum deoxycholic acid in patients with acromegaly. *Gut* 54:630-635.

[66] Berr, F., Kullak-Ublick, G.A., Paumgartner, G., Munzing, W., and Hylemon, P.B. 1996. 7 alpha-dehydroxylating bacteria enhance deoxycholic acid input and cholesterol saturation of bile in patients with gallstones. *Gastroenterology* 111:1611-1620.

[67] van Erpecum, K.J., Wang, D.Q., Lammert, F., Paigen, B., Groen, A.K., and Carey, M.C. 2001. Phenotypic characterization of Lith genes that determine susceptibility to

cholesterol cholelithiasis in inbred mice: soluble pronucleating proteins in gallbladder and hepatic biles. *J Hepatol* 35:444-451.

[68] DiMagno, E.P., Hendricks, J.C., Go, V.L., and Dozois, R.R. 1979. Relationships among canine fasting pancreatic and biliary secretions, pancreatic duct pressure, and duodenal phase III motor activity--Boldyreff revisited. *Dig Dis Sci* 24:689-693.

[69] Stolk, M.F., van Erpecum, K.J., Smout, A.J., Akkermans, L.M., Jansen, J.B., Lamers, C.B., Peeters, T.L., and vanBerge-Henegouwen, G.P. 1993. Motor cycles with phase III in antrum are associated with high motilin levels and prolonged gallbladder emptying. *Am J Physiol* 264:G596-600.

[70] Stolk, M.F., Van Erpecum, K.J., Peeters, T.L., Samsom, M., Smout, A.J., Akkermans, L.M., and Vanberge-Henegouwen, G.P. 2001. Interdigestive gallbladder emptying, antroduodenal motility, and motilin release patterns are altered in cholesterol gallstone patients. *Dig Dis Sci* 46:1328-1334.

[71] Attili, A.F., Scafato, E., Marchioli, R., Marfisi, R.M., and Festi, D. 1998. Diet and gallstones in Italy: the cross-sectional MICOL results. *Hepatology* 27:1492-1498.

[72] Wang, D.Q., Zhang, L., and Wang, H.H. 2005. High cholesterol absorption efficiency and rapid biliary secretion of chylomicron remnant cholesterol enhance cholelithogenesis in gallstone-susceptible mice. *Biochim Biophys Acta* 1733:90-99.

[73] DenBesten, L., Connor, W.E., and Bell, S. 1973. The effect of dietary cholesterol on the composition of human bile. *Surgery* 73:266-273.

[74] Lee, D.W., Gilmore, C.J., Bonorris, G., Cohen, H., Marks, J.W., Cho-Sue, M., Meiselman, M.S., and Schoenfield, L.J. 1985. Effect of dietary cholesterol on biliary lipids in patients with gallstones and normal subjects. *Am J Clin Nutr* 42:414-420.

[75] Nervi, F., Covarrubias, C., Bravo, P., Velasco, N., Ulloa, N., Cruz, F., Fava, M., Severin, C., Del Pozo, R., Antezana, C., et al. 1989. Influence of legume intake on biliary lipids and cholesterol saturation in young Chilean men. Identification of a dietary risk factor for cholesterol gallstone formation in a highly prevalent area. *Gastroenterology* 96:825-830.

[76] Andersen, E., and Hellstrom, K. 1979. The effect of cholesterol feeding on bile acid kinetics and biliary lipids in normolipidemic and hypertriglyceridemic subjects. *J Lipid Res* 20:1020-1027.

[77] 1988. The epidemiology of gallstone disease in Rome, Italy. Part II. Factors associated with the disease. The Rome Group for Epidemiology and Prevention of Cholelithiasis (GREPCO). *Hepatology* 8:907-913.

[78] Bennion, L.J., and Grundy, S.M. 1978. Risk factors for the development of cholelithiasis in man (second of two parts). *N Engl J Med* 299:1221-1227.

[79] Liddle, R.A., Goldstein, R.B., and Saxton, J. 1989. Gallstone formation during weight-reduction dieting. *Arch Intern Med* 149:1750-1753.

[80] Attili, A.F., Capocaccia, R., Carulli, N., Festi, D., Roda, E., Barbara, L., Capocaccia, L., Menotti, A., Okolicsanyi, L., Ricci, G., et al. 1997. Factors associated with gallstone disease in the MICOL experience. Multicenter Italian Study on Epidemiology of Cholelithiasis. *Hepatology* 26:809-818.

[81] Shaffer, E.A. 2005. Epidemiology and risk factors for gallstone disease: has the paradigm changed in the 21st century? *Curr Gastroenterol Rep* 7:132-140.

[82] Cuevas, A., Miquel, J.F., Reyes, M.S., Zanlungo, S., and Nervi, F. 2004. Diet as a risk factor for cholesterol gallstone disease. *J Am Coll Nutr* 23:187-196.

[83] Eckel, R.H., Grundy, S.M., and Zimmet, P.Z. 2005. The metabolic syndrome. *Lancet* 365:1415-1428.

[84] Grundy, S.M. 2004. Cholesterol gallstones: a fellow traveler with metabolic syndrome? *Am J Clin Nutr* 80:1-2.

[85] Honda, A., Yoshida, T., Tanaka, N., Matsuzaki, Y., He, B., Osuga, T., Kobayashi, N., and Ozawa, K. 1993. Hepatic cholesterol and bile acid synthesis in Japanese patients with cholesterol gallstones. *Gastroenterol Jpn* 28:406-414.

[86] Tsunoda, K., Shirai, Y., and Hatakeyama, K. 2004. Prevalence of cholesterol gallstones positively correlates with per capita daily calorie intake. *Hepatogastroenterology* 51:1271-1274.

[87] Johnston, D.E., and Kaplan, M.M. 1993. Pathogenesis and treatment of gallstones. *N Engl J Med* 328:412-421.

[88] Caroli-Bosc, F.X., Deveau, C., Peten, E.P., Delabre, B., Zanaldi, H., Hebuterne, X., Hastier, P., Viudes, F., Belanger, F., Caroli-Bosc, C., et al. 1998. Cholelithiasis and dietary risk factors: an epidemiologic investigation in Vidauban, Southeast France. General Practitioner's Group of Vidauban. *Dig Dis Sci* 43:2131-2137.

[89] Maclure, K.M., Hayes, K.C., Colditz, G.A., Stampfer, M.J., Speizer, F.E., and Willett, W.C. 1989. Weight, diet, and the risk of symptomatic gallstones in middle-aged women. *N Engl J Med* 321:563-569.

[90] Tsai, C.J., Leitzmann, M.F., Willett, W.C., and Giovannucci, E.L. 2004. The effect of long-term intake of cis unsaturated fats on the risk for gallstone disease in men: a prospective cohort study. *Ann Intern Med* 141:514-522.

[91] Rewbridge, A. 1937. The disappearance of gallstone shadows following the prolonged admnistration of bile acids. *Surgery* 1:6.

[92] Shaffer, E.A. 2006. Gallstone disease: Epidemiology of gallbladder stone disease. *Best Pract Res Clin Gastroenterol* 20:981-996.

[93] Palasciano, G., Portincasa, P., Vinciguerra, V., Velardi, A., Tardi, S., Baldassarre, G., and Albano, O. 1989. Gallstone prevalence and gallbladder volume in children and adolescents: an epidemiological ultrasonographic survey and relationship to body mass index. *Am J Gastroenterol* 84:1378-1382.

[94] Kaechele, V., Wabitsch, M., Thiere, D., Kessler, A.L., Haenle, M.M., Mayer, H., and Kratzer, W. 2006. Prevalence of gallbladder stone disease in obese children and adolescents: influence of the degree of obesity, sex, and pubertal development. *J Pediatr Gastroenterol Nutr* 42:66-70.

[95] Volzke, H., Baumeister, S.E., Alte, D., Hoffmann, W., Schwahn, C., Simon, P., John, U., and Lerch, M.M. 2005. Independent risk factors for gallstone formation in a region with high cholelithiasis prevalence. *Digestion* 71:97-105.

[96] Cirillo, D.J., Wallace, R.B., Rodabough, R.J., Greenland, P., LaCroix, A.Z., Limacher, M.C., and Larson, J.C. 2005. Effect of estrogen therapy on gallbladder disease. *JAMA* 293:330-339.

[97] Maringhini, A., Ciambra, M., Baccelliere, P., Raimondo, M., Orlando, A., Tine, F., Grasso, R., Randazzo, M.A., Barresi, L., Gullo, D., et al. 1993. Biliary sludge and gallstones in pregnancy: incidence, risk factors, and natural history. *Ann Intern Med* 119:116-120.

[98] Ogden, C.L., Yanovski, S.Z., Carroll, M.D., and Flegal, K.M. 2007. The epidemiology of obesity. *Gastroenterology* 132:2087-2102.

[99] Everhart, J.E., Khare, M., Hill, M., and Maurer, K.R. 1999. Prevalence and ethnic differences in gallbladder disease in the United States. *Gastroenterology* 117:632-639.

[100] Nakeeb, A., Comuzzie, A.G., Martin, L., Sonnenberg, G.E., Swartz-Basile, D., Kissebah, A.H., and Pitt, H.A. 2002. Gallstones: genetics versus environment. *Ann Surg* 235:842-849.

[101] Heaton, K.W., Braddon, F.E., Mountford, R.A., Hughes, A.O., and Emmett, P.M. 1991. Symptomatic and silent gall stones in the community. *Gut* 32:316-320.

[102] Diehl, A.K. 1991. Epidemiology and natural history of gallstone disease. *Gastroenterol Clin North Am* 20:1-19.

[103] Heaton, K., Braddon, F., and Emmett PM, e.a. 1991. Why do men get gallstones? Roles of abdominal fat and hyperinsulinemia. *Eur J Gastroenterol Hepatol* 3:7.

[104] Friedman, G.D., Kannel, W.B., and Dawber, T.R. 1966. The epidemiology of gallbladder disease: observations in the Framingham Study. *J Chronic Dis* 19:273-292.

[105] Sama, C., Labate, A.M., Taroni, F., and Barbara, L. 1990. Epidemiology and natural history of gallstone disease. *Semin Liver Dis* 10:149-158.

[106] Hanis, C.L., Ferrell, R.E., Tulloch, B.R., and Schull, W.J. 1985. Gallbladder disease epidemiology in Mexican Americans in Starr County, Texas. *Am J Epidemiol* 122:820-829.

[107] Shaffer, E.A., and Small, D.M. 1977. Biliary lipid secretion in cholesterol gallstone disease. The effect of cholecystectomy and obesity. *J Clin Invest* 59:828-840.

[108] Amaral, J.F., and Thompson, W.R. 1985. Gallbladder disease in the morbidly obese. *Am J Surg* 149:551-557.

[109] Carey, M.C., and Small, D.M. 1978. The physical chemistry of cholesterol solubility in bile. Relationship to gallstone formation and dissolution in man. *J Clin Invest* 61:998-1026.

[110] Shiffman, M.L., Sugerman, H.J., Kellum, J.M., Brewer, W.H., and Moore, E.W. 1991. Gallstone formation after rapid weight loss: a prospective study in patients undergoing gastric bypass surgery for treatment of morbid obesity. *Am J Gastroenterol* 86:1000-1005.

[111] Shiffman, M.L., Sugerman, H.J., Kellum, J.M., and Moore, E.W. 1992. Changes in gallbladder bile composition following gallstone formation and weight reduction. *Gastroenterology* 103:214-221.

[112] Yu, P., Chen, Q., Harnett, K.M., Amaral, J., Biancani, P., and Behar, J. 1995. Direct G protein activation reverses impaired CCK signaling in human gallbladders with cholesterol stones. *Am J Physiol* 269:G659-665.

[113] Behar, J., Lee, K.Y., Thompson, W.R., and Biancani, P. 1989. Gallbladder contraction in patients with pigment and cholesterol stones. *Gastroenterology* 97:1479-1484.

[114] Vezina, W.C., Paradis, R.L., Grace, D.M., Zimmer, R.A., Lamont, D.D., Rycroft, K.M., King, M.E., Hutton, L.C., and Chey, W.Y. 1990. Increased volume and decreased emptying of the gallbladder in large (morbidly obese, tall normal, and muscular normal) people. *Gastroenterology* 98:1000-1007.

[115] Ruhl, C.E., and Everhart, J.E. 2000. Association of diabetes, serum insulin, and C-peptide with gallbladder disease. *Hepatology* 31:299-303.

[116] Nervi, F., Miquel, J.F., Alvarez, M., Ferreccio, C., Garcia-Zattera, M.J., Gonzalez, R., Perez-Ayuso, R.M., Rigotti, A., and Villarroel, L. 2006. Gallbladder disease is

associated with insulin resistance in a high risk Hispanic population. *J Hepatol* 45:299-305.

[117] Li, V.K., Pulido, N., Fajnwaks, P., Szomstein, S., Rosenthal, R., and Martinez-Duartez, P. 2009. Predictors of gallstone formation after bariatric surgery: a multivariate analysis of risk factors comparing gastric bypass, gastric banding, and sleeve gastrectomy. *Surg Endosc* 23:1640-1644.

[118] Everhart, J.E. 1993. Contributions of obesity and weight loss to gallstone disease. *Ann Intern Med* 119:1029-1035.

[119] Broomfield, P.H., Chopra, R., Sheinbaum, R.C., Bonorris, G.G., Silverman, A., Schoenfield, L.J., and Marks, J.W. 1988. Effects of ursodeoxycholic acid and aspirin on the formation of lithogenic bile and gallstones during loss of weight. *N Engl J Med* 319:1567-1572.

[120] Weinsier, R.L., Wilson, L.J., and Lee, J. 1995. Medically safe rate of weight loss for the treatment of obesity: a guideline based on risk of gallstone formation. *Am J Med* 98:115-117.

[121] Al-Jiffry, B.O., Shaffer, E.A., Saccone, G.T., Downey, P., Kow, L., and Toouli, J. 2003. Changes in gallbladder motility and gallstone formation following laparoscopic gastric banding for morbid obestity. *Can J Gastroenterol* 17:169-174.

[122] Mendez-Sanchez, N., Zamora-Valdes, D., Chavez-Tapia, N.C., and Uribe, M. 2007. Role of diet in cholesterol gallstone formation. *Clin Chim Acta* 376:1-8.

[123] Rudkowska, I., and Jones, P.J. 2008. Polymorphisms in ABCG5/G8 transporters linked to hypercholesterolemia and gallstone disease. *Nutr Rev* 66:343-348.

[124] Angelico, M., and Della Guardia, P. 2000. Review article: hepatobiliary complications associated with total parenteral nutrition. *Aliment Pharmacol Ther* 14 Suppl 2:54-57.

[125] Shaffer, E.A. 2001. Gallbladder sludge: what is its clinical significance? *Curr Gastroenterol Rep* 3:166-173.

[126] Lambou-Gianoukos, S., and Heller, S.J. 2008. Lithogenesis and bile metabolism. *Surg Clin North Am* 88:1175-1194, vii.

[127] Sun, H., Tang, H., Jiang, S., Zeng, L., Chen, E.Q., Zhou, T.Y., and Wang, Y.J. 2009. Gender and metabolic differences of gallstone diseases. *World J Gastroenterol* 15:1886-1891.

[128] Leitzmann, M.F., Rimm, E.B., Willett, W.C., Spiegelman, D., Grodstein, F., Stampfer, M.J., Colditz, G.A., and Giovannucci, E. 1999. Recreational physical activity and the risk of cholecystectomy in women. *N Engl J Med* 341:777-784.

[129] Lammert, F., and Miquel, J.F. 2008. Gallstone disease: from genes to evidence-based therapy. *J Hepatol* 48 Suppl 1:S124-135.

[130] Sarin, S.K., Negi, V.S., Dewan, R., Sasan, S., and Saraya, A. 1995. High familial prevalence of gallstones in the first-degree relatives of gallstone patients. *Hepatology* 22:138-141.

[131] Katsika, D., Grjibovski, A., Einarsson, C., Lammert, F., Lichtenstein, P., and Marschall, H.U. 2005. Genetic and environmental influences on symptomatic gallstone disease: a Swedish study of 43,141 twin pairs. *Hepatology* 41:1138-1143.

[132] Bertomeu, A., Ros, E., Zambon, D., Vela, M., Perez-Ayuso, R.M., Targarona, E., Trias, M., Sanllehy, C., Casals, E., and Ribo, J.M. 1996. Apolipoprotein E polymorphism and gallstones. *Gastroenterology* 111:1603-1610.

[133] Mella, J.G., Schirin-Sokhan, R., Rigotti, A., Pimentel, F., Villarroel, L., Wasmuth, H.E., Sauerbruch, T., Nervi, F., Lammert, F., and Miquel, J.F. 2007. Genetic evidence that apolipoprotein E4 is not a relevant susceptibility factor for cholelithiasis in two high-risk populations. *J Lipid Res* 48:1378-1385.

[134] Grunhage, F., Acalovschi, M., Tirziu, S., Walier, M., Wienker, T.F., Ciocan, A., Mosteanu, O., Sauerbruch, T., and Lammert, F. 2007. Increased gallstone risk in humans conferred by common variant of hepatic ATP-binding cassette transporter for cholesterol. *Hepatology* 46:793-801.

[135] Rosmorduc, O., Hermelin, B., Boelle, P.Y., Parc, R., Taboury, J., and Poupon, R. 2003. ABCB4 gene mutation-associated cholelithiasis in adults. *Gastroenterology* 125:452-459.

[136] Nakken, K.E., Labori, K.J., Rodningen, O.K., Nakken, S., Berge, K.E., Eiklid, K., and Raeder, M.G. 2009. ABCB4 sequence variations in young adults with cholesterol gallstone disease. *Liver Int* 29:743-747.

[137] Buch, S., Schafmayer, C., Volzke, H., Becker, C., Franke, A., von Eller-Eberstein, H., Kluck, C., Bassmann, I., Brosch, M., Lammert, F., et al. 2007. A genome-wide association scan identifies the hepatic cholesterol transporter ABCG8 as a susceptibility factor for human gallstone disease. *Nat Genet* 39:995-999.

[138] Puppala, S., Dodd, G.D., Fowler, S., Arya, R., Schneider, J., Farook, V.S., Granato, R., Dyer, T.D., Almasy, L., Jenkinson, C.P., et al. 2006. A genomewide search finds major susceptibility loci for gallbladder disease on chromosome 1 in Mexican Americans. *Am J Hum Genet* 78:377-392.

[139] Jackson, C.E., and Gay, B.C. 1959. Inheritance of gall-bladder disease. *Surgery* 46:853-857.

[140] Jorgensen, T. 1988. Gallstones in a Danish population: familial occurrence and social factors. *J Biosoc Sci* 20:111-120.

[141] Barbara, L., Sama, C., Morselli Labate, A.M., Taroni, F., Rusticali, A.G., Festi, D., Sapio, C., Roda, E., Banterle, C., Puci, A., et al. 1987. A population study on the prevalence of gallstone disease: the Sirmione Study. *Hepatology* 7:913-917.

[142] Progetto, S., Barbara, L., and Festi, D., et al. 1984. The Sirmone Study: Familial frequency of gallstone disease. *Hepatology* 4.

[143] Nurnberg, D., Berndt, H., and Pannwitz, H. 1989. [Familial incidence of gallstones]. *Dtsch Med Wochenschr* 114:1059-1063.

[144] Vanderlinden, W., and Lindeloef, G. 1965. The Familial Occurrence of Gallstone Disease. *Acta Genet Stat Med* 15:159-164.

[145] van der Linden, W., and Westlin, N. 1966. The familial occurrence of gallstone disease. II. Occurrence in husbands and wives. *Acta Genet Stat Med* 16:377-382.

[146] van der Linden, W., and Simonson, N. 1973. Familial occurrence of gallstone disease. Incidence in parents of young patients. *Hum Hered* 23:123-127.

[147] Gilat, T., Feldman, C., Halpern, Z., Dan, M., and Bar-Meir, S. 1983. An increased familial frequency of gallstones. *Gastroenterology* 84:242-246.

[148] Antero Kesaniemi, Y., Koskenvuo, M., Vuoristo, M., and Miettinen, T.A. 1989. Biliary lipid composition in monozygotic and dizygotic pairs of twins. *Gut* 30:1750-1756.

[149] Duggirala, R., Mitchell, B.D., Blangero, J., and Stern, M.P. 1999. Genetic determinants of variation in gallbladder disease in the Mexican-American population. *Genet Epidemiol* 16:191-204.

[150] Acalovschi, M., Badea, R., Dumitrascu, D., and Varga, C. 1988. Prevalence of gallstones in liver cirrhosis: a sonographic survey. *Am J Gastroenterol* 83:954-956.

[151] Conte, D., Barisani, D., Mandelli, C., Bodini, P., Borzio, M., Pistoso, S., Segala, M., Aimo, G.P., Fraquelli, M., and Bianchi, P.A. 1991. Cholelithiasis in cirrhosis: analysis of 500 cases. *Am J Gastroenterol* 86:1629-1632.

[152] Conte, D., Fraquelli, M., Fornari, F., Lodi, L., Bodini, P., and Buscarini, L. 1999. Close relation between cirrhosis and gallstones: cross-sectional and longitudinal survey. *Arch Intern Med* 159:49-52.

[153] Alvaro, D., Angelico, M., Gandin, C., Ginanni Corradini, S., and Capocaccia, L. 1990. Physico-chemical factors predisposing to pigment gallstone formation in liver cirrhosis. *J Hepatol* 10:228-234.

[154] Acalovschi, M., Blendea, D., Feier, C., Letia, A.I., Ratiu, N., Dumitrascu, D.L., and Veres, A. 2003. Risk factors for symptomatic gallstones in patients with liver cirrhosis: a case-control study. *Am J Gastroenterol* 98:1856-1860.

[155] Acalovschi, M., Buzas, C., Radu, C., and Grigorescu, M. 2009. Hepatitis C virus infection is a risk factor for gallstone disease: a prospective hospital-based study of patients with chronic viral C hepatitis. *J Viral Hepat* 16:860-866.

[156] Loria, P., Lonardo, A., Lombardini, S., Carulli, L., Verrone, A., Ganazzi, D., Rudilosso, A., D'Amico, R., Bertolotti, M., and Carulli, N. 2005. Gallstone disease in non-alcoholic fatty liver: prevalence and associated factors. *J Gastroenterol Hepatol* 20:1176-1184.

[157] Whorwell, P.J., Hawkins, R., Dewbury, K., and Wright, R. 1984. Ultrasound survey of gallstones and other hepatobiliary disorders in patients with Crohn's disease. *Dig Dis Sci* 29:930-933.

[158] Vitek, L., and Carey, M.C. 2003. Enterohepatic cycling of bilirubin as a cause of 'black' pigment gallstones in adult life. *Eur J Clin Invest* 33:799-810.

[159] Kennedy, T.M., and Jones, R.H. 2000. Epidemiology of cholecystectomy and irritable bowel syndrome in a UK population. *Br J Surg* 87:1658-1663.

[160] Trendle, M.C., Moertel, C.G., and Kvols, L.K. 1997. Incidence and morbidity of cholelithiasis in patients receiving chronic octreotide for metastatic carcinoid and malignant islet cell tumors. *Cancer* 79:830-834.

[161] Bickford, C.L., and Spencer, A.P. 2005. Biliary sludge and hyperbilirubinemia associated with ceftriaxone in an adult: case report and review of the literature. *Pharmacotherapy* 25:1389-1395.

[162] Tsai, C.J., Leitzmann, M.F., Willett, W.C., and Giovannucci, E.L. 2009. Statin use and the risk of cholecystectomy in women. *Gastroenterology* 136:1593-1600.

[163] Reshetnyak, V.I. 2012. Concept of the pathogenesis and treatment of cholelithiasis. *World J Hepatol* 4:18-34.

[164] Marschall, H.U., and Einarsson, C. 2007. Gallstone disease. *J Intern Med* 261:529-542.

[165] Carey, M.C. 1993. Pathogenesis of gallstones. *Am J Surg* 165:410-419.

[166] He, J., Nishida, S., Xu, M., Makishima, M., and Xie, W. 2011. PXR prevents cholesterol gallstone disease by regulating biosynthesis and transport of bile salts. *Gastroenterology* 140:2095-2106.

[167] Dikkers, A., and Tietge, U.J. 2010. Biliary cholesterol secretion: more than a simple ABC. *World J Gastroenterol* 16:5936-5945.

[168] Claudel, T., Zollner, G., Wagner, M., and Trauner, M. 2011. Role of nuclear receptors for bile acid metabolism, bile secretion, cholestasis, and gallstone disease. *Biochim Biophys Acta* 1812:867-878.
[169] Small, D. 1981. *The staging of cholesterol gallstones with respect to nucleation and growth.* England: MTP Press Limited. 10 pp.
[170] Carey, M., and Cohen, D. 1987. *Biliary transport of cholesterol in ves¬icles, micelles and liquid crystals.* England: MTP Press Limited. 14 pp.
[171] Cohen, D.E., Kaler, E.W., and Carey, M.C. 1993. Cholesterol carriers in human bile: are "lamellae" involved? *Hepatology* 18:1522-1531.
[172] Loginov, A.S., Chebanov, S.M., Marakhovskii, I., and Goncharik, II. 1989. [Microstructure of vesicular agglomerates of the lithogenic bile]. *Biull Eksp Biol Med* 108:251-254.
[173] Been, J.M., Bills, P.M., and Lewis, D. 1979. Microstructure of gallstones. *Gastroenterology* 76:548-555.
[174] Chijiiwa, K., Hirota, I., and Noshiro, H. 1993. High vesicular cholesterol and protein in bile are associated with formation of cholesterol but not pigment gallstones. *Dig Dis Sci* 38:161-166.
[175] Holan, K.R., Holzbach, R.T., Hermann, R.E., Cooperman, A.M., and Claffey, W.J. 1979. Nucleation time: a key factor in the pathogenesis of cholesterol gallstone disease. *Gastroenterology* 77:611-617.
[176] Konikoff, F.M., Cohen, D.E., and Carey, M.C. 1994. Phospholipid molecular species influence crystal habits and transition sequences of metastable intermediates during cholesterol crystallization from bile salt-rich model bile. *J Lipid Res* 35:60-70.
[177] Loginov, A.S., Chebanov, S.M., Saparin, G.V., and Obyden, S.K. 1998. The morphology and composition of cholesterol, protein, and bilirubin deposits in dried human bile: cathodoluminescence and backscattered electron imaging. *Scanning* 20:442-446.
[178] Jungst, C., Sreejayan, N., Eder, M.I., von Stillfried, N., Zundt, B., Spelsberg, F.W., Kullak-Ublick, G.A., Jungst, D., and von Ritter, C. 2007. Lipid peroxidation and mucin secretagogue activity in bile of gallstone patients. *Eur J Clin Invest* 37:731-736.
[179] Hofmann, A.F. 2007. Biliary secretion and excretion in health and disease: current concepts. *Ann Hepatol* 6:15-27.
[180] Uchiyama, K., Kawai, M., Tani, M., Terasawa, H., Tanimura, H., and Yamaue, H. 2007. Pathogenesis of hepatolithiasis based on the analysis of components of intrahepatic stones. *Hepatogastroenterology* 54:1798-1804.
[181] Kim, H.J., Kim, S.H., Chae, G.B., Lee, S.J., and Kang, C.D. 2008. Increased expression of mucin 5AC mRNA and decreased expression of epidermal growth-factor receptor mRNA in gallstone patients. *Tohoku J Exp Med* 214:139-144.
[182] Wu, S.D., Yu, H., and Sun, J.M. 2006. Bacteriological and electron microscopic examination of primary intrahepatic stones. *Hepatobiliary Pancreat Dis Int* 5:228-231.
[183] Manolis, E.N., Filippou, D.K., Papadopoulos, V.P., Kaklamanos, I., Katostaras, T., Christianakis, E., Bonatsos, G., and Tsakris, A. 2008. The culture site of the gallbladder affects recovery of bacteria in symptomatic cholelithiasis. *J Gastrointestin Liver Dis* 17:179-182.

[228] Krawczyk, M., Lutjohann, D., Schirin-Sokhan, R., Villarroel, L., Nervi, F., Pimentel, F., Lammert, F., and Miquel, J.F. 2012. Phytosterol and cholesterol precursor levels indicate increased cholesterol excretion and biosynthesis in gallstone disease. *Hepatology* 55:1507-1517.

[229] de Bari, O., Neuschwander-Tetri, B., Liu, M., Portincasa, P., and Wang, D. 2012. Ezetimibe: its novel effects on the prevention and the treatment of cholesterol gallstones and nonalcoholic fatty liver disease. *J Lipids* 2012:17.

[230] Wang, H.H., Portincasa, P., Afdhal, N.H., and Wang, D.Q. 2010. Lith genes and genetic analysis of cholesterol gallstone formation. *Gastroenterol Clin North Am* 39:185-207, vii-viii.

[231] Wang, H.H., Portincasa, P., Mendez-Sanchez, N., Uribe, M., and Wang, D.Q. 2008. Effect of ezetimibe on the prevention and dissolution of cholesterol gallstones. *Gastroenterology* 134:2101-2110.

[232] Davis, H.R., Jr., Zhu, L.J., Hoos, L.M., Tetzloff, G., Maguire, M., Liu, J., Yao, X., Iyer, S.P., Lam, M.H., Lund, E.G., et al. 2004. Niemann-Pick C1 Like 1 (NPC1L1) is the intestinal phytosterol and cholesterol transporter and a key modulator of whole-body cholesterol homeostasis. *J Biol Chem* 279:33586-33592.

[233] Katsika, D., Magnusson, P., Krawczyk, M., Grunhage, F., Lichtenstein, P., Einarsson, C., Lammert, F., and Marschall, H.U. 2010. Gallstone disease in Swedish twins: risk is associated with ABCG8 D19H genotype. *J Intern Med* 268:279-285.

[234] Wang, D.Q., Tazuma, S., Cohen, D.E., and Carey, M.C. 2003. Feeding natural hydrophilic bile acids inhibits intestinal cholesterol absorption: studies in the gallstone-susceptible mouse. *Am J Physiol Gastrointest Liver Physiol* 285:G494-502.

[235] Zuniga, S., Molina, H., Azocar, L., Amigo, L., Nervi, F., Pimentel, F., Jarufe, N., Arrese, M., Lammert, F., and Miquel, J.F. 2008. Ezetimibe prevents cholesterol gallstone formation in mice. *Liver Int* 28:935-947.

[236] Smit, J.W., van Erpecum, K.J., Stolk, M.F., Geerdink, R.A., Cluysenaer, O.J., Erkelens, D.W., and van Berge Henegouwen, G.P. 1992. Successful dissolution of cholesterol gallstone during treatment with pravastatin. *Gastroenterology* 103:1068-1070.

[237] Bodmer, M., Brauchli, Y.B., Krahenbuhl, S., Jick, S.S., and Meier, C.R. 2009. Statin use and risk of gallstone disease followed by cholecystectomy. *JAMA* 302:2001-2007.

[238] Turley, S.D., and Dietschy, J.M. 1981. The contribution of newly synthesized cholesterol to biliary cholesterol in the rat. *J Biol Chem* 256:2438-2446.

[239] Smit, J.W., van Erpecum, K.J., Renooij, W., Stolk, M.F., Edgar, P., Doornewaard, H., and Vanberge-Henegouwen, G.P. 1995. The effects of the 3-hydroxy, 3-methylglutaryl coenzyme A reductase inhibitor pravastatin on bile composition and nucleation of cholesterol crystals in cholesterol gallstone disease. *Hepatology* 21:1523-1529.

[240] Smit, J.W., Van Erpecum, K.J., Portincasa, P., Renooij, W., Erkelens, D.W., and Van Berge-Henegouwen, G.P. 1995. Effects of simvastatin and cholestyramine on bile lipid composition and gall bladder motility in patients with hypercholesterolaemia. *Gut* 37:654-659.

[241] Davis, K.G., Wertin, T.M., and Schriver, J.P. 2003. The use of simvastatin for the prevention of gallstones in the lithogenic prairie dog model. *Obes Surg* 13:865-868.

[242] Tazuma, S., Kajiyama, G., Mizuno, T., Yamashita, G., Miura, H., Kajihara, T., Hattori, Y., Miyake, H., Nishioka, T., Hyogo, H., et al. 1998. A combination therapy with simvastatin and ursodeoxycholic acid is more effective for cholesterol gallstone

dissolution than is ursodeoxycholic acid monotherapy. *J Clin Gastroenterol* 26:287-291.

[243] Sackmann, M., Koelbl, R., Pauletzki, J., Cremer, P., Klueppelberg, U.G., von Ritter, C., Sauter, G., Holl, J., Seidel, D., and Paumgartner, G. 1995. Simvastatin added to ursodeoxycholic acid does not enhance disappearance of gallstone fragments after shock wave therapy. *Z Gastroenterol* 33:585-589.

[244] Attili, A.F., Carulli, N., Roda, E., Barbara, B., Capocaccia, L., Menotti, A., Okoliksanyi, L., Ricci, G., Capocaccia, R., Festi, D., et al. 1995. Epidemiology of gallstone disease in Italy: prevalence data of the Multicenter Italian Study on Cholelithiasis (M.I.COL.). *Am J Epidemiol* 141:158-165.

[245] Simonen, P., Kotronen, A., Hallikainen, M., Sevastianova, K., Makkonen, J., Hakkarainen, A., Lundbom, N., Miettinen, T.A., Gylling, H., and Yki-Jarvinen, H. 2011. Cholesterol synthesis is increased and absorption decreased in non-alcoholic fatty liver disease independent of obesity. *J Hepatol* 54:153-159.

[246] Acton, S., Rigotti, A., Landschulz, K.T., Xu, S., Hobbs, H.H., and Krieger, M. 1996. Identification of scavenger receptor SR-BI as a high density lipoprotein receptor. *Science* 271:518-520.

[247] Lammert, F., and Wang, D.Q. 2005. New insights into the genetic regulation of intestinal cholesterol absorption. *Gastroenterology* 129:718-734.

[248] Altmann, S.W., Davis, H.R., Jr., Zhu, L.J., Yao, X., Hoos, L.M., Tetzloff, G., Iyer, S.P., Maguire, M., Golovko, A., Zeng, M., et al. 2004. Niemann-Pick C1 Like 1 protein is critical for intestinal cholesterol absorption. *Science* 303:1201-1204.

[249] Berge, K.E., Tian, H., Graf, G.A., Yu, L., Grishin, N.V., Schultz, J., Kwiterovich, P., Shan, B., Barnes, R., and Hobbs, H.H. 2000. Accumulation of dietary cholesterol in sitosterolemia caused by mutations in adjacent ABC transporters. *Science* 290:1771-1775.

[250] Lee, M.H., Lu, K., Hazard, S., Yu, H., Shulenin, S., Hidaka, H., Kojima, H., Allikmets, R., Sakuma, N., Pegoraro, R., et al. 2001. Identification of a gene, ABCG5, important in the regulation of dietary cholesterol absorption. *Nat Genet* 27:79-83.

[251] Miettinen, T.A., Tilvis, R.S., and Kesaniemi, Y.A. 1990. Serum plant sterols and cholesterol precursors reflect cholesterol absorption and synthesis in volunteers of a randomly selected male population. *Am J Epidemiol* 131:20-31.

[252] Kempen, H.J., Glatz, J.F., Gevers Leuven, J.A., van der Voort, H.A., and Katan, M.B. 1988. Serum lathosterol concentration is an indicator of whole-body cholesterol synthesis in humans. *J Lipid Res* 29:1149-1155.

[253] Berge, K.E., von Bergmann, K., Lutjohann, D., Guerra, R., Grundy, S.M., Hobbs, H.H., and Cohen, J.C. 2002. Heritability of plasma noncholesterol sterols and relationship to DNA sequence polymorphism in ABCG5 and ABCG8. *J Lipid Res* 43:486-494.

[254] Krawczyk, M., Wang, D.Q., Portincasa, P., and Lammert, F. 2011. Dissecting the genetic heterogeneity of gallbladder stone formation. *Semin Liver Dis* 31:157-172.

[255] Acalovschi, M., Ciocan, A., Mostean, O., Tirziu, S., Chiorean, E., Keppeler, H., Schirin-Sokhan, R., and Lammert, F. 2006. Are plasma lipid levels related to ABCG5/ABCG8 polymorphisms? A preliminary study in siblings with gallstones. *Eur J Intern Med* 17:490-494.

[256] Gylling, H., Hallikainen, M., Pihlajamaki, J., Agren, J., Laakso, M., Rajaratnam, R.A., Rauramaa, R., and Miettinen, T.A. 2004. Polymorphisms in the ABCG5 and ABCG8

genes associate with cholesterol absorption and insulin sensitivity. *J Lipid Res* 45:1660-1665.

[257] Lutjohann, D., Bjorkhem, I., Beil, U.F., and von Bergmann, K. 1995. Sterol absorption and sterol balance in phytosterolemia evaluated by deuterium-labeled sterols: effect of sitostanol treatment. *J Lipid Res* 36:1763-1773.

[258] Fassbender, K., Lutjohann, D., Dik, M.G., Bremmer, M., Konig, J., Walter, S., Liu, Y., Letiembre, M., von Bergmann, K., and Jonker, C. 2008. Moderately elevated plant sterol levels are associated with reduced cardiovascular risk--the LASA study. *Atherosclerosis* 196:283-288.

[259] Miettinen, T.A., Vuoristo, M., Nissinen, M., Jarvinen, H.J., and Gylling, H. 2000. Serum, biliary, and fecal cholesterol and plant sterols in colectomized patients before and during consumption of stanol ester margarine. *Am J Clin Nutr* 71:1095-1102.

[260] Kuipers, F., van Ree, J.M., Hofker, M.H., Wolters, H., In't Veld, G., Havinga, R., Vonk, R.J., Princen, H.M., and Havekes, L.M. 1996. Altered lipid metabolism in apolipoprotein E-deficient mice does not affect cholesterol balance across the liver. *Hepatology* 24:241-247.

[261] Gurantz, D., Laker, M.F., and Hofmann, A.F. 1981. Enzymatic measurement of choline-containing phospholipids in bile. *J Lipid Res* 22:373-376.

[262] Miquel, J.F., Covarrubias, C., Villaroel, L., Mingrone, G., Greco, A.V., Puglielli, L., Carvallo, P., Marshall, G., Del Pino, G., and Nervi, F. 1998. Genetic epidemiology of cholesterol cholelithiasis among Chilean Hispanics, Amerindians, and Maoris. *Gastroenterology* 115:937-946.

[263] Lammert, F., and Miquel, J. 2008. Gallstone disease: from genes to evidence-based therapy. *J Hepatol* 48:12.

[264] Empen, K., Lange, K., Stange, E.F., and Scheibner, J. 1997. Newly synthesized cholesterol in human bile and plasma: quantitation by mass isotopomer distribution analysis. *Am J Physiol* 272:G367-373.

[265] Yu, L., Li-Hawkins, J., Hammer, R.E., Berge, K.E., Horton, J.D., Cohen, J.C., and Hobbs, H.H. 2002. Overexpression of ABCG5 and ABCG8 promotes biliary cholesterol secretion and reduces fractional absorption of dietary cholesterol. *J Clin Invest* 110:671-680.

[266] Buch, S., Schafmayer, C., Volzke, H., Seeger, M., Miquel, J.F., Sookoian, S.C., Egberts, J.H., Arlt, A., Pirola, C.J., Lerch, M.M., et al. 2010. Loci from a genome-wide analysis of bilirubin levels are associated with gallstone risk and composition. *Gastroenterology* 139:1942-1951 e1942.

[267] Kosters, A., Frijters, R.J., Schaap, F.G., Vink, E., Plosch, T., Ottenhoff, R., Jirsa, M., De Cuyper, I.M., Kuipers, F., and Groen, A.K. 2003. Relation between hepatic expression of ATP-binding cassette transporters G5 and G8 and biliary cholesterol secretion in mice. *J Hepatol* 38:710-716.

[268] Kamisako, T., and Ogawa, H. 2003. Regulation of biliary cholesterol secretion is associated with abcg5 and abcg8 expressions in the rats: effects of diosgenin and ethinyl estradiol. *Hepatol Res* 26:348-352.

[269] Yu, L., von Bergmann, K., Lutjohann, D., Hobbs, H.H., and Cohen, J.C. 2004. Selective sterol accumulation in ABCG5/ABCG8-deficient mice. *J Lipid Res* 45:301-307.

[270] Cohen, J.C., Pertsemlidis, A., Fahmi, S., Esmail, S., Vega, G.L., Grundy, S.M., and Hobbs, H.H. 2006. Multiple rare variants in NPC1L1 associated with reduced sterol absorption and plasma low-density lipoprotein levels. *Proc Natl Acad Sci USA* 103:1810-1815.

[271] Ramirez, R., Cohen, J.C., Hobbs, H.H., and Browning, J.D. 2011. Hepatic triglyceride content in individuals with reduced intestinal cholesterol absorption due to variants in Nieman Pick C1-like 1. *Hepatology* 54:736-737.

[272] Cuevas, A., Molina, A., Rigotti, A., Miquel, J.F., Marshall, G., Reyes, S., and Nervi, F. 2008. Trends in obesity and diabetes prevalence in a Chilean urban population: 1993-2001. *Metab Syndr Relat Disord* 6:219-222.

[273] Lindenthal, B., Sudhop, T., Schiedermaier, P., Agnan, M., Sauerbruch, T., and von Bergmann, K. 2002. Serum plant sterols and biliary cholesterol secretion in humans: studies with ursodeoxycholic acid. *J Lipid Res* 43:1072-1077.

[274] Miettinen, T.E., Kesaniemi, Y.A., Gylling, H., Jarvinen, H., Silvennoinen, E., and Miettinen, T.A. 1996. Noncholesterol sterols in bile and stones of patients with cholesterol and pigment stones. *Hepatology* 23:274-280.

[275] Koivusalo, A.I., Pakarinen, M.P., Sittiwet, C., Gylling, H., Miettinen, T.A., Miettinen, T.E., and Nissinen, M.J. 2010. Cholesterol, non-cholesterol sterols and bile acids in paediatric gallstones. *Dig Liver Dis* 42:61-66.

[276] Krawczyk, M., Bonfrate, L., and Portincasa, P. 2010. Nonalcoholic fatty liver disease. *Best Pract Res Clin Gastroenterol* 24:695-708.

Chapter III

Etiology and Pathogenesis of Pigment Gallstones

I. New Pathophysiological Concepts Underlying Pathogenesis of Pigment Gallstones [1]

Pigment gallstones, which are much less frequent than cholesterol stones, are classified descriptively as "black" or "brown". They are composed mostly of calcium hydrogen bilirubinate, Ca (HUCB) 2, which is polymerized and oxidized in "black" stones but remains unpolymerized in "brown" stones. Black stones form in sterile gallbladder bile but brown stones form secondary to stasis and anaerobic bacterial infection in any part of the biliary tree, including the gallbladder. Other calcium salts coprecipitate in both stone types; crystalline calcium phosphate and/or carbonate in the case of "black" stones and amorphous calcium salts of long chain saturated fatty acids ("soaps") in the case of "brown" stones. Cholesterol is present in variable proportions in "brown" more than "black" stones and in the latter, the bile sterol may be totally absent. The "scaffolding" of both stone types is a mixed mucin glycoprotein matrix secreted by epithelial cells lining the biliary tree. The critical pathophysiological prerequisite for "black" stone formation is "hyperbilirubinbilia" (biliary hypersecretion of bilirubin conjugates). It is due principally to hemolysis, ineffective erythropoiesis, or pathologic enterohepatic cycling of unconjugated bilirubin. Endogenous biliary β-glucuronidase hydrolysis of bilirubin conjugates in gallbladder bile provides $HUCB^-$ molecules that precipitate as insoluble salts with ionized Ca. Putatively, reactive oxygen species secreted by an inflamed gallbladder mucosa are responsible for transforming the initial soft yellow precipitates into hard black $[Ca(HUCB)_2]n$ polymers. Despite "brown" gallstones being soft and amenable to mechanical removal, chronic anaerobic infection of the biliary tree is often markedly resistant to eradication.

Although cholesterol gallstones can contain as much as 30% calcium bilirubinate and are sometimes called "mixed" stones advocated by Schafmeyer et al., [2] pigment gallstones are distinct containing calcium bilirubinate, Ca(HUCB)2, as the principal component. They are classified descriptively as "black" stones, which are hard, and "brown" stones, which are soft suggested by Cahalane et al. [3] True prevalence as opposed to clinical, autopsy or surgical prevalence in free-living populations has not been determined. Black stones are mostly amorphous, containing primarily polymerized calcium monoacidic unconjugated bilirubin, $Ca(HUCB)_2$. They often contain crystalline salts of calcium phosphate and/or calcium carbonate in one of its polymorphic forms, calcite, aragonite or valerite and may also contain many metals found in bile by Suzuki et al. [4] They form in sterile gallbladder bile, and the principal risk factor is "hyperbilirubinbilia"1 (secretion of excess bilirubin conjugates into bile). This results particularly from hemolysis from any cause, ineffective erythropoiesis or induced enterohepatic cycling (EHC) of unconjugated bilirubin (UCB), which we focus on in this review. Other causes of "black" stones are gallbladder hypomotility, secondary to diabetes mellitus by Cahalane et al., [3] total parenteral nutrition by Cahalane et al. [3] and truncal vagotomy byTsunoda et al. [5] Neither intensive blue-light phototherapy for hyperbilirubinemia in neonates and Crigler-Najjar syndrome Type 1 patients Strauss et al., [6] nor excessive sun exposure has been proven to cause black pigment gallstone formation Pavel et al. [7] Blue light leads to biliary and urinary excretion of water-soluble configurationally as well as structural UCB photoisomers. These rapidly revert to the more stable but insoluble natural Z-Z photoisomer in bile by Lund and Agati et al. [8, 9] It is not surprising therefore that cholestasis can result from phototherapy due to massive precipitation of bile pigment in the small intrahepatic bile ducts by Wolkoff and Ostrow et al. [10, 11] The "bronze baby syndrome" is due to retention of the geometric isomer, photobilirubin II in the skin of infants with phototherapy-induced cholestasis by Onishi et al. [12] "Brown" gallstones are invariably laminated, contain unpolymerized $Ca(HUCB)_2$ co-precipitated with amorphous calcium salts of palmitate and stearate (calcium "soaps") derived from bacterial phospholipase A1 hydrolysis of biliary phosphatidylcholines by Robins et al. [13] They also contain unconjugated (free) bile acids [3] and Ca bile salts and variable amounts of cholesterol. This contrasts with "black" stones, in which the bile sterol is often absent. [3] "Brown" stones may occur anywhere in the biliary tree but rarely in the gallbladder. They are associated with anaerobic bacterial infection secondary to obstruction and/or stasis of any etiology by Kaufman et al, [14] including parasitic infestation from nematodes and flukes by Rana et al. [15] Thick section electron microscopy reveals bacterial cytoskeletons within the stones' structures by Stewart et al. [16] migratory cholesterol/ black pigment gallstone that escapes the gallbladder and becomes impacted in the bile duct is frequently the cause of stasis and secondary bacterial infection by Sauerbruch et al. [17] An often overlooked cause of biliary stasis-associated brown stones is a juxtapapillary duodenal diverticulum harboring anaerobes by Sandstad et al. [18] In developing and tropical countries, the bile-seeking worms that are initiating factors are *Ascaris lumbricoides, Clonorchis sinensis by* Jang et al. [19] and *Opisthorchis viverrini by Sripa* et al. [20] In contrast to black pigment stones that are usually radiopaque, brown pigment gallstones are radiolucent. For brown gallstones to form, the biliary tree must become infected with colonic anaerobic microbiota producing β-glucuronidase, an enzyme that hydrolyzes bisglucuronosyl bilirubin to UCB. Bacterial production of detergent-resistant phospholipase A1 produces free palmitic and stearic acids, the products of hydrolysis of the sn-1 ester linkage of biliary phosphatidylcholines by Robins et al. [13]. These precipitate with calcium counter-ions as long-chain insoluble soaps. [3] The amide linkage of conjugated bile salts is hydrolyzed by cholylglycylamidase, which is secreted by many anaerobic strains of bacteria (e.g. *Streptococcus faecalis, Clostridium spp., Bacteroides spp.*) by Akiyoshi et al., [21] forming free i.e. unconjugated bile acids. These are capable of precipitating as insoluble bile acids *per se* or less likely as calcium bile salts by Gu et al. [22] Provided marked stasis is present, "brown" pigment gallstones may develop exceptionally under apparently "sterile" conditions, such as throughout the biliary tree in patients with Caroli's syndrome or in isolated choledochal cysts by Nakanuma et al. [23] Because hyperbilirubinbilia is the critical risk factor, black stones are associated frequently with all major hemolytic anemias e.g. spherocytosis by del Giudice et al. [24] sickle cell disease by Chaar et al., [25] thalassemia by Premawardhena et al., [26] and also with subclinical hemolysis from prosthetic valve replacements Azemoto et al., [27] malaria by Chawla et al., [28] hypersplenism from hepatic cirrhosis by Diehl et al., [29] and foot trauma in long-distance runners by Weight et al. [30] Ineffective erythropoiesis typically secondary to folate and vitamin B12 deficiencies by Aydogdu et al. [31] is now rare but can complicate thalassemia as well as sickle cell disease. Other conditions associated with increased prevalence of black pigment gallstones are Gilbert's syndrome by Buch et al., [32] associated with enhanced biliary secretion of monoglucuronosyl bilirubin, and hyperparathyroidism by Broulik et al., [33] associated with higher levels of ionized calcium in bile. Acquired EHC of UCB as a cause of hyperbilirubinbilia and black pigment stone formation is a newly described pathophysiological and clinical entity by Vitek and Carey.(34) Its principal causes are ileal dysfunction, disease, resection or bypass, and various dietary influences on ileal function, such as high carbohydrate or cholesterol intake, or alcohol abuse by Vitek and Carey. [34] Although absence of biliary infection has always been the basic prerequisite for black pigment gallstone formation, recent data suggest that they might also be primed by biles infected with "nanobacteria" that produce hydroxyapatite by Wang et al. [35] as was also suggested for nephrolithiasis by Ostrow et al. [36] These claims have not been further elucidated clinically or experimentally. Figure 3.1.1 summarizes the proven concepts underlying the pathobiology of black (A) and brown (B) pigment stone formation in humans.

Physical-Chemistry of "Black" and "Brown" Pigment Gallstone Formation

UCB, the end product of heme catabolism, is an open-chain tetrapyrrole molecule whose outer monopyrroles are interconnected by rigid —CH= linkages and the dipyrrole units by a flexible central —CH2— bridge. The central pyrrole rings subtend two carboxyethyl side-chains, which in aqueous systems ionize only at alkaline pH values.[37] Because of six intramolecular hydrogen bonds by Ostrow et al., [37] UCB, which is in the H2UCB form at physiological pH values, is highly insoluble in aqueous media (< 70 nM) by Ostrow et al. [38] Nevertheless, at pH values of human hepatic (7.3—8.7) and gallbladder (6.2—7.8) biles, [3] UCB is a monoacidic species ($HUCB^-$) principally because of the presence of high concentrations of bile salts. Nevertheless, it is exquisitely sensitive to precipitation as the monoacid salt with typical biliary concentrations of ionized Ca by Ostrow et al. [3, 39] In contrast, mono- and bisglucuronosyl bilirubins, the predominant conjugated bile pigment species in human and most laboratory animal biles, bind ionized calcium as soluble salts and are not precipitated with physiological calcium concentrations. [40] Increased plasma ionized calcium concentrations, a hallmark of hyperparathyroidism, also seems to be a risk factor for black pigment gallstone disease by Broulik et al. [33] due to the rapid equilibration of ionized calcium, which has a small hydrated radius, between intravascular and biliary compartments. Several physiological and biochemical mechanisms solubilize UCB in aqueous environments: binding to albumin or HDL in plasma; binding to bile salt monomers, dimers and micelles by

Smith et al., [41] mucin glycoproteins in bile and intestinal lumen by McDonagh et al.; [42] covalent linkage of one or both —COOH groups with glucuronic acid catalyzed by hepatic bilirubin UDP-glucuronosyl transferase (UGT1A1) producing monoglucuronosyl bilirubins and bisglucuronosyl bilirubins; disruption of internal hydrogen bonding by phototherapy induced isomerization of UCB forming water-soluble structural and configurationally isomers by Goresky et al. [43] or; binding to unilamellar vesicles in cholesterol supersaturated bile by Cohalane et al. [3] Increased proportions of biliary monoglucuronosyl bilirubin to bisglucuronosyl bilirubin are the rule in biles of patients with black pigment gallstones by Goresky and Boonyapisit et al. [44, 45] Monoglucuronosyl bilirubin can more easily be deconjugated in bile by endogenous acidic β-glucuronidase that is secreted by hepatic parenchymal cells by Whiting et al., [46] or less frequently by biliary epithelial β-glucuronidase and non-enzymatic hydrolysis by Spivak et al. [47] An increase in the absolute concentration of biliary UCB has been reported in humans and animals with black pigment gallstones, as well as early calcium bilirubinate precipitates by Donovan and Malet et al. [48, 49] Calcium bilirubinate precipitates may also serve as seed nuclei during the initiation of cholesterol cholelithiasis by Malet and LaMont et al. [49, 50] In addition, human "biliary sludge" consists of calcium, monoconjugated and unconjugated bilirubins plus mucin glycoproteins, and may serve as a matrix in which pigment or cholesterol stones develop by Malet et al. [50] Because human pigment gallstones invariably contain a mucin glycoprotein matrix, or "scaffolding" by Malet et al, [51] it is likely that hypersecretion of mucin by the gallbladder, as observed in animal models of pigment gallstones by LaMont et al., [52] leads to mucin gel—Ca-HUCB− interactions. Similar association of pigment gallstones has also been reported for osteopontin, a lithogenic Ca binding glycoprotein secreted by human gallbladder mucosa by LaMont et al. [53].

Intestinal Pathobiology of Bile Salts and Bilirubin in Relation to "Black" Pigment Gallstone Formation

Important pathophysiological perturbations in the gut-liver axis controlling the homeostasis of both bilirubin and bile salts may lead to hyperbilirubinbilia, the critical risk factor in formation of "black" pigment gallstones by Vitek et al. [34] In all of these scenarios, the common denominator appears to be ileal dysfunction from any cause with spillage of malabsorbed bile salts into the cecum and large intestine. Under physiological conditions, the bile salt pool enjoys a very efficient EHC. Bile salt molecules are retrieved from the gut via the sodium-coupled apical membrane co-transporters (SLC10A2) in the distal ileum, which is responsible for greater than 96% of bile salt conservation within the enterohepatic axis. In health, an EHC of UCB does not exist or is negligible. [3] The conjugates are too bulky and polar, intestinal deconjugation of bilirubin conjugates to UCB is rapid by Cahalane et al., [3] and efficient reduction of bilirubin to urobilinoids prevents passive resorption of UCB by Vitek et al. [34] Deconjugation in the gut can occur via a β- glucuronidase of bacterial origin but also by the mammalian enzyme of sloughed enterocytes, which contain a neutral β - glucuronidase. Luminal solubilization is crucial for induced resorption of UCB. This can occur with: higher rates of bilirubin deconjugation due to prolonged intestinal transit time such as during calorie deprivation with overgrowth of β-glucuronidase producing bacteria, or a supply of β-glucuronidase from extraintestinal sources, such as breast milk, resulting in "breast milk jaundice" in premature infants; slow or absent intestinal reduction of UCB by bacteria such as present in neonates or in adults during oral antibiotic therapy; more alkaline luminal pH, higher bile salt concentrations, or agents preventing complexing of UCB with Ca^{2+} in the intestinal lumen. Malabsorbed bile salts are the most obvious cause of an induced EHC of UCB. They elevate colonic detergent levels that solubilize UCB promoting its passive resorption from the intestine. [54] Even in the absence of ileal disease, ileal resorption of conjugated bile salts via SLC10A2 is dependent on intraluminal pH. A 0.5 pH unit decrease in ileal luminal pH diminishes sodium taurocholate transport by 9% per enterohepatic cycle by LaMont et al. [55]. Finally, complexing of UCB with Ca^{2+} in the intestinal lumen blocks its resorption and a diminution in Ca^{2+} concentration may lead to higher UCB levels. Bile salts also bind intraluminal calcium forming soluble calcium complexes with similar results on elevating soluble UCB levels.(56) Another example of insoluble calcium salt formation depleting intraluminal Ca^{2+} ions occurs in the setting of dietary fat malabsorption. In this regard, intraluminal calcium precipitates as calcium long-chain fatty acid soaps in the proximal small intestine and becomes unavailable to bind cation-sensitive anions, such as UCB in the distal intestine, thereby increasing its solution levels. It has been proposed by Brink et al. (54) that hyperbilirubinbilia from an induced EHC of UCB represents a parallel pathophysiology to that of enteric hyperoxaluria in the setting of fat malabsorption by Chadwick et al. [57] Apart from its primary lithogenic effect, hyperbilirubinbilia may lead to "uncoupling" of biliary lipids from bile salts at the canalicular level with diminution in their biliary secretion rates. [58] Diminished biliary secretion of biliary phosphatidylcholine and cholesterol molecules leads in turn to a lessening of their protective role on bile salt detergency. As a result, there is a higher likelihood of bile salt-induced injury to the mucosa of the bile ducts and gallbladder, further facilitating pigment gallstone formation via production of mucosal β-glucuronidase from biliary epithelial cells, and possibly also mucin glycoproteins and reactive oxygen species (ROS) [54, 55].

The Intestinal Microflora, Dietary Factors and Pigment Gallstone Formation

Intestinal bacterial overgrowth occurs in several pathologic conditions and may result in increased bile salt and bilirubin deconjugation in the small intestine. This could contribute further to bile salt malabsorption and enhanced solubilization and EHC of UCB from the colon by Vitek et al. [34] This is exemplified by intestinal hypomotility from any cause including chronic constipation,(34) total parenteral nutrition by Vitek et al., [34] cystic fibrosis by Vitek et al., [34] and spinal cord injury by Apstein et al. [59] Further, bile salt malabsorption may also be caused by undigested starch and α-cyclodextrin, a starch degradation product in subjects ingesting high carbohydrate diets.(60) Likewise, high intake of refined sugars affect metabolism of intestinal microflora and prolongs intestinal transit time, [61] again potentially affecting an EHC of UCB. Moreover, hypertonic solutions of sucrose increase intestinal mucosa permeability by Laker et al. [62] In fact, high sucrose diets induce pigment gallstones in prairie dogs by Conter et al., [63] a species known otherwise as a facile model of cholesterol gallstone formation by Holzbach et al. [64] Contrariwise, high dietary fiber may prevent pigment gallstone formation, because of the production of abundant short chain fatty acids from bacterial fermentation by Conter et al. [63] These diminish distal intestinal pH, precipitate UCB and sequester bile acids as insoluble species in the large intestine. Such a scenario is common in subjects where an abundance of dietary fiber is a food staple, such as with vegetarians and sub-Saharian Africans known to have very low prevalences of gallstone disease. [65, 66] Resorption of UCB may be impaired additionally because of bulk-induced increases in colonic transit times by Cummings and Waters et al. [67, 68] Besides direct effects of bile salts on UCB solubilization, secondary bile salt production from bacterial overgrowth may also promote release of intracellular microbiotal β-glucuronidase by enhancing plasma membrane permeability of bacteria by Fujisawa et al. [69] Decreased concentrations of biliary β-glucuronolactone, an inhibitor of β-glucuronidase by Nagase et al., [70] was reported to be associated with black pigment gallstone disease in post- WWII Japan because of low-protein diets. A role for impaired intestinal barrier function has been proposed as playing a role in passive UCB resorption during experimental pigment lithogenesis in hamsters by Fan et al., [71] as is also evidenced by high serum endotoxin levels and indices of immune cell activation in the intestinal mucosa by Fan and Su et al. [71, 72]. In germ-free Swiss Webster, intestinal barrier dysfunction may also be a critical factor facilitating an EHC of UCB, which in the germ-free state cannot be degraded to urobilinoids by Phary et al. [73] In black pigment gallstone formation, another potential lithogenic factor is slow or absent bacterial reduction of intestinal UCB as evidenced by the dearth of intestinal microflora in neonates and in patients requiring prolonged oral antibiotic therapy. Absence of UCB reduction in the intestinal lumen is both a contributing factor to neonatal jaundice by Vitek et al. [74] but also for pigment gallstone disease as well as the hyperbilirubinemia associated with oral antibiotic therapy by Vitek et al. [75] As alluded to above, Germfree Swiss Webster mice exhibit extremely high prevalences of black pigment gallstone formation spontaneously by Phary and Leonard et al. [73, 76] apparently secondary to what appears to be at least four factors; inability to degrade UCB to urobilinoids, decreased intestinal motility, gallbladder hypomotility from a pre-diabetic state, and diminution in intestine mucosal barrier function. [73, 76] Since gallbladder inflammation is implicated in black pigment gallstone formation, it is tempting to speculate that UCB *per se* might be specifically involved in the immune response ultimately leading to pigment cholelithiasis. In fact, UCB has been shown to be involved in regulatory T-cell differentiation by Quintana et al. [77].

Putative Role of ROS in "Black" Stone Polymerization and Oxidation

It is likely that polymerization of the HUCB− tetrapyrrole, a key event in the transition of soft yellow to hard black pigment gallstones, is initiated by free radicals or singlet oxygen species and occurs in the solid or semisolid state. A hepatic source of ROS is unlikely since $Ca(HUCB)_2$ in "brown" stones remains unpolymerized. [3] ROS are more likely products of mucosal macrophages or neutrophils from an inflamed gallbladder that accompanies pigment stone disease by Phary and Leonard et al. [3, 73, 76] This is consistent with observations of bacterially-derived oxysterols in human bile as well as in black pigment gallstones by Haigh et al. [78]

In addition, oxidative stress induces formation of bilirubin-free radicals, which are prone to polymerize easily, as evidenced by ESR and NMR studies of human pigment stones by Liu et al. [79] Indeed, administration of the free radical scavenger melatonin (N-acetyl-5-methoxytryptamine) is reported to prevent pigment gallstone formation in bile duct-ligated guinea pigs by Shiesh et al. [80] In addition, this appears to be the case for methionine, which acts also as a free radical scavenger. Methionine deficiency in the diet of domestic dogs is associated with increased formation of black pigment gallstones, whereas methionine supplementation counteracts lithogenesis by Christan et al., [81] Moreover, as inferred from *ex vivo* studies by Braganza et al., [82] suppression of oxidative stress in the gallbladder may well play a role in ameliorating cholesterol gallstone formation also.

Conclusion

"Black" pigment gallstones form only in the gallbladder and are due to "hyperbilirubinbilia" usually from three conditions: hemolysis from any cause including unsuspected conditions such as malaria, hypersplenism and prosthetic neovasculalure; ineffective erythropoiesis from vitamin B12 and folate deficiencies which are now rare in humans; induced EHC of UCB, a new pathophysiologic concept which has multiple predisposing factors highlighted in this review. With respect to the latter, any or all of the factors that make more UCB soluble and available in the large intestine facilitate its resorption to return to the liver, for reconjugation and resecretion into bile. UCB resorption may be aided by an increased permeability and residence time of UCB in the gut as well as low levels of ionized Ca^{2+}.

The primary source of free UCB in gallbladder bile is from endogenous biliary β-glucuronidase hydrolysis of bilirubin conjugates. This enzyme is of hepatic origin but with gallbladder inflammation can also be secreted from a biliary mucosal source. In the concentrated bile salt milieu of hepatic and gallbladder bile, UCB at biliary pH values is a monoacid, HUCB−. Two molecules of HUCB− bind with ionized biliary Ca2+, to form a divalent salt that has miniscule solubility in aqueous systems and precipitates from solution in bile. The ROS secreted by an inflamed gallbladder mucosa apparently causes $Ca(HUCB)_2$ polymerization and oxidationby Baig et al. [83]

The germ-free Swiss Webster mouse, a newly described animal model of "black" pigment gallstone formation, [73, 76] promises to answer many of the vexing questions regarding the pathophysiology and physical-chemistry of this disease. "Brown" stones are a phase-separated artifact of bile that can form in any part of the biliary tree secondary to chronic stasis from any cause and anaerobic bacterial infection. The anaerobes secrete multiple enzymes that hydrolyze ester and amide linkages of all biliary lipids and lipopigments into calcium-sensitive anions that phaseseparate as insoluble protonated anions or calcium salts. These precipitates deposit on obstructing "nuclei" such as small migratory cholesterol or "black" stones formed in the gallbladder, parasite eggs and dead worms or flukes.

The Oriental hepatolithiasis syndrome is the most serious manifestation of "brown" pigment stone disease. Beginning in early life, it is initiated by nematode or fluke infestation within the extrahepatic and intrahepatic bile ducts usually favoring the left lobe of the liver; worldwide, *Ascaris lumbricoides*, *Clonorchis sinensis* and *Opisthorchis viverrini* appear to be the principal parasites involved.

II. Pathogenesis of Calcium Bilirubinate Gallstone: Role of E. Coli, β-Glucuronidase and Coagulation by Inorganic Ions, Polyelectrolytes and Agitation [84]

From the practical viewpoint, especially in Japan, gallstones can be classified into three main types, that is gallstones of cholesterol line, those of bilirubin line and rare ones including inorganic stones (Table 1). Gallstones of bilirubin line are characterized by their relatively high bilirubin content and low cholesterol content and are divided into two subtypes; one is the so-called calcium bilirubinate stone or pigmented calcium stone and the other is usually referred to as the pure pigment stone.10 39 Calcium bilirubinate stones are prevalent in Asia and are very rare in Europe and the United States. In Japan, however, the incidence of these stones seems to have decreased in recent years. [85] Today, the incidence in Japan is estimated to be about 30 or 40 per cent of all gallstones, significantly lower than the 70 or 80 per cent in the period during and shortly after the Second World War. The typical calcium bilirubinate stones (Figure 1) are dark or reddish brown and usually very fragile. The cut surface is sometimes amorphous and sometimes stratified in structure. The stones are formed not only in the gallbladder but also fairly commonly in every portion of the biliary system, including the intrahepatic biliary tree. The number and size of these stones differ considerably from case to case. Besides concrements of definite shapes, that is gallstones, bile often contains a muddy substance consisting chiefly of numerous fine particles of calcium bilirubinate which can be identified microscopically. According to our investigations, [86] the bilirubin content of these calcium bilirubinate stones varied from 40.2 to 57.1 per cent including ammonia-extractable fractions and the cholesterol content from 2.9 to 25.6 per cent.

In contrast, analysis of gallstones of cholesterol line Miyaki and Ishiyama [87] showed the cholesterol content to be 96 per cent or more in pure cholesterol stones and over 71.3 per cent even in mixed stones. Bilirubin content was only 0.02 to 5.0 per cent in gallstones of this kind. Thus, calcium bilirubinate stones differ from cholesterol stones not only in clinical manifestations but also in composition, implying a difference in pathogenesis. Miyake and Ishiyama [88] proposed that the peculiarities of gallstones in the Japanese might be based on the difference of food and race between the Japanese and the Western people. At any rate, the difference in the varieties of cholelithiasis between Asian and Western countries-in other words the reason for a higher incidence of calcium bilirubinate stones in Asia by Digby and Miyake [85, 89, 90] is a matter of great interest for medical scientists of Asian countries. Despite many theories concerning development of gallstones, little is known about the separation mechanism of stone constituents from bile. No theory systematically elucidates how the separated gallstone constituents coagulate and solidify in bile to form a solid concrement, although some speculations such as theory of Liesegang phenomenon by Lichwitz [91] and coacervation theory [92, 93] have been presented. Recently, we studied characteristics of calcium bilirubinate stones, both clinically and biochemically, to clarify the mechanism of separation of calcium bilirubinate in bile and the mechanism of coagulation of the separated calcium bilirubinate, two major steps involved in pathogenesis of calcium bilirubinate stones. So-called pure pigment stones are different from calcium bilirubinate stones in many aspects. They are occasionally encountered in conditions without any biliary infection, especially in hemolytic jaundice in which bile is abnormally concentrated and in other conditions with metabolic imbalances. The site of production of these gallstones is usually the gallbladder. They are usually greenish dark or almost black appearance and chemically are compounds of bilirubin or its derivatives with calcium and other inorganic elements. Further discussions on the so-called pure pigment stones will be made elsewhere. Inducement to Formation of Calcium Bilirubinate Stone.

Although the incidence of calcium bilirubinate stone was quite high in the general population of Japan, farmers and fishermen of low income and poor living circumstances were more likely to be involved than better class patients. Laboratory examinations revealed that the bile of patients with calcium bilirubinate stones had almost invariably been infected with Escherichia coli. Eggs or fragments of cuticles of Ascaris lumbricoides were also identified in 55 per cent of pigmented calcium stones collected from many hospitals at the time directly after the Second World War.

Tung et al. [94] reported from Vietnam that they found roundworm elements in 70 per cent of examined gallstones as a kernel of gallstone formation. These facts indicate that contamination of the biliary tract may induce formation of this kind of gallstones. Accordingly, local factors such as intracholedochal migration of the roundworm or other parasites and duodenitis of unknown origin, which causes papillitis, might be responsible for the development of calcium bilirubinate stones. Should papillitis occur in consequence of these conditions, stag-nation of bile, and ascending infection to the biliary system and backflow of pancreatic juice would result in formation of gallstones in the stagnated and dilated bile ducts. Details of these facts were described previously by Maki. [85] Although it has been claimed by some authors [95, 96] that the cause of cholangiohepatitis in Southeast Asia is on most occasions Escherichia coli and these bacilli may reach the liver through the portal vein, we believe that "ascending infection" as outlined above is more likely as the route of infection to the biliary system. The relatively common atrophic gastritis which occurs in Japan and is associated with hypo-achlorhydria may facilitate bacterial growth in the duodenum and also promote ascending infection to the biliary infection. Stock and Tinckler [97] in Hong Kong presumed that clonorchiasis sinensis, another parasitic disease of the biliary tract, would be a common cause of the calcium bilirubinate stone in Southeast Asia where heavy infestation of the worm is not rare. In Japan, clonorchiasis is less commonly associated with gallstones than is invasion of Ascaris lumbricoides into the common bile duct. One reason for this may be that in Japan infestation of Clonorchis sinensis is usually not severe, and another may be the fact that Clonorchis sinensis migrates from the papilla of Vater into the intrahepatic ducts at the time of metacercaria which is too small to induce significant irritation to the papilla of Vater. A solid calcium bilirubinate stone was experimentally formed by Sato [98] in their laboratory by keeping an ascarid carcass for about 10 months in the gallbladder of a living dog. Following this experiment, Atsumi,1 also of our department, demonstrated that calcium bilirubinate was precipitated easily in the form of sporadic dots on the eggshell of the roundworm within 4 to 5 days after introduction of a saline suspension of the eggs into the gallbladder of a dog. At any rate, the fact that the parasite gallstones are exclusively calcium bilirubinate stones is an enigma. As to the biochemical aspect of bile in cholelithiasis, it was revealed that not only cholesterol but also bilirubin were unexpectedly lower in concentration in cases with calcium bilirubinate stones than in those with cholesterol stones, although the content in bile of bile acids generally decreased in cholelithiasis and showed no noteworthy difference according to the kind of gallstones. On the other hand, the fact that Japanese residing in Honolulu or in California, unlike those residing in Japan, rarely develop calcium bilirubinate stones [85] gives some interesting suggestions as to the mechanism of formation of these gallstones. The average daily per capita intake of fat and animal protein by Asians is generally lower than that by Europeans and Americans by Maki. [99] From laboratory and clinical data, it seems likely that food, which influences the metabolism of bilirubin, is also related to formation of calcium bilirubinate stones. The recent decrease in incidence of calcium bilirubinate stones in Japan is presumed due to both improvement of diet and a decrease of infestation by intestinal parasites.

Separation Mechanism of Calcium Bilirubinate in Bile Hypothesis of Combination of Bilirubin with Calcium in Bile

With recent progress in assay methods in biochemistry, many research workers have dealt with chemical constitution of bile and gallstones, and the mechanism of precipitation of gallstone constituents from bile is more clear. [100] In 1954, Isaksson [101] reported on the dissolving power of cholesterol in human bile and advocated that a decrease in lecithin-bile salt complexes might promote separation of cholesterol in bile; this theory has been supported by others. [102] However, no theory has elucidated precipitation of calcium bilirubinate on the basis of chemical experiments. The bilirubin moiety of the calcium bilirubinate stone has been identified to be free, non-esterified bilirubin since it is chloroform-extractable after treatment with dilute hydrochloric acid. [103] Therefore, bilirubin is presumed to be present in the stone in water-insoluble compounds with inorganic elements, mostly with calcium. In other words the main ingredient of so-called pigmented calcium stones is bilirubinate of calcium. Little has been known of the mechanism leading to the combination of bilirubin with calcium. In the last decade Billing and Lathe, [104] Schmidt [105] and Talafant [106] reported that bilirubin in the circulating blood is esterified in the liver to form water-soluble glucuronide before it is excreted into bile. In further studies, including some in our department, [101, 107-109]it has been pointed out that pigments in bile are mostly glucuronides of bilirubin but approximately [110] per cent is non-glucuronide bilirubin. The latter fraction includes salts of bilirubin and pigments that, on electrophoresis, move with proteins, phospholipids or bile acids. Bilirubin glucuronide is known to undergo hydrolysis into free bilirubin and glucuronic acid in the presence of the enzyme β-glucuronidase. The activity of figlucuronidase in bile was studied primarily in a variety of biliary disorders. [89] Normal bile was always free of β-glucuronidase activity, whereas bile infected with E. coli, especially specimens obtained from patients with calcium bilirubinate stones, exhibited intense activity of this enzyme. The activity was maximal at about pH 7.0 which was near the optimal pH for β-glucuronidase from E. coli. This indicates that the bile in the case of calcium bilirubinate stone is under the influence of β-glucuronidase of bacterial origin. According to Sasaki, [111] β-glucuronidase from a group of coli bacilli showed the most intense activity of various other bacteria tested. It is presumed that bilirubin glucuronide in bile is hydrolyzed into free bilirubin and glucuronic acid by enzymatic activity, and calcium, which increases in the biliary tract in inflammatory conditions, 6 combines with the liberated free bilirubin at its free carboxyl radical, yielding the water-insoluble calcium bilirubinate. This hypothesis is outlined in Table 2. A precipitate of calcium bilirubinate was prepared when free bilirubin (Daiichi Chemical Co.) was dissolved in water in the form of sodium or potassium salts and calcium hydroxide added to the solution, or when calcium hydroxide was immediately added to a water suspension of the bilirubin preparation.'3 In Vitro Precipitation of Calcium Bilirubinate Miyake [112] and Westphal et al. [95] observed that fine concrements of bile pigments were produced in the gallbladder of dog by prolonged bile stasis combined with injection of E. coli. It has long been known that human bile sometimes produces precipitates when it is left standing in an upright vessel. Bacmeister [113] observed over 50 years ago that a sediment of cholesterol formed in bile from patients who had cholesterol stones. Recently, Tera [114] observed a similar phenomenon and advocated that precipitation of cholesterol from bile could occur without a simultaneous change in lecithin bile salts concentration, contrary to the opinion of Isaksson. [101] Such precipitation in bile seems to represent an initial stage of gallstone formation but investigations have been limited to bile obtained from patients who had cholesterol stones. A similar experiment was undertaken by Saito with bile obtained at laparotomy from various patients who had calcium bilirubinate stones, cholesterol stones and no biliary disorders. Collected samples were centrifuged and incubated at 38° C. for 48 hours and observed for precipitation. Bilirubin and glucuronic acid contents of the samples were determined before and after incubation, and the resulting precipitates were subjected to physical and chemical analyses. Control bile samples developed no precipitation nor appreciable change in concentration of bilirubin or glucuronic acid. The bile from patients with cholesterol stones occasionally produced precipitates even in non-infected specimens; the precipitates showed about the same appearance as in Tera's experiment, i.e., a large quantity of cholesterol crystals. Bile from patients with calcium bilirubinate stones, mostly infected with E. coli, invariably yielded a precipitate of spherical particles which consisted mainly of calcium bilirubinate and resembled a suspension of powdered pigmented calcium stone. After incubation, the content of bilirubin decreased and that of free glucuronic acid increased in the supernatant, demonstrating that bilirubin glucuronide in bile was hydrolyzed by the enzymatic activity of β-glucuronidase of bacterial origin into free bilirubin and glucuronic acid, and the former combined with inorganic elements to form the spherical particles of calcium bilirubinate. Chemical and physical analyses, especially paper electrophoresis and infrared spectroscopy, of the precipitate showed the presence of calcium bilirubinate and substances such as phospholipids, polysaccharides, bile acids and insoluble proteins which are all common ingredients of calcium bilirubinate stones. Thus, such precipitation of infected bile is considered an initial stage of pigmented calcium stone formation. When a large amount (50 mg./ ml.) of a bacterial preparation of β-glucuronidase (Sigma Chemical Co.) was added to normal bile, the incubation procedure resulted in formation of precipitates similar to those from infected specimens. Three test tubes contain a control bile sample, a bile sample of a case of pigmented calcium stone and a normal bile sample supplemented with β-glucuronidase, respectively, after incubation. Precipitates are seen in the latter two samples but not in the first. It should be noted that precipitates of bile in patients with gallstones are quite different, not only in mechanism of formation but also in composition, between patients with cholesterol stones and those with pigmented calcium stones that are invariably infected with E. coli. Substances inhibiting the β-glucuronidase Activity Although β-glucuronidase of bacterial origin plays an essential role in the development of calcium bilirubinate stones, biliary infection with E. coli does not always give rise to gallstones. It is presumed that bile contains substances that inhibit the f8- glucuronidase activity. Matsushiro [115] demonstrated that normal bile considerably inhibited the activity of bacterialβ-glucuronidase; glucuronic acid and copper ion among usual constituents of bile had some inhibitory effects. Effects were almost negligible at concentrations in the ranges found in bile, and the inhibitory effect of bile seemed not to be ascribable to these substances. [116] In 1963, Marsh [117] elucidated a pathway through which glucuronic acid is metabolized into glucaro-1,4-lactone, a powerful inhibitor of β-glucuronidase. This substance is partly excreted in urine as confirmed by Marsh and later by Ishidate. Recently, Matsushiro qualitatively identified this substance for the first time in bile by means of paper chromatography. A successful method was devised for quantitative estimation of glucaro-1,4-lactone (as glucaric acid) in bile by means of column chromatography by Yamaguchi et al. [118] Oral administration of this substance was followed by a marked reduction in the f8-glucuronidase activity in bile. In in vitro experiments, precipitation of calcium bilirubinate from infected bile was prevented by adding glucaro-1,4-lactone to the specimen. Precipitation of calcium bilirubinate onto ascarid eggs in infected bile was prevented by application of glucaro-1,4-lactone. [119] These facts indicate that inhibitors of ft-glucuronidase in bile, especially glucaro-1,4-lactone, control separation of calcium bilirubinate in bile by depressing the activity of bacterial f-glucuronidase. According to determinations, the content in bile of inhibitory substances is subject to considerable individual variation. Although the reason for this is not known, we believe that diet may be a significant factor. It may be significant that the separation mechanism of ingredients of calcium bilirubinate stones has been clarified and that one can experimentally produce, or inhibit, precipitation of calcium bilirubinate from bile, unlike ingredients of cholesterol stones. Coagulation Mechanism of Calcium Bilirubinate Particles Sedimented in Bile The above-mentioned theory explains the separation mechanism of calcium bilirubinate as insoluble particles in bile. Nevertheless, the mechanism by which these particles coagulate and solidify to form a gallstone is not clear. Most previous work on gallstone formation, both cholesterol and bilirubin, have left this subject untouched. Recently, Yusa and Gaudin [120] succeeded in preparing pellet-like flocks from a suspension of kaolinate. The mechanism of coagulation of bile sediment has been investigated by Maki and Suzuki, who produced a gallstone-like concrement in vitro from a suspension of human bile sediment consisting chiefly of calcium bilirubinate. Experimental results are described in the following. Coagulation of a colloidal substance may first require elimination of hydrophilic layers on colloidal particles to bring the particles close to each other. Adequate energy is necessary to coagulate particles firmly, as pointed out by Yusa and Gaudin [120]. These conditions can be brought about by the following procedures: 1) addition of electrolytes which approximate the colloidal particles by shrinking the ionic atmospheres around them, 2) addition of a high-molecular- weight substance that promotes aggregation of the particles by its bridging action, and 3) application of physical movement to supply kinetic energy required for consolidation of the aggregate. An outline of the experimental procedures is described below.

Coagulating Effects of Inorganic Substances

Bile was collected from patients with calcium bilirubinate stones through a T-tube inserted in the common bile duct, and the sediment of calcium bilirubinate was prepared by incubating it. To simplify the condition, the experiment was performed with a suspension of the sedimented calcium bilirubinate in distilled water. The C-potential of suspending particles of calcium bilirubinate measured approximately -20 mV in distilled water when determined with a microscopic electrophoresis apparatus. When inorganic cations, such as calcium ion, which are opposite in electric charge to the particles of bile sediment were added to the suspension, the absolute value of the c-potential was lowered and the suspending particles coagulated. The larger the valence of the cation, the more remarkable the coagulating effect, agreeing with Schultz-Hardy's law. Hydrogen ion concentration appeared to significantly influence the above mechanism, the coagulation being more remarkable at an acid pH than in the alkaline range.

The coagulate thus obtained by addition of an inorganic electrolyte was gel-like flocks which were hydrophilic and did not drain well. Such a hydrophilic nature of the flocks is due to a hydrated layer surrounding each particle, and this must be removed to transform the flocks into well drained coagulates. This was attained to some extent by adding calcium carbonate to the suspension. The dehydrating effect of calcium carbonate may be that fine particles of this compound adsorb colloid particles on their surfaces and thus disintegrate the gel structure of the flocks of the colloid particles. Coagulating Effects of Organic Substances A group of high-molecular-weight organic compounds are also effective as coagulating agents for colloidal substances and a study was made of their effects on the suspension of bile sediments. Konanfloc 1250 and Konanfloc 2000 (Konan Chemical Co.) are both linear polyelectrolytes of positive charge, exhibiting marked coagulating effects. It was found that the effect of such a polyelectrolyte was enhanced by simultaneous addition of an inorganic electrolyte such as calcium chloride or aluminum chloride; on such occasions the coagulation of particles was more remarkable and the supernatant became more transparent than in the suspension coagulated with a polyelectrolyte alone. The effect of linear high-molecular-weight organic compounds on coagulation of bile sediment is probably due to two factors. One is its remarkable adsorption characteristics and the other a bridging action by which molecules of a high-molecular-weight substance combine many colloid particles. The bridging action is apparently due to the large number of function groups arranged around a linear skeleton in the molecule.

Application of Physical Movement to the Sample

On the basis of experiment by Yusa and Gaudin, the suspension of bile sediment was subjected to slow rotation with the inorganic and organic reagents that proved most effective for coagulation of the sample. In the course of rotation, visible coagulates were formed in the suspension, and the coagulates increased in size and finally formed solid concrements in about 30 minutes.

The progress of change is shown in Figure 4 which consists of fragments of a movie film taken during the rotating movement of bile supplemented with calcium carbonate, calcium chloride and Konanfloc 2000. Although the role of rotation in the formation of gallstone-like concrements has not yet been established, a probable interpretation is that an adequate form of agitation must be supplied to over- whelm the potential energy barrier (Figure 5) that may increase with increase in the size of the particles as coagulation progresses.

These experiments may provide a model for study of the coagulation mechanism of calcium bilirubinate stones in vivo. In the human being, many inorganic ions such as Na, K,

Ca, Fe, Cu, Mg, Al etc. are present in bile, and high-molecular-weight organic substances that act as bridging agents may be increased in inflammatory processes. But it is not yet clear which inorganic ions and high-molecular-weight substances are actually promoting coagulation of particles of calcium bilirubinate in the biliary tract.

The physical energy required for the last step of consolidation may be supplied by motility of the gallbladder and by bile flow due to pressure of bile secretion or movement of the body as a whole. The capability of the biliary system to absorb water provides an additional favorable condition.

The fact that solid concrements resembling genuine calcium bilirubinate stones were actually produced in vitro on the basis of our hypothesis would justify our view concerning the initiation of calcium bilirubinate stones which are in many instances amorphous. However the reason stratified structure is occasionally seen in gallstones of this type and the coagulation mechanism of cholesterol stones remain unsolved. The theory by Maki and Suzuki may also apply to coagulation mechanisms of other substances separated from a colloidal solution in the living organism.

In conclusion, the pathogenesis of gallstones should be discussed from three aspects, inducement, separation and precipitation of gallstone ingredients in bile and consolidation of these constituents. The problem has hitherto been dealt with vaguely without differentiating these three aspects.

Summary

Both stagnation and infection of bile, especially with Escherichia coli, together with dietary deficiencies, appear to induce formation of calcium bilirubinate stones which are common in the Asian area. As to the mechanism by which calcium bilirubinate separates out of bile, the activity of β-glucuronidase of bacterial origin is presumed to play an essential role; the enzyme hydrolyzes bilirubin glucuronide into free bilirubin and glucuronic acid, and calcium in bile combines at the carboxyl radical of liberated bilirubin to form calcium bilirubinate.

On the other hand, bile usually has an inhibitory effect on the glucuronidase activity. This is mainly due to glucaro-1,4-lactone which is present in bile and known to be the most powerful inhibitor of this enzyme. Glucaro-1,4-lactone in bile was identified both qualitatively and quantitatively as glucaric acid. A new hypothesis has been presented on the mechanism of consolidation of calcium bilirubinate stones: Particles separated from bile, consisting mainly of calcium bilirubinate, are negatively charged and undergo loose coagulation as a result of electrostatic effect of inorganic ions and bridging action of high-molecular-weight organic substances.

The coagulate then consolidates more tightly under influence of physical movement. In support of this hypothesis, solid stone-like concrements which resembled the amorphous pigmented calcium stones in man were produced in a model experiment.

III. Role of Parietal (Gallbladder Mucosa) Factors in the Formation of Black Pigment Gallstones [121]

In a recent number of *Clinics and Research in Hepatology and Gastroenterology* very interesting article of Vitek and Carey about the pathogenesis of black pigment gallstones has been published. [1] In the conclusion, authors stated that endogenous biliary β-glucuronidase hydrolysis of bilirubin conjugates provides hydrogen bilirubinate that precipitates with ionized calcium and that inflamed gallbladder mucosa secretes reactive oxygen species that transform the initial precipitates into hard black pigment gallstones with the participation of a mixed mucin glycoprotein matrix acting as the gallstones scaffolding. In Cariati et al.'s previous ultrastructural studies by Cariati and Cetta, [122] they demonstrated that parietal (gallbladder mucosa) factors play an important role in black pigment gallstones formation. In fact, hard black pigment microstones can form on gallbladder mucosal surface and in particular in Rokitansky-Aschoff sinuses of the gallbladder were the effects of β-glucuronidase, reactive oxygen species and mucin glycoprotein matrix are amplified. Gallbladder mucosa surface is irregular with deep cleft (Rokitansky-Aschoff sinuses) that can facilitate black microstones formation (Figure 1). In our series, nearly the 34% of the patients with black pigment gallstones and Rokitansky-Aschoff sinuses (or adenomyomatosis) had none of the typical risk factors of black pigment gallstones as hemolysis, ineffective erythropoiesis, pathologic enterohepatic cycling of unconjugated bilirubin by Vitek and Brink et al. [34, 54] chronic hepatitis or cirrhosis by Alvaro et al. [123] Adenomyomatosis patients with black pigment gallstones have usually a sterile bile (infection was present only in the 8% of the cases). In conclusion, parietal factors as mucosal secretion of β-glucuronidase, mixed mucin glycoprotein, reactive oxygen species and the microenvironments of Rokitansky-Aschoff sinuses play a basic role in black pigment gallstones formation as the hyperbilirubinbilia factors (hemolysis, chronic hepatitis, ineffective erythropoiesis and pathologic enterohepatic cycling of unconjugated bilirubin).

IV. Enterohepatic Cycling of Bilirubin As a Cause of "Black" Pigment Gallstones in Adult Life [71]

In Contrast To Bile Salts, Which Undergo A Highly Efficient Enterohepatic circulation with multiple regulatory and physiologic functions, glucuronic acid conjugates of bilirubin are biliary excretory molecules that in health do not have a continuing biologic life. Intestinal absorptive cells are devoid of recapture transporters for bilirubin conjugates, and their large size and polarity prevent absorption by passive diffusion. However, unconjugated bilirubin, the B-glucuronidase hydrolysis product of bilirubin glucuronides can be absorbed passively from any part of the small and large intestines. This can occur only if unconjugated bilirubin is kept in solution and does not undergo rapid bacterial reduction to form urobilinoids. Here we collect, and in some cases reinterpret, experimental and clinical evidence to show that in addition to the well-known occurrence in newborns, enterohepatic cycling of unconjugated bilirubin can reappear in adult life. This happens as a result of several common conditions, particularly associated with bile salt leakage from the small intestine, the most notable ileal dysfunction resulting from any medical or surgical cause. Vitek and Carey propose that when present in excess, colonic bile salts solubilize unconjugated bilirubin, delay urobilinoid formation, prevent calcium complexing of unconjugated bilirubin and promote passive absorption of unconjugated bilirubin from the large intestine. Following uptake, reconjugation, and resecretion into bile, this source of 'hyperbilirubinbilia' may be the important pathophysiological risk factor for 'black' pigment gallstone formation in predisposed adult humans.

The enterohepatic circulation (EHC) of bile salts (Figure 1) is a highly efficient internal circulation of water-soluble hydroxylated derivatives of cholanoic acid, the principal catabolic products of cholesterol and the major solutes of bile by Carey and Duane. [124] Bile salts are potent steroidal detergents that solubilize biliary as well as dietary lipids, thereby facilitating their hepatic secretion and intestinal absorption, respectively. Maintenance of bile salts within this circulation is governed by sodium-coupled co-transporters on hepatic sinusoidal membranes as well as apical plasma membranes of ileal enterocytes by Love and Dawson. [125] In contrast, the natural glucuronic acid conjugates of bilirubin IX A , the principal catabolic product of Fe-protoporphyrin IX, do not recycle enterohepatically, as intestinal cells lack transporters for their recapture. However, resorption of unconjugated bilirubin (UCB) can occur passively by nonionic diffusion from any part of the small and large intestine Carey and Duane. [124] This resorption and recycling of UCB occurs commonly in human newborns and results from (i) deficiency in the intestinal microflora capable of reducing UCB to urobilinoids, [74] (ii) high β-glucuronidase activity in human milk, which hydrolyzes bilirubin conjugates to UCB Gourly and Arend(126) and (iii) bile salt malabsorption [127] associated with intestinal immaturity. Here we collect and critically collate a large body of literature, including our own work, to show that enterohepatic recycling of UCB can re-emerge in adult life. This recycling of UCB may be caused by a number of common pathophysiological conditions, which have in common principally, but not exclusively, increased bile salt loss into the large intestine. Vitek and Carey have marshaled evidence to show that the clinical manifestations of recycling UCB from the intestines are distinct in adults compared with neonates. In adults, recycling UCB molecules elevate biliary levels of bilirubin conjugates, simply because of physiologic maturity of uptake, conjugation, transport and secretory mechanisms of the adult liver. In contrast, because of immaturity of these hepatic steps as well as the lack of urobilinoid production in the neonatal intestinal lumen, recycling UCB contributes to hyperbilirubinaemia in newborns. The adult syndrome would be otherwise benign, were it not for the knowledge that sustained 'hyperbilirubinbilia', even of modest proportions, places patients at risk for 'black' pigment (calcium bilirubinate) gallstones [127]. Vitek and Caey have classified three conditions that render intestinal resorption of UCB possible: 1) Higher rates of bilirubin deconjugation in the small intestine. The proposed causes include prolonged intestinal transit time, colonization with β –glucuronidase producing bacteria, or a supply of β -glucuronidase from extraintestinal sources. 2) Deficiency of bacteria capable of reducing UCB in the large intestine. Typically, this category is physiologic in neonates and possibly acquired in some adults receiving broad-spectrum antibiotics for gut 'sterilization' or as an adverse effect of prolonged systemic antibiotic therapy. 3) Augmented solubilization of UCB in the large intestine. Vitek and Carey propose that high bile salt concentrations in the proximal large intestine increase solubilization of UCB, delay urobilinoid formation and also prevent calcium bilirubinate formation.

Association of Pigment Cholelithiasis with Enterohepatic Cycling of Bilirubin

Several lines of evidence support the proposal that 'black' pigment gallstones can be caused by an acquired EHC of bilirubin. Increased prevalence of black pigment cholelithiasis is known to occur in Crohn's disease by Brink, Heaton and Lapidus et al., [127-129] ileal resection by Brink and Magnuson et al. [127, 130] or bypass by Buchwald et al., [131] oral bile acid administration by Frabboni, Raedsch, Freilich, Ros and Peirera et al., [132-136] high cholesterol by Dam and LaMorte et al., [137, 138] and carbohydrate-containing diets,(63) total parenteral nutrition by Bolondi and Roslyn et al. [139, 140] alcoholism by Schwesinger et al., [141] and cystic fibrosis by Angelico et al., [142] Vitek and Carey show now that the common denominator in all of these appears to be hyperbilirubinbilia caused by bile salt malabsorption with resorption of UCB from the distal small and large intestines.

Diagnosing and Preventing Enterohepatic Cycling of Bilirubin

Unfortunately, no simple diagnostic tool is currently available to identify subjects with an EHC of UCB and thereby the risk for hyperbilirubinbilia and 'black' pigment gallstones. At the research level, studies with radiolabelled or stable isotope-labelled bilirubin conjugates would be essential to prove an intestinal source of resorbed bilirubin and its role in mild hyperbilirubinaemia and hyperbilirubinbilia. Furthermore, these studies would be important to directly prove and quantify an EHC of bilirubin in ileal dysfunctional states. At the clinical level, one is left with no choice but to rule in the diagnosis of EHC of UCB, only by excluding the two other major causes of hyperbilirubinbilia, which are hemolysis and shunt/dyserythropoiesis. Indirect diagnostic tests for excess biliary secretion of bilirubin conjugates, such as a challenge with Phenobarbital or nicotinic acid, which have been widely used in patients with unconjugated hyperbilirubinaemia, would be of little quantitative value, as biliary levels cannot easily be assayed except at the research level. A test of prolonged fasting might be useful for EHC-induced hyperbilirubinnaemia, as its effect is based on decreased gut motility; however, the specificity and sensitivity of such a test might be difficult to establish without investigations on a large cohort of humans.

V. Melatonin Prevents Pigment Gallstone Formation Induced by Bile Duct Ligation in Guinea Pigs [80]

Free radical-mediated oxidative stress has been implicated in the genesis of gallstone *in vitro*. Shiesh et al.'s study was designed to examine the oxidative stress changes during pigment gallstone formation and to investigate whether melatonin (MLT) could act as a chemopreventive agent for cholelithiasis in a guinea pig model. The common bile duct of guinea pigs was ligated with or without MLT pretreatment. Animals were studied on day 7, 9, 12, and 14 after surgery. Stone and/or sludge developed in ligated guinea pigs without MLT. Fourier transform infrared spectra of the sludge showed the presence of calcium bilirubinate, whose peak height per milligram of sludge gradually increased with time after ligation. Total antioxidant activity (TAA) in bile of guinea pigs at day 14 after ligation reduced to one third of the level in sham-operated controls ($P < .001$). In addition, the bile of ligated guinea pigs had increased pH ($P < .001$), bile salts ($P < .01$), and malondialdehyde (MDA) ($P < .05$), compared to sham controls. Pretreatment of guinea pigs with MLT at a dose of 1,000 mg/kg significantly decreased the incidence of pigment gallstone formation at day 14 after ligation, as compared to no pretreatment (0/7 vs. 8/10). MLT also reverted the ligation-induced changes in biliary bile salts, pH, MDA, and TAA to control levels. These *in vivo* findings support a causative role of oxidative stress in the bile duct ligation–induced pigment gallstone formation. Antioxidants may prove useful in preventing pigment gallstone formation in humans.

Oxidative stress has been implicated in the pathogenesis and pathophysiology of more than 100 disease states advocated by Hale et al. [143] Only a few studies have implicated oxidative stress in pigment gallstone. Hydroxyl radical was reported to stimulate a rapid release of glycoprotein from gallbladder epithelium in organ culture [143] and to be a promotor of cholesterol crystallization in model bile.[144] An *in vitro* experiment showed that an oxygen-free radical oxidized unconjugated bilirubin and led to the formation of a brown-black precipitation by Tiribelli and Ostrow. [145] The presence of an oxygen-free radical has been reported in fresh pigment gallstone suggested by Elek and Rockenbouer. [146]. Moreover, increased F2-isoprostanes and 4-hydroxynonenal, products of lipid peroxidation, were observed in the bile of stone patients. [147] However, the role of oxidative stress in pigment gallstone formation is not fully understood. Gallbladder stasis resulting from mechanical obstruction is an important antecedent to the development of pigment gallstones and sludge. Changes in biliary content may facilitate the precipitation of calcium salts of bilirubinate or fatty acid and lead to the stone formation. Animal studies on bile duct ligation showed the effects of ligation on the increase of gallbladder mucins content by Bernhoft et al,(148) liver mitochondrial lipid peroxidation by Sokol and Krahenbuhl et al., [149, 150] and serum malondialdehyde (MDA) by Krahenbuhl et al., [150] and the decrease of liver vitamin E concentration and glutathione reductase activity by Krahenbuhl and and Singh et al. [150, 151] Yet, no study has assessed the oxidative stress in bile during the course of sludge and stone formation and the feasibility of antioxidant administration in the prevention of cholelithiasis *in vivo*. Melatonin (N-acetyl-5-methoxytryptamine, MLT), a lipophilic indole amine derived from tryptophan, was for years thought to be produced exclusively in the pineal gland as a hormone. It is now clear that MLT can be found in a number of other cells and organs by Brzezinski et al. [152]. MLT is known to regulate circadian rhythms, sleep, and immune system activity, as well as to scavenge oxygen-centered free radicals, which may contribute to the prevention of cancer and aging by Reiter and Montifla et al. [153, 154].The potency of MLT is at least 10 times more than that of vitamin C and α-tocopherol in breaking the lipid peroxidation chain reaction.14 In this study, we used a guinea pig model of pigment gallstone15 to examine how oxidative stress changes during the formation of pigment gallstone and to test whether MLT, a scavenger of free radicals, protects against its formation. The parameters analyzed to evaluate oxidative stress included changes of lipoperoxides (MDA) and total antioxidant activity (TAA) in bile and serum. The effects of pretreatment with 2 doses of MLT on ligation-induced gallstone and oxidative stress were determined.

The serial changes in the concentrations of bile salts, protein, and conjugated and unconjugated bilirubins were observed, as well as the activity of free calcium and pH to assess the mechanism of MLT in the prevention of pigment gallstone.

In the **materials and methods** section, male Hartley guinea pigs, weighing 400 g to 600 g were purchased from National Taiwan University Medical Center (Taipei, Taiwan) and maintained at the Animal Center of National Cheng Kung University (Tainan, Taiwan). Animals were fed with a standard chow (Laboratory Rodent Diet; PMI Feeds Inc., Brentwood, MO) and water *ad libitum*. MLT was administered daily by intraperitoneal injection at a dose of 100 or 1,000 mg/kg, starting from 3 days before the ligation and ending at the day of sacrifice (Table 1). Pigment gallstones were induced by incomplete bile duct ligation under ketamine and xylocaine anesthesia. A 19-gauge catheter was placed beside the common bile duct and tied together with a 3-0 cat gut ligature. After withdrawing the 19-gauge catheter, an incomplete bile duct was achieved. On day 7, 9, 12, or 14 after ligation, the guinea pigs were killed after a 24-hour fast (water allowed). The abdomen was then exposed and the gallbladder was examined visually for the presence of sludge and/or gallstones. The gallbladder was then disinfected with povidone solution and punctured with a 22-gauge syringe to aspirate bile. Blood samples were obtained by cardiac puncture for the determination of TAA and MDA. Guinea pigs that underwent laparotomy without bile duct ligation were used as controls. Their bile and blood were sampled 2 weeks after the sham operation by the same procedure described previously.

Analysis of Sludge And Gallstones

The sludge and stones were washed in distilled water to remove residual bile. Gallstones were examined by transform infrared spectroscopy and scanning electron microscopy as reported previously by Chen et al. [155]. The sludge was dried by vacuum centrifugation. One milligram of dried sludge was mixed with 200 mg of spectral grade potassium bromide (Merck, Darmstadt, Germany). The mixture was pelleted in a 13-mm-diameter evacuable pellet die under a pressure of 750 MPs. Transmission spectra of sludge pellets were determined with a Fourier Transform Infrared Spectroscopy FTS-60 (Bio-Rad, Cambridge, MA) for wave number 4,000 to 400 cm [156] and a spectral resolution of 8 cm [156, 15] Potassium bromide pellets were used to generate the background spectra. The chemical compositions of the sludge were compared to the spectra of calcium bilirubinate, calcium carbonate, calcium palmitate, and human gallstones obtained at surgery.

Analysis of Bile and Serum

Sampling and handling of bile were performed in dimmed light as much as possible to avoid photoisomerization of bile pigments. Bile samples were immediately analyzed for ionized calcium (Ciba Corning 634 analyzer, Ciba Corning Diagnostics Corp., Medfield,

MA) and pH (PHM82 standard pH meter; Radiometer, Bagsvaerd, Denmark) using ion-selective electrodes at 37°C. The bile was then centrifuged at 7,500 rpm for 10 minutes, and the supernatant was aspirated and stored at 270°C until analysis within 4 weeks. The major oxidation damage product of polyunsaturated fatty acid, MDA, was measured to reflect the level of lipoperoxide. A modified method for the measurement of MDA as thiobarbituric acid reacting substance was performed by reversed-phase high-performance liquid chromatography with spectrophotometric detection by Fukunaga et al. [158]. The bile and serum samples were pretreated with zinc sulfate to avoid substances, such as protein and bilirubin from reacting with thiobarbituric acid. The MDA concentration in one bile with undetectable bilirubin was 1.45 mmol/L and changed to 0.57 mmol/L with zinc sulfate treatment. By adding 100 mmol/L of bilirubin to the bile, the MDA increased to 3.15mmol/L, but returned to 0.64mmol/L with zinc sulfate treatment. In brief, an aliquot of 200 mL of bile or serum was mixed with 1/20 volume of 30% zinc sulfate. After centrifugation at 10,000*g* for 10 minutes, 20 mL of supernatant was mixed with 20 mL of 5% butylhydroxytoluene and 2.0 mL of 42 mmol/L thiobarbituric acid in 2 mol/L sodium acetate buffer (pH 3.5). The mixture was heated at 95°C for 45 minutes. After cooling, the MDA-thiobarbituric acid complex was extracted with n-butanol and chromatographed on a Beckman high-performance liquid chromatography System Gold (Beckman Instruments, Inc., Irvine, CA) equipped with a visible detector monitoring the peak at 532 nm. The analytical column (Waters Corp., Milford, MA) used was a mBondapack C18 10-mm reversed-phase column. 1,1,3,3-tetraethoxypropane was used to generate a standard curve on each run. The within-day and day-to-day precision, expressed as coefficient of variation, was 1.9% and 2.8%, respectively, with the mean value of 1.173 mmol/L. The average recovery of MDA assay was 101.9% (range 92.5%-107.5%, n 5 5).

The total antioxidant activity in serum and bile was determined on an AutoLumat LB 953 Luminometer (EG & G Berthold, Bad Wildbad, Germany) as described by Whitehead et al.18 In brief, chemiluminescent reaction was generated in a test tube by carefully mixing 800 mL of distilled water, 100 mL of signal reagent (luminol and p-iodophenol in buffer solution), and 50 mL of 1:200 diluted horseradish peroxidase solution (Sigma, St. Louis, MO). Then, 10 mL of sample was added to inhibit the luminescence. The duration of the quenching was measured and compared with that of a water-soluble α-tocopherol analogue, trolox (6-hydroxy-2,5,7,8-tetra-methylchroman- 2-carboxylic acid). The precision of the assay (coefficient of variation) was 2.3% and 5.1% for within-day and day-to-day variation, respectively. The average recovery of trolox added in bile was 103.3% (range 97.6%-106.2%, n 5 5). Conjugated and unconjugated bilirubins were assayed by the high-performance liquid chromatography method of Alvaro et al. 19 To prevent bilirubin degradation during storage, aliquots of bile were mixed with sodium ascorbate (100 mg/mL of bile) and ethylenediaminetetraacetic acid (5 mg/mL of bile) and kept in the dark at270°C until analysis. Unconjugated bilirubin and bilirubin monoglucuronide are the major components of guinea pig bile with trace amounts of bilirubin diglucuronide. The retention time for these bilirubins was 5.0, 12.5, and 14.2 minutes, respectively. Bile salts concentration was determined using the 3a-hydroxysteroid dehydrogenase enzymatic method described by Mashige et al. [159]. Bile salts concentrations were obtained by calculating the difference between the test and blank (without 3a-hydroxysteroid dehydrogenase) reaction at 530 nm. The protein concentration was determined based on bicinchoninic acid chromophore (Pierce, Rockford,

IL) with the use of albumin as a standard. The samples were pretreated with cold acetone to eliminate interfering substances [156].

Statistical Analysis

The data are reported as mean ± SD. One-way analysis of variance and unpaired *t* test were used to test for statistically significant differences among groups by the Statistical Analysis System computer program (SAS Institute Inc., Cary, NC). All statistical tests were 2-sided and significance was assumed when *P* was less than .05.

In the **results** section, the incidence of stones and sludge formation after bile duct ligation with or without MLT treatment. The mortality rate was approximately 40% in the ligated group without MLT treatment by Chen et al. [155] and 10% in the ligated group with MLT treatment. No animal died in the control group. The death was either caused by bile leakage with bile peritonitis from a severely distended gallbladder or complications associated with bile duct obstruction, such as cholangitis. All fatal events occurred within the first week of the experiment. Stone and/or sludge were present in all bile duct ligated guinea pigs without MLT treatment. At day 7 after ligation, all animals developed sludge but without stone formation, the average percentage of sludge in bile volume was 20%. The incidence of "sludge only" gradually decreased and "sludge with stone formation" increased thereafter. At day 14 after ligation, all animals had sludge and 80% of the animals had gallstones. Intraperitoneal administration of MLT reduced the ligation-induced formation of biliary sludge and stones in a dose-dependent manner. MLT treatment at 100 and 1,000 mg/kg reduced the incidence of sludge to 60% (6/ 10) and 28% (2/7), respectively. MLT at a dose of 1,000 mg/kg for 17 days (group 7) prevented the stone formation. In particular, 2 of 7 MLT-treated animals had sludge less than 5% of bile volume, and the other 5 had no sludge at all.

Stone and Sludge Examination

The morphology and chemical composition of the stones displayed the characteristics of a human brown pigment gallstone as reported previously.15 Both biliary sludge and stones shared the same infrared spectra characteristics, with broad peaks corresponding to calcium bilirubinate and amide I peak of protein in the absorbency region 1,600-1,640 cm [156] and to calcium palmitate in 2,900 to 2,940 cm [156]. No carbonate (870 cm by Brown et al. [156]) was detected. The peak height in the 1,600 to 1,640 cm [156] and 2,900 to 2,940 cm [156] region per milligram of the sludge gradually increased as the ligation periods increased.

MLT Moderated Ligation-Induced Oxidative Stress in Bile

Biliary TAA decreased progressively after ligation (ANOVA, $P < .0001$). In guinea pigs subjected to 14 days of ligation, biliary TAA was reduced to 35% of that in control animals ($P < .001$). The biliary MDA was significantly increased by (1.321 vs. 0.744 mmol/L, 14-day ligation vs. control, $P < .05$). MLT treatment at a dose of 1,000 mg/kg significantly increased biliary TAA and decreased biliary MDA as compared to no treatment group (*P* =.004 and *P* =.015, respectively). Serum TAA did not change significantly during stone formation, whereas serum MDA increased 54% at day 14 after ligation (*P* , .05), but MLT treatment failed to return this increased MDA to the control level.

Biliary Contents in Bile Duct–Ligated Guinea Pigs with or without MLT

The results of administration of MLT at 100mg/kg or 1,000 mg/kg on biliary contents other than indicators of oxidative stress in bile duct–ligated guinea pigs reveals that the pH and bile salts concentration increased progressively as the duration of ligation increased (ANOVA, $P < .001$). Protein and calcium concentrations also increased significantly, but reached a maximum at day 7 and 9 after ligation, respectively. Bilirubins, on the other hand, decreased significantly at day 9 after ligation. MLT treatment reduced the protein concentration to the control level at day 7 after ligation. At a dose of 1,000 mg/kg, MLT significantly reduced the ligation-induced elevation of pH ($P < .01$) and bile salts concentration ($P < .01$) at day 14.

In the **discussion** section, Shiesh et al.'s study showed a link between oxidative stress and pigment gallstone formation induced by bile duct ligation in guinea pigs. Oxidative stress as shown by MDA and TAA in bile changed during the course of stone formation. Antioxidant treatment with MLT not only reversed the increased oxidative stress, but also prevented gallstone formation. These results indicate that oxidative stress plays a vital role in the formation of pigment gallstone. Christian and Rege [81] showed that methionine protected against pigment gallstone formation in dogs fed a lithogenic diet. The protective effect of methionine was unclear but it might be mediated in part by its antioxidant properties. Free radicals seem to play a role in both cholesterol and pigment gallstone formation. Eder et al. [144] showed that the initiation of cholesterol gallstone in model bile was induced by reactive oxygen metabolites and that hydroxyl radical reaction appeared to be a promoter of crystallization of cholesterol. The accelerated dissolution of cholesterol stone by the use of 2-mercaptoethanol and N-acetylcysteine, which are thio-compound antioxidants, [160] further indicate the importance of oxidative stress in gallstone formation. Grace et al.24 showed that bile stasis could promote gallstone formation by increasing the residence time for crystallization and stone growth in the gallbladder. Mechanical obstruction of the biliary tract may also lead to bacterial degradation of bile pigment and the deposition of calcium salts of fatty acids in human brown pigment stones. [3] Vitek and Carey's previous results showed the activity of bacterial β-glucuronidase did not increase in bile after ligation, and the infected animals died in the first week of the experiment. The induced pigment sludge and stone were therefore mainly a result of stasis and nonenzymatic hydrolysis of conjugated bilirubins by Chen et al. [155] Although guinea pig bile is quite different from human bile in the concentrations of bilirubin and lipid and in the proportions of bilirubin monoglucuronide and bilirubin diglucuronide, the induced pigment sludge and gallstones in our ligated animals were chemically and morphologically similar to the pigment stone in humans, indicating that the pathogenesis may be the same. Therefore, it is justified to use this animal model to study the effect of oxidative. In general, direct measurement of free radical is impractical because it is highly reactive and has a short half-life. Therefore, we measured MDA, one of the products formed during the radical-induced decomposition of polyunsaturated fatty acid, and used it as an indicator of oxidative damage by Valenzvela, Ohkawa and Hallwell et al. [161-163] Shiesh et al. also measured the change of antioxidant activity. Antioxidants are a defense mechanism of the body and the level of antioxidants in body fluids has been used as an indicator for the severity of oxidative stress by Hallwell et al. [163] In Shiesh et al.'s study, they measured total rather than individual antioxidant activity, because individual antioxidant has its specific role and measurement of a specific antioxidant activity may not adequately represent oxidative stress *per se*. [164] In addition, recent studies have suggested that reduction in total antioxidant activity, rather than any single plasma antioxidant, contributed to the development of diabetic vascular complications. Their results showed a significant increase of oxidative stress in bile after ligation and MLT treatment could alleviate the stress. Nevertheless, the change in serum oxidative stress was not consistent and only MDA increased significantly at day 14 after ligation. Furthermore, MLT treatment did not significantly change serum TAA and MDA levels. These results suggested that the oxidative indicators in bile were a better parameter to assess the oxidative stress in gallstone formation. A significant increase in the biliary protein concentration was seen only at day 7 but not at other time points after ligation, suggesting the involvement of proteins in the early stage of gallstone formation by Strasberg et al. [143, 165] A previous *in vitro* study has shown that oxygen radicals stimulated rapid release of mucous-type glycoproteins from guinea pig gallbladder epithelium. [143] As mucin-glycoproteins are suggested to be the initiator of gallstone, [148, 166] the excessive secretion of mucin/glycoproteins induced by oxidative stress may account for the change. MLT pretreatment reduced the ligation-induced increase in biliary protein concentration accompanying a reduction of sludge and stone formation. Thus, the effect of MLT on cholelithiasis seemed to reduce oxidative stress and interfere biliary protein release during the early stage of the process. Increased bile salts concentration was also observed in ligated guinea pigs. Bile salts are a potent nucleating agent, able to stimulate the release of gallbladder glycoproteins in gallbladder explants by O'Leary et al. [167]. The treatment of MLT in ligated guinea pigs decreased the contents of bile salts and protein in bile. Collectively, our results suggested that the mechanism of MLT in preventing gallstone formation might be through the change of bile salts and protein concentrations. MLT treatment did not protect against ligation-induced changes in ionized calcium and bilirubins of the bile. The time course study of sludge suggested that the decrease in bile pigment in bile after ligation was probably caused by the incorporation of the pigments into the sludge or stones. The reason why MLT treatment decreased biliary bilirubins below the control levels is unknown. However, the interpretation of bilirubin or calcium in bile might be difficult because of their coprecipitation in the sludge and stones. Therefore, the determination of bilirubins or calcium in bile alone might not sufficiently elucidate the gallstone states.

Bile duct obstruction resulted in an enhanced oxidative stress in gallbladder associated with an increased incidence of pigment gallstone formation in guinea pigs. The role of oxidative stress in the pigment gallstone was probably related to its role in promoting the formation of a mucin-glycoprotein layer in gallbladder that would allow the precipitation of calcium bilirubinate and the oxidation of unconjugated bilirubin to form stones. MLT treatment, on the other hand, was associated with a significant decrease in oxidative stress and the incidence of gallstone formation. Collectively, these results suggest prophylactic and therapeutic roles of antioxidant defense on pigment gallstone. Further studies are needed to examine the potential of MLT in preventing pigment stone formation in patients with bile duct stenosis or the prevention of stent occlusion.

VI. Possible Relationship between Intestinal Barrier Function and Formation of Pigment Gallstones in Hamsters [70]

The presence of bacteria in bile is an important factor in the formation of pigment gallstones. The bile of healthy people is sterile and bacteria in the biliary system come from endogenous infection from the gut. Yet, the route of bacterial translocation into the bile duct is still unclear. Theoretically, two routes exist: one is through the intestinal barrier and the other is by direct reflux from the sphincter of Oddi. This study was undertaken to explore the relationship between the effectiveness of intestinal barrier and the formation of pigment gallstones in hamsters.

In the **methods** section, thirty-two hamsters were divided into an experimental and a control group, with 16 hamsters in each group. A low protein and high cellulose diet was given for 6 weeks to induce the formation of pigment gallstones in the experimental group (PS) and a normal diet was given to the control group (CON). Morphological changes, changes in the levels of serum endotoxin and diamine oxidase, and changes in the numbers of B lymphocytes, plasma cells and secretory immunoglobin A (sIgA) in the intestinal mucosa were assessed after 6 weeks. The results showed four hamsters died during lithogenesis and body weight decreased in the PS group. Pigment gallstones were found in 11 hamsters at the end of the experiment, giving a lithogenesis rate of 91.67%. The serum endotoxin level before and after gallstone formation in the PS group was 0.2960±0.1734 U/ml and 8.2964±4.6268 U/ml, respectively ($P<0.05$). The blood diamine oxidase level before and after gallstone formation in the PS group was 2.6333±0.8037 U/ml and 3.3642±0.9545 U/ml, respectively ($P<0.05$). The numbers of B lymphocytes, plasma cells and sIgA in the intestinal mucosa in the PS group were 71.56± 2.89, 68.65±2.09 and 27.56±1.07, respectively, and were significantly decreased compared with the corresponding values in the CON group (94.25±3.69, 93.47±3.98 and 42.57±1.96, respectively, $P<0.05$).

Conclusion

A low protein and high cellulose diet can markedly reduce intestinal barrier function and facilitate the formation of pigment gallstones. The decrease of intestinal barrier function may take part in the formation of pigment gallstone.

Bile duct pigment stone still represents a high proportion of cholelithiasis, and the mortality rate of acute obstructive suppurative cholangitis remains high. [168] Although improved endoscopic or laparoscopic surgery has been minimal invasive to patients in the treatment of this disease, the high postoperative recurrence rate is still an obstacle for the attainment of long-term satisfactory results. Thus, it is necessary to study the etiology of biliary pigment stones. The presence of bacteria in the bile duct is an important factor in the formation of pigment gallstones by Swidsinski, Stewart and Wu et al. [169-174] Yet, the route of bacterial translocation into the duct is still a question. Is there a relationship between intestinal barrier and pigment gallstone formation? And, if so, how does it work? To further test this notion and ascertain the potential mechanism, hamsters fed on a low protein and high cellulose diet were studied, and the serum levels of endotoxin and diamine oxidase and number of B lymphocytes, plasma cells and secretory immunoglobin A (sIgA) in the intestinal mucosa, which reflect intestinal barrier function, were measured.

Thirty-two female hamsters, 15 weeks old with body weight 130 to 150 g were supplied by the Laboratory Animal Center of China Medical University Shenyang, China. They were randomly assigned to a pigment gallstones group (PS) and a control group (CON), with 16 hamsters in each group. A low protein and high cellulose diet and a standard diet were fed to the PS and CON groups, respectively under the same living conditions for 6 weeks. Blood samples of 1.5 ml were collected by puncture of the orbital vein with a mini tube before and 6 weeks after the administration of the lithogenic diet in the PS group. After the blood samples were centrifuged at 3500 rpm, a supernatant of 0.5 ml from each sample was collected and stored at -20°C for analysis. The low protein and high cellulose diet was given to induce gallstone formation. Six weeks later, cholecystectomy was performed to search for gallstones. If stones were found, they were washed with water, dried naturally and stored carefully. The concentrations of serum endotoxin and diamine oxidase before and after stone formation in the PS group were measured by the dynamic turbidity method and the flicker photometer method, respectively by Klebtsov and Sun et al. [175, 176] The mucosal structure of the terminal ileum in each group was studied after HE staining. The numbers of B lymphocytes, plasma cells and sIgA in the mucosa of the terminal ileum in each group were assessed by immunohistochemistry. The data were expressed as mean ± standard error. The SPSS 14.0 software was applied to the analysis of the data by paired-samples t test and independent samples t test. A P value less than 0.05 was considered statistically significant.

In the **results section,** four hamsters died during lithogenesis, giving a mortality rate of 25%. Body weight decreased during the experiment, with loss of hair in some malnourished hamsters in the PS group. Pigment gallstones were found in 11 hamsters at the end of the experiment, giving a lithogenesis rate of 91.67% in the PS group. In the CON group, the hamsters were healthy and no gallstones were found at the end of 6 weeks. The serum endotoxin levels before and after gallstone formation in the PS group were 0.296 0.1734 U/ml and 8.2964±4.6268 U/ml, respectively. The blood diamine oxidase levels before and after gallstone formation in the PS group were 2.6333± 0.8037 U/ml and 3.3642±0.9545 U/ml, respectively. Both increased after stone formation with statistically significant differences (t=6.0596, P<0.001 and t=4.1984, P=0.002, respectively). Compared with that of the CON group, the structure of intestinal mucosa cells of the PS group showed some signs of disorder: unevenness in microvilli with reduced surface area. The distribution of cells in the mucosa became concentrated with massive infiltration of inflammatory cells. The numbers of B lymphocytes, plasma cells and sIgA in the intestinal mucosa of the terminal ileum in the PS group were 71.56±2.89, 68.65±2.09 and 27.56± 1.07, respectively, which were significantly decreased compared with the corresponding numbers in the CON group (94.25±3.69, 93.47±3.98 and 42.57±1.96, respectively, t=17.6072, P<0.001, t=19.6082, P<0.001 and t=23.9175, P<0.001, respectively).

In the **discussion** section, the bile of healthy people is sterile. Infection of the biliary system arises from endogenous infection of the gut. Theoretically, the bacteria in the gut can enter the bile duct in two ways: one is through intestinal barrier and the other is by reflux from the sphincter of Oddi. The intestinal barrier serves as an effective defense to limit systemic contamination by intraluminal microbes or their products. Changes of the intestinal barrier are associated with many events, such as burns, wounds, and pancreatitis. One of the key pathological factors leading to these changes is bacterial translocation and endotoxemia due to intestinal hyperpermeability. This study demonstrated increased intestinal permeability after the formation of pigment gallstones in an animal model. Endotoxin is lipid polysaccharide on the cell wall of gram-negative bacilli, especially intestinal bacilli. Under normal conditions, it cannot enter the circulation because of the integrity of the intestinal barrier. When the function of the intestinal barrier is in disorder, endotoxin can penetrate into the mucosa and lead to endotoxemia. Measurement of the endotoxin level in serum is an important method of assessing the functional status of the intestinal barrier. [10] This study found that the level of serum endothelin increased markedly after formation of pigment gallstones in hamsters, indicating that a low protein and high cellulose diet increases intestinal permeability and facilitates stone formation. Diamine oxidase occurs in the mucosa or villus layer of mammals and is regarded as the marker enzyme of the intestinal mucosa. Its activity is closely related to the synthesis of nucleic acids and proteins in cells. Normally, the activity of diamine oxidase in serum is very low. In case of intestinal barrier dysfunction, diamine oxidase released from cells of the intestinal mucosa enters the blood, leading to a rise in its concentration by Hilsden et al. [177]. Thus, serum diamine oxidase activity is an ideal index reflecting the integrity of intestinal mucosal structure. In Fan et al.'s study, the level of serum diamine oxidase increased after formation of pigment gallstones in hamsters, also indicating that a low protein and high cellulose diet increases intestinal permeability and facilitates stone formation. In Fan et al.'s study, morphological analysis of the intestinal mucosa showed that part of the epithelium in the PS group exhibited signs of degeneration and inflammation, which were almost absent in the CON group, further suggesting that the intestinal mechanical barrier is disturbed in animals with gallstone formation. B lymphocytes, plasma cells and sIgA constitute a major part of the intestinal immunity barrier: humoral immunity by Czyczewska-Buczynska et al. [178] A close relationship exists between the number of lymphocytes and their function. [179] In this study, we found that the numbers of B lymphocytes, plasma cells and sIgA in the intestinal mucosa of the terminal ileum in the PS group decreased compared with the corresponding numbers in the CON group. This finding indicates that the intestinal immunity barrier is disrupted and the generation of an effective immune chain is interrupted. These changes can lead to increased bacterial translocation.(180) Just as in the animal model, the occurrence of hyperpermeability of the intestine in patients who have undergone choledocholithotomy may play a role in the high recurrence rate of choledocholithiasis. Intestinal bacteria and endotoxin reach the hepatobiliary system more easily in patients with hyperpermeability. Some bacteria in the hepatobiliary system can produce β-glucuronidase and phospholipase, which can respectively hydrolyze conjugated bilirubin and lecithin. The products, unconjugated bilirubin and palmitic acid, precipitate with calcium to form gallstones. Endotoxin can activate the hepatocytes, biliary epithelial cells or leukocytes in the bile to release endogenous β-glucuronidase by a cytotoxic effect or other mechanisms by Osnes and Wu et al. [181, 182] The hyperpermeability and impaired local immunity of the intestine we demonstrated in an animal model provide indirect evidence that bacteria can pass through the intestinal mucosa barrier into the hepatobiliary system due to bacterial translocation. Clinically, we find that the poor and malnourished are more vulnerable to choledocholithiasis or intrahepatic lithiasis. One reason may be the lack of glucaro-1, 4-lactone, a β-glucuronidase inhibitor, which facilitates the deconjugation reaction of bilirubin by Sacco et al. [183] Another reason is that low protein and malnutrition decreases resistance, causing decreased regeneration of epithelium in the bile duct and increasing the incidence of infection of the bile duct. [184] From this study, we think that a low intake of protein and fat may negatively affect the growth and development of the intestinal mucosa. As a result, mucosal integrity is damaged and hyperpermeability together with impaired local immunity occurs. Then intestinal bacteria translocate into the hepatobiliary system, playing a role in gallstone formation. Agents that protect the intestinal mucosa may be effective in the prevention of the formation and recurrence of gallstones by Ding and Li et al. [185-187].

In summary, there is a relationship between decreased intestinal barrier function and pigment gallstones in hamsters. A low protein and high cellulose diet significantly can reduce intestinal barrier function and facilitate the formation of pigment gallstones. We conclude that dysfunction of the intestinal barrier may play a role in the process of gallstone formation via the mechanism of secondary bacterial translocation, endotoxemia, and the activity of endogenous and exogenous β-glucuronidase.

VII. Effects of Variant UDP-Glucuronosyltransferase 1A1 Gene Glucose-6-Phosphate Dehydrogenase Deficiency and Thalassemia on Cholelithiasis [188, 189]

To test the hypothesis that the variant UDPglucuronosyltransferase 1A1 (UGT1A1) gene, glucose-6- phosphate dehydrogenase (G6PD) deficiency, and thalassemia influence bilirubin metabolism and play a role in the development of cholelithiasis. A total of 372 Taiwan Chinese with cholelithiasis who had undergone cholecystectomy and 293 healthy individuals were divided into case and control groups, respectively. PCR and restriction fragment length polymorphism were used to analyze the promoter area and nucleotides 211, 686, 1 091, and 1 456 of the UGT1A1 gene for all subjects and the gene variants for thalassemia and G6PD deficiency. Variation frequencies for the cholelithiasis patients were 16.1%, 25.8%, 5.4%, and 4.3% for A(TA)6 TAA/A(TA)7TAA (6/7), heterozygosity within the coding region, compound heterozygosity, and homozygosity of the UGT1A1 gene, respectively. Comparing the case and control groups, a statistically significant difference in frequency was demonstrated for the homozygous variation of the UGT1A1 gene ($P = 0.012$, $\chi 2$ test), but not for the other variations. Further, no difference was demonstrated in a between-group comparison of the incidence of G6PD deficiency and thalassemia (2.7% vs. 2.4% and 5.1% vs. 5.1%, respectively). The bilirubin levels for the cholelithiasis patients with the homozygous variant-UGT1A1 gene were significantly different from the control analog (18.0±6.5 and 12.7±2.9 μmol/L, respectively; $P<0.001$, Student's t test).

Conclusion

Our results show that the homozygous variation in the UGT1A1 gene is a risk factor for the development of cholelithiasis in Taiwan Chinese. The life span of erythrocytes in individuals with chronic hemolytic disease is short relative to normal subjects. The accelerated red-cell turnover produces more bilirubin and is probably a risk factor for the development of gallstones. Cholelithiasis has been detected in 38% of subjects with chronic hemolytic anemia due to glucose-6-phosphate dehydrogenase (G6PD) deficiency. [190]. It has been demonstrated that G6PD-deficient subjects without chronic hemolytic anemia also have a higher frequency of cholelithiasis development than normal individuals [1]. Because the enzyme UDP-glucuronosyltransferase 1A1 (UGT1A1) catalyzes unconjugated bilirubin into the diglucuronidated and conjugated forms, UGT1A1 defects decrease the elimination of bilirubin [2]. Genetic variation in the *UGT1A1* gene promoter, A(TA)7TAA, instead of A(TA)6TAA influences bilirubin levels causing hyperbilirubinemia, which is associated with Gilbert's syndrome in Caucasians. [191] Further, it has been determined that *UGT1A1* gene expression is a major modifying factor for bilirubin levels in heterozygous β-thalassemia [192] and that cholelithiasis is one of the manifestations of thalassemia. [193] In a previous study of the *UGT1A1* gene in Taiwan Chinese,(194) they found that occurrence of the A(TA)7TAA allele in the promoter area was relatively rare (14.3% *vs.* 40%) and that the variation rate within the coding region was much higher (29.3% *vs.* 0.1%) relative to Caucasians, [191] respectively. The aim of this study was to analyze variations in the promoter area and coding region in the *UGT1A1* gene in Taiwan Chinese patients with cholelithiasis. The incidence and genetic expression of G6PD deficiency in these subjects was also investigated. Additionally, Huang et al. studied the genetic alteration of thalassemia. Variations in the *UGT1A1*, *G6PD* and thalassemia genes were compared with those of normal subjects. To our knowledge, this is the first report elucidating the relationship between these three genes and cholelithiasis.

In the **materials and methods** section, the study subjects (157 males and 215 females) were selected from Taiwan Chinese adults who had undergone cholecystectomy for symptomatic gallstone. Healthy controls (135 males and 158 females) were selected from adults who had undergone physical examination at Cathay General Hospital as previously described. The control subjects were investigated for cholelithiasis by abdominal ultrasonography (model SSD-1700, Aloka Co., Tokyo, Japan) and no change in abdomen was determined with respect to gallstones. Blood samples were collected from all subjects in the morning after 10-12 h of fasting. An automatic cell-counter (NE 9000, Sysmex Co., Kobe, Japan) was used for hematology testing, and erythrocyte G6PD activity was quantitatively measured using the enzyme-coupled method. G6PD deficiency was confirmed by polymerase chain reaction-restriction fragment length polymorphism (PCR-RFLP).(195) The 15 single-nucleotide mutations, restriction enzymes, and restriction-fragment results are listed in Table 3.7.1 and Table 3.7.2, with priority arranged in descending order of mutation frequency of our Taiwan Chinese sample population by Huang et al. [195]. The promoter area and nucleotides 211, 686, 1 091, and 1 456 of the *UGT1A1* gene were amplified by PCR and analyzed using RFLP by Huang et al. [196] The restriction enzymes and restriction-fragment results are listed in Table 3.7.2. Mean corpuscular volume 80 fL, the gene variants for α- and β-thalassemia were identified using PCR-RFLP. [197, 198].

Comparison of Bilirubin Values

Serum bilirubin levels were measured using an autoanalyzer (model 747, Hitachi Co., Tokyo, Japan). The bilirubin values in cholelithiasis patients with statistically significant differences in gene frequency relative to controls were obtained from the records made 2-3 months after cholecystectomy and compared with that in the control group.

Statistical Analysis

The χ^2 test, with or without Yate's correction, and Student's *t* test were used to analyze the data as appropriate. A *P* value less than 0.05 was defined as statistically significant.

In the **results** section, 6PD deficiency was confirmed for 4 of the 157 males (2.5%) and 6 of the 215 females (2.8%) cholelithiasis patients, with respective gender distribution as follows: hemizygous 493, 871, 1 024, and 1 388 (n = 1 each), and heterozygous 1 376 (n = 5) and heterozygous 1 388 (n = 1) (data not shown in Tables).

Table 3.7.1. Fifteen single nucleotide mutations of G6PD deficiency in Taiwan Chines

		Restriction	fragment (bp)
Mutation site	Restriction enzyme	Normal	Mutant
1 376 G T	*Afl*II	214	194, 202
1 388 G A	*Nde*I	227	06, 21
		120, 11	
493 A G	*Ava*II	187	87, 33, 11
1 024 C T	*Mbo*II	142, 45	150, 37
		198	
1 360 C T	*Hha*I	188	27 187, 27
95 A G	*Mlu*I	157, 83	174, 24
		134	
392 G	T *Bst*EII	49	15 203
592 C T	*Pst*I1	105	57, 63, 20
517 T C	*Xho*I		114, 20
1 004 C A	*Hha*I		20 69
1 387 C T	*Hha*I		22 127

Table 3.7.2. Variations of the UGT1A1 gene

		Restriction	fragment (bp)
Variation site	Restriction enzyme	Normal	Variant
211 G A	*Ava*II	128	18 146
686 C A	*Bsr*I	374, 51	242, 132, 51
1 091 C T	*Bcl*I	209	190, 19
1 456 T G	*Ava*II	270	197, 73
		77	
Promoter			

There was no significant between-gender difference in incidence of G6PD deficiency. Analysis of pooled data showed an overall incidence of G6PD deficiency of 2.7% (10/372) for the cholelithiasis group. The frequencies of the *UGT1A1* genotypes are presented in Table 3. Less than half (48.4%) of the cholelithiasis patients carried the wild genotype. The variation frequencies for A(TA)6TAA/A(TA)7TAA (6/7), heterozygosity within the coding region, compound heterozygosity, and homozygosity were 16.1%, 25.8%, 5.4%, and 4.3%, respectively. The incidence of thalassemia in the cholelithiasis patients was 5.1% (19/372) [heterozygous α-thalassemia 2.7% (*n* = 10); heterozygous β-thalassemia 1.6% (*n* = 6); homozygous β-thalassemia 0.53% (*n* = 2); and heterozygous α-thalassemia plus heterozygous β-thalassemia 0.27% (*n* = 1)] (detailed data not shown in Tables). Analysis for the combination of G6PD deficiency, homozygous variation in the *UGT1A1* gene, and presence of thalassemia revealed that two cholelithiasis patients carried the 211 G A/211 G A *UGT1A1* and the heterozygous α-thalassemia genes (data not shown in Tables). Clinical data for the cholelithiasis patients and healthy controls are compared in Table 3.7.3. There was no difference in gender distribution, neither in the mean of age, comparing the two groups. A significant difference was demonstrated comparing the frequency of homozygous variation (7/7, 211 G A/211 G A, and 686 C A plus 7/7) of the *UGT1A1* gene for the case and control groups ($P = 0.012$, χ^2 test), while those for the other three variation types were not statistically meaningful. There was no significant between-group difference in the incidence of G6PD deficiency and thalassemia (2.7% *vs.* 2.4% and 5.1% *vs.* 5.1%, with the homozygous variant-*UGT1A1* gene had bilirubin levels 17.1 μmol/L (upper limit of normal reference value) with significant difference between means in comparing the 16 patients with the controls [18.0±6.5 μmol/L (range 6.8-32.5 μmol/L) and 12.7±2.9 μmol/L (range 6.8-17.1 μmol/L), respectively; $P<0.001$, Student's *t* test] (data not shown in Tables).

In the **discussion** section, no gender difference has been demonstrated in the incidence of variant *UGT1A1* gene and thalassemia, while G6PD deficiency is X-linkage transmitted by Beutler et al. [199] In this study, as the male/female ratio was approximately equal for the case and control groups, the genders were pooled for analysis. More than 50% of the members of both groups had at least one heterozygous variation in the *UGT1A1* gene, while the frequency of homozygous variation differed between groups. The 686 C A variation was associated with the 6/7 or 7/7 variation for both study subjects and the controls, as observed in our previous studies. [194-196, 200, 201]. In the present investigation, however, the 7/7 and 686 C A plus 7/7 variations were found only in the case group (Table 3.7.2). Since bilirubin may be affected by cholelithiasis status, bilirubin values were obtained for cholelithiasis patients with the homozygous variant-*UGT1A1* gene from the records which were made 2-3 months post cholecystectomy. UGT1A1 enzyme activity was found to be 18-33% of normal in individuals with the 7/7 variation of the *UGT1A1* gene.(191) In another *in vitro* gene-expression study,(202) subjects bearing the homozygous 211 G A variant-*UGT1A1* gene were demonstrated to have 32.2% of the UGT1A1 enzyme activity of normal analogs. Moreover, coinheritance of heterozygous α-thalassemia gene was observed in two of our four cholelithiasis patients who carried the homozygous 211 G A variation. These findings may account for the significant difference in serum bilirubin levels in cholelithiasis patients with the homozygous variant-*UGT1A1* gene (7/7, 211 G A/211 G A, and 686 C A plus 7/7) related to controls. Although it has been determined that G6PD deficiency and thalassemia are risk factors for cholelithiasis development in Caucasians by Meloni and Tunaci et al., [190, 193] these associations were not observed in our sample, with no between-group difference in incidences of these two factors were noted. This discrepancy may be due to the ethnic differences between the sample populations. Co-inheritance of the homozygous variant-*UGT1A1* gene and G6PD deficiency may lead to pronounced hyperbilirubinemia in adults, [201] and coinheritance of Gilbert's syndrome and hereditary spherocytosis may increase the risk for developing gallstones [24]. However, these co-inheritances were not noted in this study. Structural analysis of gallstones from a sample of Taiwan Chinese patients revealed that a relatively small proportion of the gallstones were composed of bilirubin (pure cholesterol 35%, combination 12%, mixed 17%, black 25%, calcium bilirubinate 8%, and unclassified 3%) by Kiu et al. [203]. It is not surprising, therefore, that only 4.3% of our cholelithiasis patients carried the homozygous variant-*UGT1A1* gene, which leads to the bilirubin accumulation and is a risk factor for cholelithiasis. We suggest that investigation of cholelithiasis status and carriage of variant *UGT1A1* gene for specific subpopulations, such as G6PD-deficient or thalassemic Taiwan Chinese, is a superior alternative in genetic research for gallstones. A research program of this type is ongoing at the Cathay General Hospital.

References

[1] Vitek, L., and Carey, M.C. 2012. New pathophysiological concepts underlying pathogenesis of pigment gallstones. *Clin Res Hepatol Gastroenterol* 36:122-129.

[2] Schafmayer, C., Hartleb, J., Tepel, J., Albers, S., Freitag, S., Volzke, H., Buch, S., Seeger, M., Timm, B., Kremer, B., et al. 2006. Predictors of gallstone composition in 1025 symptomatic gallstones from Northern Germany. *BMC Gastroenterol* 6:36.

[3] Cahalane, M.J., Neubrand, M.W., and Carey, M.C. 1988. Physical-chemical pathogenesis of pigment gallstones. *Semin Liver Dis* 8:317-328.

[4] Suzuki, N., Nakamura, Y., Kobayashi, N., and Sato, T. 1975. On metal elements in pure pigment gallstones. *Tohoku J Exp Med* 116:233-240.

[5] Tsunoda, K., Shirai, Y., Wakai, T., Yokoyama, N., Akazawa, K., and Hatakeyama, K. 2004. Increased risk of cholelithiasis after esophagectomy. *J Hepatobiliary Pancreat Surg* 11:319-323.

[6] Strauss, K.A., Robinson, D.L., Vreman, H.J., Puffenberger, E.G., Hart, G., and Morton, D.H. 2006. Management of hyperbilirubinemia and prevention of kernicterus in 20 patients with Crigler-Najjar disease. *Eur J Pediatr* 165:306-319.

[7] Pavel, S., Thijs, C.T., Potocky, V., and Knipschild, P.G. 1992. Fair, and still a sun lover: risk of gallstone formation. *J Epidemiol Community Health* 46:425-427.

[8] Lund, H., and Jacobsen, J. 1972. Influence of phototherapy on unconjugated bilirubins in duodenal bile of newborn infants with hyperbilirubinemia. *Acta Pædiatrica* 61:693-696.

[9] Agati, G., Fusi, F., Pratesi, S., Galvan, P., and Donzelli, G. 1998. Bilirubin photoisomerization products in serum and urine from a Crigler-Najjar type I patient treated by phototherapy. *J Photochem Photobiol* 47:9.

[10] Wolkoff, A.W., Chowdhury, J.R., Gartner, L.A., Rose, A.L., Biempica, L., Giblin, D.R., Fink, D., and Arias, I.M. 1979. Clinical conference. Crigler-Najjar syndrome (type I) in an adult male. *Gastroenterology* 76:840-848.

[11] Ostrow, J.D. 1971. Photocatabolism of labeled bilirubin in the congenitally jaundiced (Gunn) rat. *J Clin Invest* 50:707-718.

[12] Onishi, S., Itoh, S., Isobe, K., Togari, H., Kitoh, H., and Nishimura, Y. 1982. Mechanism of development of bronze baby syndrome in neonates treated with phototherapy. *Pediatrics* 69:273-276.

[13] Robins, S.J., Fasulo, J.M., and Patton, G.M. 1982. Lipids of pigment gallstones. *Biochim Biophys Acta* 712:21-25.

[14] Kaufman, H.S., Magnuson, T.H., Lillemoe, K.D., Frasca, P., and Pitt, H.A. 1989. The role of bacteria in gallbladder and common duct stone formation. *Ann Surg* 209:584-591; discussion 591-582.

[15] Rana, S.S., Bhasin, D.K., Nanda, M., and Singh, K. 2007. Parasitic infestations of the biliary tract. *Curr Gastroenterol Rep* 9:156-164.

[16] Stewart, L., Smith, A.L., Pellegrini, C.A., Motson, R.W., and Way, L.W. 1987. Pigment gallstones form as a composite of bacterial microcolonies and pigment solids. *Ann Surg* 206:242-250.

[17] Sauerbruch, J., Stellaard, F., Soehendra, N., and Paumgartner, G. 1980. Cholesterol content of bile-duct stones. *Disch Med Wochenschr* 122:4.

[18] Sandstad, O., Osnes, T., Skar, V., Urdal, P., and Osnes, M. 1994. Common bile duct stones are mainly brown and associated with duodenal diverticula. *Gut* 35:1464-1467.

[19] Jang, J.S., Kim, K.H., Yu, J.R., and Lee, S.U. 2007. Identification of parasite DNA in common bile duct stones by PCR and DNA sequencing. *Korean J Parasitol* 45:301-306.

[20] Sripa, B., Kanla, P., Sinawat, P., and Haswell-Elkins, M.R. 2004. Opisthorchiasis-associated biliary stones: light and scanning electron microscopic study. *World J Gastroenterol* 10:3318-3321.

[21] Akiyoshi, T., and Nakayama, F. 1990. Bile acid composition in brown pigment stones. *Dig Dis Sci* 35:27-32.

[22] Gu, J.J., Hofmann, A.F., Ton-Nu, H.T., Schteingart, C.D., and Mysels, K.J. 1992. Solubility of calcium salts of unconjugated and conjugated natural bile acids. *J Lipid Res* 33:635-646.

[23] Nakanuma, Y., Terada, T., Nagakawa, T., Kakita, A., Yoshikawa, T., Ohta, G., Yamaguchi, K., and Yamamoto, K. 1988. Pathology of hepatolithiasis associated with biliary malformation in Japan. *Liver* 8:287-292.

[24] del Giudice, E.M., Perrotta, S., Nobili, B., Specchia, C., d'Urzo, G., and Iolascon, A. 1999. Coinheritance of Gilbert syndrome increases the risk for developing gallstones in patients with hereditary spherocytosis. *Blood* 94:2259-2262.

[25] Chaar, V., Keclard, L., Diara, J.P., Leturdu, C., Elion, J., Krishnamoorthy, R., Clayton, J., and Romana, M. 2005. Association of UGT1A1 polymorphism with prevalence and age at onset of cholelithiasis in sickle cell anemia. *Haematologica* 90:188-199.

[26] Premawardhena, A., Fisher, C.A., Fathiu, F., de Silva, S., Perera, W., Peto, T.E., Olivieri, N.F., and Weatherall, D.J. 2001. Genetic determinants of jaundice and gallstones in haemoglobin E beta thalassaemia. *Lancet* 357:1945-1946.

[27] Azemoto, R., Tsuchiya, Y., Ai, T., Murayama, H., Nakagawa, Y., Saisho, H., and Ohto, M. 1996. Does gallstone formation after open cardiac surgery result only from latent hemolysis by replaced valves? *Am J Gastroenterol* 91:2185-2189.

[28] Chawla, L.S., Sidhu, G., Sabharwal, B.D., Bhatia, K.L., and Sood, A. 1989. Jaundice in Plasmodium falciparum. *J Assoc Physicians India* 37:390-391.

[29] Diehl, A.K., Schwesinger, W.H., Holleman, D.R., Jr., Chapman, J.B., and Kurtin, W.E. 1995. Clinical correlates of gallstone composition: distinguishing pigment from cholesterol stones. *Am J Gastroenterol* 90:967-972.

[30] Weight, L.M., Byrne, M.J., and Jacobs, P. 1991. Haemolytic effects of exercise. *Clin Sci (Lond)* 81:147-152.

[31] Aydogdu, I., Sari, R., Ulu, R., and Sevinc, A. 2001. The frequency of gallbladder stones in patients with pernicious anemia. *J Surg Res* 101:120-123.

[32] Buch, S., Schafmayer, C., Volzke, H., Seeger, M., Miquel, J.F., Sookoian, S.C., Egberts, J.H., Arlt, A., Pirola, C.J., Lerch, M.M., et al. 2010. Loci from a genome-wide analysis of bilirubin levels are associated with gallstone risk and composition. *Gastroenterology* 139:1942-1951 e1942.

[33] Broulik, P.D., Haas, T., and Adamek, S. 2005. Analysis of 645 patients with primary hyperparathyroidism with special references to cholelithiasis. *Intern Med* 44:917-921.

[34] Vitek, L., and Carey, M.C. 2003. Enterohepatic cycling of bilirubin as a cause of 'black' pigment gallstones in adult life. *Eur J Clin Invest* 33:799-810.

[35] Wang, L., Shen, W., Wen, J., An, X., Cao, L., and Wang, B. 2006. An animal model of black pigment gallstones caused by nanobacteria. *Dig Dis Sci* 51:1126-1132.

[36] Shiekh, F.A., Khullar, M., and Singh, S.K. 2006. Lithogenesis: induction of renal calcifications by nanobacteria. *Urol Res* 34:53-57.

[37] Ostrow, J.D., and Mukerjee, P. 2007. Revalidation and rationale for high pKa values of unconjugated bilirubin. *BMC Biochem* 8:7.

[38] Ostrow, J., Pascolo, L., Brites, D., and Tiribelli, C. 2004. Molecular basis of bilirubin-induced neurotoxicity. *Trend Mol Med* 10:6.

[39] Ostrow, J.D., and Celic, L. 1984. Bilirubin chemistry, ionization and solubilization by bile salts. *Hepatology* 4:38S-45S.

[40] Ostrow, J.D., and Murphy, N.H. 1970. Isolation and properties of conjugated bilirubin from bile. *Biochem J* 120:311-327.

[41] Ostrow, J.D., Celic, L., and Mukerjee, P. 1988. Molecular and micellar associations in the pH-dependent stable and metastable dissolution of unconjugated bilirubin by bile salts. *J Lipid Res* 29:335-348.

[42] Smith, B.F., and LaMont, J.T. 1983. Bovine gallbladder mucin binds bilirubin in vitro. *Gastroenterology* 85:707-712.

[43] McDonagh, A.F., and Lightner, D.A. 1988. Phototherapy and the photobiology of bilirubin. *Semin Liver Dis* 8:272-283.

[44] Goresky, C.A., Gordon, E.R., Hinchey, E.J., and Fried, G.M. 1995. Bilirubin conjugate changes in the bile of gallbladders containing gallstones. *Hepatology* 21:373-382.

[45] Boonyapisit, S.T., Trotman, B.W., and Ostrow, J.D. 1978. Unconjugated bilirubin, and the hydrolysis of conjugated bilirubin, in gallbladder bile of patients with cholelithiasis. *Gastroenterology* 74:70-74.

[46] Whiting, J.F., Narciso, J.P., Chapman, V., Ransil, B.J., Swank, R.T., and Gollan, J.L. 1993. Deconjugation of bilirubin-IX alpha glucuronides: a physiologic role of hepatic microsomal beta-glucuronidase. *J Biol Chem* 268:23197-23201.

[47] Spivak, W., DiVenuto, D., and Yuey, W. 1987. Non-enzymic hydrolysis of bilirubin mono- and diglucuronide to unconjugated bilirubin in model and native bile systems. Potential role in the formation of gallstones. *Biochem J* 242:323-329.

[48] Donovan, J.M., and Carey, M.C. 1991. Physical-chemical basis of gallstone formation. *Gastroenterol Clin North Am* 20:47-66.

[49] Ostrow, J.D. 1990. Unconjugated bilirubin and cholesterol gallstone formation. *Hepatology* 12:219S-224S; discussion 224S-226S.

[50] Malet, P.F., Williamson, C.E., Trotman, B.W., and Soloway, R.D. 1986. Composition of pigmented centers of cholesterol gallstones. *Hepatology* 6:477-481.

[51] LaMont, J.T., Ventola, A.S., Trotman, B.W., and Soloway, R.D. 1983. Mucin glycoprotein content of human pigment gallstones. *Hepatology* 3:377-382.

[52] LaMont, J.T., Turner, B.S., Bernstein, S.E., and Trotman, B. 1983. Gallbladder glycoprotein secretion in mice with hemolytic anemia and pigment gallstones. *Hepatology* 3:198-200.

[53] Imano, M., Satou, T., Itoh, T., Takeyama, Y., Yasuda, A., Peng, Y.F., Shinkai, M., Haji, S., Yasuda, C., Nakai, T., et al. 2010. An immunohistochemical study of osteopontin in pigment gallstone formation. *Am Surg* 76:91-95.

[54] Brink, M.A., Mendez-Sanchez, N., and Carey, M.C. 1996. Bilirubin cycles enterohepatically after ileal resection in the rat. *Gastroenterology* 110:1945-1957.

[55] Freudenberg, F., Broderick, A.L., Yu, B.B., Leonard, M.R., Glickman, J.N., and Carey, M.C. 2008. Pathophysiological basis of liver disease in cystic fibrosis employing a DeltaF508 mouse model. *Am J Physiol Gastrointest Liver Physiol* 294:G1411-1420.

[56] Donovan, J.M., Leonard, M.R., Batta, A.K., and Carey, M.C. 1994. Calcium affinity for biliary lipid aggregates in model biles: complementary importance of bile salts and lecithin. *Gastroenterology* 107:831-846.

[57] Chadwick, V.S., Modha, K., and Dowling, R.H. 1973. Mechanism for hyperoxaluria in patients with ileal dysfunction. *N Engl J Med* 289:172-176.

[58] Verkade, H., Havinga, R., Kuipers, F., and Padbury, R.T. 1995. *Mechanism of biliary lipid secretion*: Dordrecht: Kluwer Academic Publishers. 17 pp.

[59] Apstein, M.D., and Dalecki-Chipperfield, K. 1987. Spinal cord injury is a risk factor for gallstone disease. *Gastroenterology* 92:966-968.

[60] Abadie, C., Hug, M., Kubli, C., and Gains, N. 1994. Effect of cyclodextrins and undigested starch on the loss of chenodeoxycholate in the faeces. *Biochem J* 299 (Pt 3):725-730.

[61] Kruis, W., Forstmaier, G., Scheurlen, C., and Stellaard, F. 1991. Effect of diets low and high in refined sugars on gut transit, bile acid metabolism, and bacterial fermentation. *Gut* 32:367-371.

[62] Laker, M.F., and Menzies, I.S. 1977. Increase in human intestinal permeability following ingestion of hypertonic solutions. *J Physiol* 265:881-894.

[63] Conter, R.L., Roslyn, J.J., Pitt, H.A., and DenBesten, L. 1986. Carbohydrate diet-induced calcium bilirubinate sludge and pigment gallstones in the prairie dog. *J Surg Res* 40:580-587.

[64] Holzbach, R.T. 1984. Animal models of cholesterol gallstone disease. *Hepatology* 4:191S-198S.

[65] Parekh, D., Lawson, H., and Kuyl, J. 1987. Gallstone disease among black South Africans. *S Afr Med J* 72:4.

[66] Rahman, G.A. 2005. Cholelithiasis and cholecystitis: changing prevalence in an African community. *J Natl Med Assoc* 97:1534-1538.

[67] Cummings, J.H., Southgate, D.A., Branch, W.J., Wiggins, H.S., Houston, H., Jenkins, D.J., Jivraj, T., and Hill, M.J. 1979. The digestion of pectin in the human gut and its effect on calcium absorption and large bowel function. *Br J Nutr* 41:477-485.

[68] Walters, R.L., Baird, I.M., Davies, P.S., Hill, M.J., Drasar, B.S., Southgate, D.A., Green, J., and Morgan, B. 1975. Effects of two types of dietary fibre on faecal steroid and lipid excretion. *Br Med J* 2:536-538.

[69] Fujisawa, T., and Mori, M. 1996. Influence of bile salts on betaglucuronidase activity of intestinal bacteria. *Appl Microbiol* 22:4.

[70] Nagase, M., Hikasa, Y., Soloway, R.D., Tanimura, H., Setoyama, M., and Kato, H. 1980. Gallstones in Western Japan. Factors affecting the prevalence of intrahepatic gallstones. *Gastroenterology* 78:684-690.

[71] Fan, Y., Wu, S.D., Sun, L., Fu, B.B., and Su, Y. 2008. Possible relationship between intestinal barrier function and formation of pigment gallstones in hamsters. *Hepatobiliary Pancreat Dis Int* 7:529-532.

[72] Su, Y., Wu, S., Fan, Y., Jin, J., and Zhang, Z. 2009. The preliminary experimental and clinical study of the relationship between the pigment gallstone and intestinal mucosal barrier. *J Gastroenterol Hepatol* 24:1451-1456.

[73] Whary, M., Woods, S., Muthupalani, S., and Fox, J. 2010. Pigment gallstones in germfree Swiss Webster mice. *Gastroenterology* 138(Suppl 1).

[74] Vitek, L., Kotal, P., Jirsa, M., Malina, J., Cerna, M., Chmelar, D., and Fevery, J. 2000. Intestinal colonization leading to fecal urobilinoid excretion may play a role in the pathogenesis of neonatal jaundice. *J Pediatr Gastroenterol Nutr* 30:294-298.

[75] Vitek, L., Zelenka, J., Zadinova, M., and Malina, J. 2005. The impact of intestinal microflora on serum bilirubin levels. *J Hepatol* 42:238-243.

[76] Leonard, M., Andrade, J., Whary, M., Fox, J., and MC., C. 2011. Striking alterations in bilirubin and bile salt solution chemistry of gallbladder bile in a germ-free mouse model of "black" pigment gallstones. . *Gastroenterology* 140(Suppl 1).

[77] Quintana, F.J., Basso, A.S., Iglesias, A.H., Korn, T., Farez, M.F., Bettelli, E., Caccamo, M., Oukka, M., and Weiner, H.L. 2008. Control of T(reg) and T(H)17 cell differentiation by the aryl hydrocarbon receptor. *Nature* 453:65-71.

[78] Haigh, W.G., and Lee, S.P. 2001. Identification of oxysterols in human bile and pigment gallstones. *Gastroenterology* 121:118-123.

[79] Liu, X.T., and Hu, J. 2002. Relationship between bilirubin free radical and formation of pigment gallstone. *World J Gastroenterol* 8:413-417.

[80] Shiesh, S.C., Chen, C.Y., Lin, X.Z., Liu, Z.A., and Tsao, H.C. 2000. Melatonin prevents pigment gallstone formation induced by bile duct ligation in guinea pigs. *Hepatology* 32:455-460.

[81] Christian, J.S., and Rege, R.V. 1996. Methionine, but not taurine, protects against formation of canine pigment gallstones. *J Surg Res* 61:275-281.

[82] Braganza, J.M., and Worthington, H. 1995. A radical view of gallstone aetiogenesis. *Med Hypotheses* 45:510-516.

[83] Baig, S.J., Biswas, S., Das, S., Basu, K., and Chattopadhyay, G. 2002. Histopathological changes in gallbladder mucosa in cholelithiasis: correlation with chemical composition of gallstones. *Trop Gastroenterol* 23:25-27.

[84] Maki, T. 1966. Pathogenesis of calcium bilirubinate gallstone: role of E. coli, beta-glucuronidase and coagulation by inorganic ions, polyelectrolytes and agitation. *Ann Surg* 164:90-100.

[85] Maki, T. 1961. Cholelithiasis in the Japanese. *Arch Surg* 82:599-612.

[86] Sato, T. 1961. Chemical Analysis of Gallstones. II.

[87] On Some Results of the Chemical Analysis of the Pigment Calcium Stones. *Hirosaki Med. J. (Jap.)* 12.

[88] Nakajima, H. 1960. Chemical Analysis of Gallstones. III. Results of the Chemical Analysis of Cholesterol Gallstones. *Hirosaki Med. J.* 11:. Miyake, H., and Ishiyama, F. 1930. Statistische und klinische Studien auf Grund von 754.

[89] Fallen von Cholelithiasisoperationen bei Japanem. *Deutsch. Z. Chir.* 225.

[90] Digby, K.H. 1930. Common Duct Stones of Liver Origin. *Brit. J. Surg* 17.

[91] Miyake, H. 1913. Statistische, klinische und chemische Studien zur Aetiologie der Gallenstein, mit besondered Beriicksichtigung der japanischen und deutschen Verhaltnisse. *Arch. Klin. Chir* 101.

[92] Lichtwitz, L. 1908. Zur Genese der Gallensteine. *Munch. Med. Wschr* 12.

[93] Miyake, H. 1965. Studies on Etiology and Treatment of Gallstones. *J. Jap. Med. Ass. (Jap.)* 53.

[94] Sweet, J. 1929. The Liesegang Phenomenon in Gallstones. *Colloid Sympos. Annual* 7.

[95] Tung, T., Schmauss, A., Co, N., and Lang, T. 1960. Aetiologie, Diagnose und Therapie der Leberabscesse in Nordvietnam. *Deutsch. Gesundh* 15.

[96] Cook, J., Hou, P.C., Ho, H.C., and Mc, F.A. 1954. Recurrent pyogenic cholangeitis. *Br J Surg* 42:188-203.

[97] Ong, G.B. 1962. A study of recurrent pyogenic cholangitis. *Arch Surg* 84:199-225.

[98] Stock, F.E., and Tinckler, L.F. 1955. Choledochoduodenostomy in the treatment of cholangiohepatitis. *Surg Gynecol Obstet* 101:599-606.

[99] Sato, G. 1955. Progress of Decomposition of the Dead Bodies of Ascarides in the Biliary Tract; Experimental Formation of So-called Roundworm Gallstones. *Hirosaki Med. J.* 6.

[100] Maki, T., Sato, T., Yamaguchi, I., and Saito, Y. 1964. Autopsy Incidence of Gallstones in Japan. *Tohoku J Exp Med* 84:37-45.

[101] Rains, A.J. 1962. Researches concerning the formation of gallstones. *Br Med J* 2:685-691.

[102] Isaksson, B. 1954. On the Dissolving Power of Lecithin and Bile Salts for Cholesterol in Human Bladder Bile. *Acta Soc. Med. Upsal* 59.

[103] Miyake, H., Kuwatsuka, K., Nakamura, Y., Matsuo, H., Tamesue, N., Kodama, M., Ozasa, G., Murakoshi, T., and Yoshimuta, S. 1959. On the Mechanism of Formation of Gallstones with Special Reference to Bacilli of Welch. *Saishin Igaku (Jap.)* 14.

[104] Sato, T. 1962. A study on bilirubin in pigmented calcium stones. *Tohoku J Exp Med* 77:83-95.

[105] Billing, B.H., Cole, P.G., and Lathe, G.H. 1957. The excretion of bilirubin as a diglucuronide giving the direct van den Bergh reaction. *Biochem J* 65:774-784.

[106] Schmid, R. 1956. Direct-reacting bilirubin, bilirubin glucuronide, in serum, bile and urine. *Science* 124:76-77.

[107] Talafant, E. 1956. Properties and composition of the bile pigment giving a direct diazo reaction. *Nature* 178:312.

[108] Isselbacher, K.J., and Mc, C.E. 1959. Studies on bilirubin sulfate and other nonglucuronide conjugates of bilirubin. *J Clin Invest* 38:645-651.

[109] Sato, T., and Saitoh, T. 1965. A Quantitative Fractionation Method for Bilirubin in Human Bile. *Tohoku J Exp Med* 84:329-338.

[110] Shimada, Y. 1954. Studies on the Bile Pigment in Bile. Chapter 3. Partition of 3 Bilirubin Fractions from the Bile, Especially Bilirubin Ester. *Igaku Kenkyu (Jap.)* 24.

[111] Matsushiro, T. 1965. Identification of Glucaro-1,4-Lactone in Bile as a Factor Responsible for Inhibitory Effect of Bile on Bacterial Beta-Glucuronidase. *Tohoku J Exp Med* 85:330-339.

[112] Sasaki, A. 1959. Studies on Bacterial Beta-glucuronidase. *Tohoku Igaku Zassi (Jap.)* 59.

[113] Miyake, H. 1900. Zur experimentelle Erzeugung der Gallensteine mit besonderer Beriicksichtigung des bakteriellen Verhaltens der Gallenwege. *Grenzgebreit,* 6.

[114] Bacmeister, A. 1908. Der Ausfall des Cholesterins in der Galle und seine Bedeutung fur die Pathogenese der Gallensteine. *Munch. Med. Wschr* 55.

[115] Tera, H. 1963. Sedimentation of bile constituents. *Ann Surg* 157:468-472.

[116] Matsushiro, T. 1963. Inhibitory Effect of Bile Constituents Upon Bacterial Beta-Glucuronidase Activity. I. Effect of Normal Bile. *Tohoku J Exp Med* 80:175-181.

[117] Matsushiro, T. 1965. Effect of Known Constituents of Bile on the Activity of Bacterial Beta-Glucuronidase. *Tohoku J Exp Med* 85:210-220.

[118] Marsh, C.A. 1963. Metabolism of d-glucuronolactone in mammalian systems. Identification of d-glucaric acid as a normal constituent of urine. *Biochem J* 86:77-86.

[119] Yamaguchi, I., Sato, T., Matsushiro, T., and Sato, H. 1965. Quantitative determination of D-glucaric acid in bile in relation to inhibitory effect of bile on bacterial beta-glucuronidase. *Tohoku J Exp Med* 87:123-132.

[120] Matsushiro, T., Oikawa, T., and Sato, H. 1964. Relation between Bacterial p-glucuronidase Activity and Deposition of Calcium Bilirubinate to Ascarid Eggs Inserted in Bile. *Tohoku Igaku Zassi (Jap.)* 69.

[121] Yusa, M., and Gaudin, A. 1964. Formation of Pellet-like Flocs of Kaolinate by Polymer. *Chains. Amer. Ceram. Soc. Bull.* 43.

[122] Cariati, A., and Piromalli, E. 2012. Role of parietal (gallbladder mucosa) factors in the formation of black pigment gallstones. *Clin Res Hepatol Gastroenterol* 36:e50-51.

[123] Cariati, A., and Cetta, F. 2003. Rokitansky-Aschoff sinuses of the gallbladder are associated with black pigment gallstone formation: a scanning electron microscopy study. *Ultrastruct Pathol* 27:265-270.

[124] Alvaro, D., Angelico, M., Gandin, C., Ginanni Corradini, S., and Capocaccia, L. 1990. Physico-chemical factors predisposing to pigment gallstone formation in liver cirrhosis. *J Hepatol* 10:228-234.

[125] Carey, M., and Duane, W. 1994. *Enterohepatic circulation.* New York: Raven Press. 49 pp.

[126] Love, M.W., and Dawson, P.A. 1998. New insights into bile acid transport. *Curr Opin Lipidol* 9:225-229.

[127] Gourley, G.R., and Arend, R.A. 1986. beta-Glucuronidase and hyperbilirubinaemia in breast-fed and formula-fed babies. *Lancet* 1:644-646.

[128] Brink, M.A., Slors, J.F., Keulemans, Y.C., Mok, K.S., De Waart, D.R., Carey, M.C., Groen, A.K., and Tytgat, G.N. 1999. Enterohepatic cycling of bilirubin: a putative mechanism for pigment gallstone formation in ileal Crohn's disease. *Gastroenterology* 116:1420-1427.

[129] Heaton, K.W., and Read, A.E. 1969. Gall stones in patients with disorders of the terminal ileum and disturbed bile salt metabolism. *Br Med J* 3:494-496.

[130] Lapidus, A., Bangstad, M., Astrom, M., and Muhrbeck, O. 1999. The prevalence of gallstone disease in a defined cohort of patients with Crohn's disease. *Am J Gastroenterol* 94:1261-1266.

[131] Magnuson, T.H., Lillemoe, K.D., and Pitt, H.A. 1989. How many Americans will be eligible for biliary lithotripsy? *Arch Surg* 124:1195-1199; discussion 1199-1200.

[132] Buchwald, H., Varco, R.L., Matts, J.P., Long, J.M., Fitch, L.L., Campbell, G.S., Pearce, M.B., Yellin, A.E., Edmiston, W.A., Smink, R.D., Jr., et al. 1990. Effect of partial ileal bypass surgery on mortality and morbidity from coronary heart disease in patients with hypercholesterolemia. Report of the Program on the Surgical Control of the Hyperlipidemias (POSCH). *N Engl J Med* 323:946-955.

[133] Frabboni, R., Bazzoli, F., Sapio, C., Mazzella, G., Festi, D., and Malavolti, M.e.a. 1985,. *Acquired calcification of radiolucent gallstones during cholelitholytic treatment with bile acids*. New York: Raven Press. 3 pp.

[134] Raedsch, R., Stiehl, A., and Czygan, P. 1981. Ursodeoxycholic acid and gallstone calcification. *Lancet* 2:1296.

[135] Freilich, H.S., Malet, P.F., Schwartz, J.S., and Soloway, R.D. 1986. Chemical and morphologic characteristics of cholesterol gallstones that failed to dissolve on chenodiol. The National Cooperative Gallstone Study. *Gastroenterology* 91:713-718.

[136] Ros, E., Navarro, S., Fernandez, I., Reixach, M., Ribo, J.M., and Rodes, J. 1986. Utility of biliary microscopy for the prediction of the chemical composition of gallstones and the outcome of dissolution therapy with ursodeoxycholic acid. *Gastroenterology* 91:703-712.

[137] Pereira, S.P., Veysey, M.J., Kennedy, C., Hussaini, S.H., Murphy, G.M., and Dowling, R.H. 1997. Gallstone dissolution with oral bile acid therapy. Importance of pretreatment CT scanning and reasons for nonresponse. *Dig Dis Sci* 42:1775-1782.

[138] Dam, H. 1968. Prange, I, Sondergaard E. Alimentary production of gallstones in hamsters. Influence of dietary cholesterol on gallstone formation. *Ernahrungswiss* 9:6.

[139] LaMorte, W.W., Brotschi, E.A., Scott, T.E., and Williams, L.F., Jr. 1985. Pigment gallstone formation in the cholesterol-fed guinea pig. *Hepatology* 5:21-27.

[140] Bolondi, L., Gaiani, S., Testa, S., and Labo, G. 1985. Gall bladder sludge formation during prolonged fasting after gastrointestinal tract surgery. *Gut* 26:734-738.

[141] Roslyn, J.J., Berquist, W.E., Pitt, H.A., Mann, L.L., Kangarloo, H., DenBesten, L., and Ament, M.E. 1983. Increased risk of gallstones in children receiving total parenteral nutrition. *Pediatrics* 71:784-789.

[142] Schwesinger, W.H., Kurtin, W.E., Levine, B.A., and Page, C.P. 1985. Cirrhosis and alcoholism as pathogenetic factors in pigment gallstone formation. *Ann Surg* 201:319-322.

[143] Angelico, M., Gandin, C., Canuzzi, P., Bertasi, S., Cantafora, A., De Santis, A., Quattrucci, S., and Antonelli, M. 1991. Gallstones in cystic fibrosis: a critical reappraisal. *Hepatology* 14:768-775.

[144] Halc, W.B., Turner, B., and LaMont, J.T. 1987. Oxygen radicals stimulate guinea pig gallbladder glycoprotein secretion in vitro. *Am J Physiol* 253:G627-630.

[145] Eder, M.I., Miquel, J.F., Jongst, D., Paumgartner, G., and von Ritter, C. 1996. Reactive oxygen metabolites promote cholesterol crystal formation in model bile: role of lipid peroxidation. *Free Radic Biol Med* 20:743-749.

[146] Tiribelli, C., and Ostrow, J.D. 1993. New concepts in bilirubin chemistry, transport and metabolism: report of the Second International Bilirubin Workshop, April 9-11, 1992, Trieste, Italy. *Hepatology* 17:715-736.

[147] Elek, G., and Rockenbouer, A. 1982. The free radical signal of pigment gallstones. *Klin Wochenschr* 60:4.

[148] Leo, M.A., Aleynik, S.I., Siegel, J.H., Kasmin, F.E., Aleynik, M.K., and Lieber, C.S. 1997. F2-isoprostane and 4-hydroxynonenal excretion in human bile of patients with biliary tract and pancreatic disorders. *Am J Gastroenterol* 92:2069-2072.

[149] Bernhoft, R.A., Pellegrini, C.A., Broderick, W.C., and Way, L.W. 1983. Pigment sludge and stone formation in the acutely ligated dog gallbladder. *Gastroenterology* 85:1166-1171.

[150] Sokol, R.J., Devereaux, M., and Khandwala, R.A. 1991. Effect of dietary lipid and vitamin E on mitochondrial lipid peroxidation and hepatic injury in the bile duct-ligated rat. *J Lipid Res* 32:1349-1357.

[151] Krahenbuhl, S., Talos, C., Lauterburg, B.H., and Reichen, J. 1995. Reduced antioxidative capacity in liver mitochondria from bile duct ligated rats. *Hepatology* 22:607-612.

[152] Singh, S., Shackleton, G., Ah-Sing, E., Chakraborty, J., and Bailey, M.E. 1992. Antioxidant defenses in the bile duct-ligated rat. *Gastroenterology* 103:1625-1629.

[153] Brzezinski, A. 1997. Melatonin in humans. *N Engl J Med* 336:186-195.

[154] Reiter, R.J., Melchiorri, D., Sewerynek, E., Poeggeler, B., Barlow-Walden, L., Chuang, J., Ortiz, G.G., and Acuna-Castroviejo, D. 1995. A review of the evidence supporting melatonin's role as an antioxidant. *J Pineal Res* 18:1-11.

[155] Montilla, P.L., Vargas, J.F., Tunez, I.F., Munoz de Agueda, M.C., Valdelvira, M.E., and Cabrera, E.S. 1998. Oxidative stress in diabetic rats induced by streptozotocin: protective effects of melatonin. *J Pineal Res* 25:94-100.

[156] Chen, C.Y., Shiesh, S.C., and Lin, X.Z. 1999. Biliary sludge and pigment stone formation in bile duct-ligated guinea pigs. *Dig Dis Sci* 44:203-209.

[157] Brown, R.E., Jarvis, K.L., and Hyland, K.J. 1989. Protein measurement using bicinchoninic acid: elimination of interfering substances. *Anal Biochem* 180:136-139.

[158] Trotman, B.W., Morris, T.A., 3rd, Sanchez, H.M., Soloway, R.D., and Ostrow, J.D. 1977. Pigment versus cholesterol cholelithiasis: identification and quantification by infrared spectroscopy. *Gastroenterology* 72:495-498.

[159] Fukunaga, K., Suzuki, T., and Takama, K. 1993. Highly sensitive high-performance liquid chromatography for the measurement of malondialdehyde in biological samples. *J Chromatogr* 621:77-81.

[160] Mashige, F., Tanaka, N., Maki, A., Kamei, S., and Yamanaka, M. 1981. Direct spectrophotometry of total bile acids in serum. *Clin Chem* 27:1352-1356.

[161] Smith, B.F., and LaMont, J.T. 1985. Identification of gallbladder mucin-bilirubin complex in human cholesterol gallstone matrix. Effects of reducing agents on in vitro dissolution of matrix and intact gallstones. *J Clin Invest* 76:439-445.

[162] Valenzvela, A. 1991. The biological significance of malondialdehyde determination in the assessment of tissue oxidative stres. *Life Sci* 48:9.

[163] Ohkawa, H., Ohishi, N., and Yagi, K. 1979. Assay for lipid peroxides in animal tissues by thiobarbituric acid reaction. *Anal Biochem* 95:351-358.

[164] Halliwell, B., and Chirico, S. 1993. Lipid peroxidation: its mechanism, measurement, and significance. *Am J Clin Nutr* 57:715S-724S; discussion 724S-725S.

[165] Whitehead, T., Thorpe, G., and Maxwell, S. 1992. Enhanced chemiluminescent assay for antioxidant capacity in biological fluids. *Clin Chim Act* 266:13.

[166] Strasberg, S.M., Toth, J.L., Gallinger, S., and Harvey, P.R. 1990. High protein and total lipid concentration are associated with reduced metastability of bile in an early stage of cholesterol gallstone formation. *Gastroenterology* 98:739-746.

[167] Lee, S.P., and Nicholls, J.F. 1986. Nature and composition of biliary sludge. *Gastroenterology* 90:677-686.

[168] O'Leary, D.P., Murray, F.E., Turner, B.S., and LaMont, J.T. 1991. Bile salts stimulate glycoprotein release by guinea pig gallbladder in vitro. *Hepatology* 13:957-961.

[169] Tazuma, S. 2006. Gallstone disease: Epidemiology, pathogenesis, and classification of biliary stones (common bile duct and intrahepatic). *Best Pract Res Clin Gastroenterol* 20:1075-1083.

[170] Swidsinski, A., and Lee, S. 2001. The role of bacteria in gallstone pathogenesis. *Front Biosci* 6:11.

[171] Stewart, L., Oesterle, A.L., Erdan, I., Griffiss, J.M., and Way, L.W. 2002. Pathogenesis of pigment gallstones in Western societies: the central role of bacteria. *J Gastrointest Surg* 6:891-903; discussion 903-894.

[172] Stewart, L., Griffiss, J.M., Jarvis, G.A., and Way, L.W. 2007. Gallstones containing bacteria are biofilms: bacterial slime production and ability to form pigment solids determines infection severity and bacteremia. *J Gastrointest Surg* 11:977-983; discussion 983-974.

[173] Stewart, L., Griffiss, J.M., Jarvis, G.A., and Way, L.W. 2007. Bacteria entombed in the center of cholesterol gallstones induce fewer infectious manifestations than bacteria in the matrix of pigment stones. *J Gastrointest Surg* 11:1298-1308.

[174] Stewart, L., Grifiss, J.M., Jarvis, G.A., and Way, L.W. 2006. Biliary bacterial factors determine the path of gallstone formation. *Am J Surg* 192:598-603.

[175] Wu, S.D., Yu, H., and Sun, J.M. 2006. Bacteriological and electron microscopic examination of primary intrahepatic stones. *Hepatobiliary Pancreat Dis Int* 5:228-231.

[176] Khlebtsov, B.N., Burygin, G.L., Matora, L.Y., Shchyogolev, S.Y., and Khlebtsov, N.G. 2004. A method for studying insoluble immune complexes. *Biochim Biophys Acta* 1670:199-207.

[177] Li, J., Sun, D., Lu, Y., Jin, H., Jiang, X., and Hu, S., et al. 2004. Change in intestinal function in sepsis in rat. *Zhongguo Wei Zhong Bing Ji Jiu Yi Xue* 16:3.

[178] Hilsden, R.J., Meddings, J.B., Hardin, J., Gall, D.G., and Sutherland, L.R. 1999. Intestinal permeability and postheparin plasma diamine oxidase activity in the prediction of Crohn's disease relapse. *Inflamm Bowel Dis* 5:85-91.

[179] Czyzewska-Buczyńska, A., Lewandowicz-Uszyńska, A., and Jankowski, A. 2007. IgA, an essential part of the immune system: selected issues. *stepy Hig Med Dosw (Online)* 61:10.

[180] Packer, M., Patterson-Kane, J.C., Smith, K.C., and Durham, A.E. 2005. Quantification of immune cell populations in the lamina propria of equine jejunal biopsy specimens. *J Comp Pathol* 132:90-95.

[181] Choudhry, M.A., Rana, S.N., Kavanaugh, M.J., Kovacs, E.J., Gamelli, R.L., and Sayeed, M.M. 2004. Impaired intestinal immunity and barrier function: a cause for

enhanced bacterial translocation in alcohol intoxication and burn injury. *Alcohol* 33:199-208.

[182] Osnes, T., Sandstad, O., Skar, V., and Osnes, M. 1997. Lipopolysaccharides and beta-glucuronidase activity in choledochal bile in relation to choledocholithiasis. *Digestion* 58:437-443.

[183] Wu, S.D., Uchiyama, K., and Fan, Y. 2007. The role and mechanism of fatty acids in gallstones. *Hepatobiliary Pancreat Dis Int* 6:399-401.

[184] Sacco, C., McEwen, W.E., and Calabrese, E.J. 1993. Selective inhibition of gastrointestinal beta-glucuronidase by polyvinylbenzyl D-glucaro(1,4)lactonate: attachment of D-glucaro(1,4)lactone to polyvinylbenzyl chloride. *Hum Exp Toxicol* 12:181-184.

[185] Lamote, J., and Willems, G. 1997. DNA synthesis, cell proliferation index in normal and abnormal gallbladder epithelium. *Microsc Res Tech* 38:609-615.

[186] Ding, L.A., Li, J.S., Li, Y.S., Liu, F.N., and Tan, L. 2004. Prophylactic treatment with growth hormone improves intestinal barrier function and alleviates bacterial translocation in stressed rats. *Chin Med J (Engl)* 117:264-269.

[187] Li, N., DeMarco, V.G., West, C.M., and Neu, J. 2003. Glutamine supports recovery from loss of transepithelial resistance and increase of permeability induced by media change in Caco-2 cells. *J Nutr Biochem* 14:401-408.

[188] Ding, L.A., and Li, J.S. 2003. Effects of glutamine on intestinal permeability and bacterial translocation in TPN-rats with endotoxemia. *World J Gastroenterol* 9:1327-1332.

[189] Yu, J., Pan, H., Huang, S., Huang, N., Yao, C., Hsiao, K., and Wu, C. 2012. Calcium content of different compositions gallstones and pathogenesis of calcium carbonate gallstones. *Asian Journal of Surgery* (In Press).

[190] Huang, Y.Y., Huang, C.S., Yang, S.S., Lin, M.S., and Huang, M.J. 2005. Effects of variant UDP-glucuronosyltransferase 1A1 gene, glucose-6-phosphate dehydrogenase deficiency and thalassemia on cholelithiasis. *World J Gastroenterol* 11:5710-5713.

[191] Meloni, T., Forteleoni, G., Noja, G., Dettori, G., Sale, M.A., and Meloni, G.F. 1991. Increased prevalence of glucose-6-phosphate dehydrogenase deficiency in patients with cholelithiasis. *Acta Haematol* 85:76-78.

[192] Bosma, P.J., Chowdhury, J.R., Bakker, C., Gantla, S., de Boer, A., Oostra, B.A., Lindhout, D., Tytgat, G.N., Jansen, P.L., Oude Elferink, R.P., et al. 1995. The genetic basis of the reduced expression of bilirubin UDP-glucuronosyltransferase 1 in Gilbert's syndrome. *N Engl J Med* 333:1171-1175.

[193] Sampietro, M., Lupica, L., Perrero, L., Comino, A., Martinez di Montemuros, F., Cappellini, M.D., and Fiorelli, G. 1997. The expression of uridine diphosphate glucuronosyltransferase gene is a major determinant of bilirubin level in heterozygous beta-thalassaemia and in glucose-6-phosphate dehydrogenase deficiency. *Br J Haematol* 99:437-439.

[194] Tunaci, M., Tunaci, A., Engin, G., Ozkorkmaz, B., Dincol, G., Acunas, G., and Acunas, B. 1999. Imaging features of thalassemia. *Eur Radiol* 9:1804-1809.

[195] Huang, C.S., Luo, G.A., Huang, M.L., Yu, S.C., and Yang, S.S. 2000. Variations of the bilirubin uridine-diphosphoglucuronosyl transferase 1A1 gene in healthy Taiwanese. *Pharmacogenetics* 10:539-544.

[196] Huang, C.S., Chang, P.F., Huang, M.J., Chen, E.S., and Chen, W.C. 2002. Glucose-6-phosphate dehydrogenase deficiency, the UDP-glucuronosyl transferase 1A1 gene, and neonatal hyperbilirubinemia. *Gastroenterology* 123:127-133.

[197] Huang, M.J., Kua, K.E., Teng, H.C., Tang, K.S., Weng, H.W., and Huang, C.S. 2004. Risk factors for severe hyperbilirubinemia in neonates. *Pediatr Res* 56:682-689.

[198] Ko, T.M., Tseng, L.H., Hsieh, F.J., Hsu, P.M., and Lee, T.Y. 1992. Carrier detection and prenatal diagnosis of alpha-thalassemia of Southeast Asian deletion by polymerase chain reaction. *Hum Genet* 88:245-248.

[199] Chang, J.G., Chen, P.H., Chiou, S.S., Lee, L.S., Perng, L.I., and Liu, T.C. 1992. Rapid diagnosis of beta-thalassemia mutations in Chinese by naturally and amplified created restriction sites. *Blood* 80:2092-2096.

[200] Beutler, E. 1994. G6PD deficiency. *Blood* 84:21.

[201] Huang, C.S., Chang, P.F., Huang, M.J., Chen, E.S., Hung, K.L., and Tsou, K.I. 2002. Relationship between bilirubin UDP-glucuronosyl transferase 1A1 gene and neonatal hyperbilirubinemia. *Pediatr Res* 52:601-605.

[202] Huang, M.J., Yang, Y.C., Yang, S.S., Lin, M.S., Chen, E.S., and Huang, C.S. 2002. Coinheritance of variant UDP-glucuronosyl transferase 1A1 gene and glucose-6-phosphate dehydrogenase deficiency in adults with hyperbilirubinemia. *Pharmacogenetics* 12:663-666.

[203] Yamamoto, K., Sato, H., Fujiyama, Y., Doida, Y., and Bamba, T. 1998. Contribution of two missense mutations (G71R and Y486D) of the bilirubin UDP glycosyltransferase (UGT1A1) gene to phenotypes of Gilbert's syndrome and Crigler-Najjar syndrome type II. *Biochim Biophys Acta* 1406:267-273.

[204] Liu, J.S., Huang, C.S., and Lien, H.H. 2002. Structural analysis of gallstones with thin-section petrographic microscopy: a study of 100 gallstones from Taiwanese patients. *J Lab Clin Med* 140:387-390.

Chapter IV

Etiology, Pathogenesis and Clinical Relevance of Calcium–Containing and Calcium Carbonate Gallstones

Abstract

Purpose: Our aim was to investigate the calcium content of different gallstone compositions and the pathogenic mechanisms of calcium carbonate gallstones.

Methods: Between August 2001 and July 2007, gallstones from 481 patients, including 68 calcium carbonate gallstones, were analyzed for total calcium content. Gallbladder (GB) bile samples from 33 cases and 6 controls were analyzed for pH, carbonate anion level, free-ionized calcium concentration and saturation index for calcium carbonate.

Findings: Total calcium content averaged 75.6 %, 11.8 % and 4.2 % for calcium carbonate, calcium bilirubinate and cholesterol gallstones. In 29.4% of patients, chronic and/or intermittent cystic duct obstructions were caused by polypoid lesions in the neck region and 70.6% by stones. Eighty-two percent of patients had chronic low-grade inflammation of the GB wall, and 18.0% had acute inflammatory exacerbations. In the bile, we found the mean pH, mean carbonate anion, free-ionized calcium concentrations and mean saturation index for calcium carbonate to be elevated in comparison to controls.

Conclusion: We found that intermittent partial cystic duct obstructions, low-grade gallbladder wall inflammation and infections might lead to dysfunctional gallbladder epithelium hydrogen secretion. Higher gallbladder bile pH, increased carbonate anion, increased free calcium ion concentrations, and raised saturation indices may influence calcium carbonate precipitation.

I. Calcium Content of Different Compositions Gallstones and Pathogenesis of Calcium Carbonate Gallstones [1]

Introduction

Although classified as a rare gallstone type by the National Institute of Health Consensus Conference, [2] calcium carbonate gallstones, resultant from so-called limy bile, compose 14.1% – 14.5% of all gallstones in Taiwan according to the literature and our present series. [3, 4] Saito reviewed 5 cases of limy bile [5] and published "Chemical and crystallographic studies on 33 cases of calcium carbonate gallstones". [5] Hashino reviewed 231 cases of calcium carbonate gallstone cases in Japan [6].

Here, we report the clinical, chemical and crystallographic studies on 68 cases of calcium carbonate gallstones. The aim of this study was to explore the calcium content of gallstones of different compositions and to investigate the pathogenesis of calcium carbonate gallstones.

Patients and Methods

Design

This is a case-control study.

Setting

The study was conducted mainly in a tertiary care setting at two medical centers, including the Veterans General Hospital of Taipei and the Chung Shan Medical University Hospital.

Participants and Intervention

Between August 2001 and July 2007, 68 cases of calcium carbonate gallstones among 481 gallstone patients (68 calcium carbonate, 252 calcium bilirubinate and 161 cholesterol) undergoing cholecystectomy and/or choledocholithotomy were collected for this study. Among the calcium bilirubinate stone group patients, 83.3% (210/252) were black pigment gallstones and 16.7% (42/252) were brown pigment gallstones, according to Stiton's criteria. [7] The clinical features, including gender, age, presence/absence of acute cholecystitis and right hypochondrium radio-opacity on KUB (kidney-ureter-bladder x-ray), were recorded and analyzed. Gallbladder (GB) bile from 33 calcium carbonate gallstone patients and 11 non-gallstone (NGS) patients were obtained. The diagnoses of the NGS patients included hepatocellular carcinoma (HCC, 3 patients), gastrointestinal stromal tumor (2 patients), pancreatic carcinoma (2 patients), GB adenocarcinomas (GBC, 2 patients) and liver trauma (2 patients). Excluding the 3 HCC and the 2 GBC, only 6 controls were obtained for comparison.

Analyses of gallstone and bile samples were carried out in triplicate. Variations of measurements were within 5% of the mean measured values of the triplicates.

Analyses of Gallstones

The total calcium content of the gallstones was chemically analyzed by atomic absorption spectrophotometry (Atomic absorption spectrophotometer, Instrumentation Laboratory, model 857, Lexington, MA, USA), and the crystal structures of the gallstones were studied by infrared absorption spectroscopy (IAS, potassium bromide-disk method, JASCO FT/IR3, Hachioji, Tokyo, Japan), polarizing microscopy (PM, Nikon, VFX-2, Kurobane Nikon Co., Lt, Otawara, Tochigi, Japan) and with/without powder X-ray diffractometry (RIGAKU diffractometer, Copper-Potassium-α radiation, Nickel-filter, RIGAKU, Japan). The details of infrared absorption spectroscopy and polarizing microscopy were previously published [2]

Powder X-ray diffractometry [7, 8]

As a quantitative crystallographic analysis, the powder X-ray diffraction method was performed on 50 mg of finely powdered samples, which were produced with an amber mortar, using nickel-filtered copper-potassium α-radiation generated from a RIGAKU X-ray diffractometer. For determination of the calcite, aragonite and vaterite ratios, the Davies' method[7] of X-ray diffraction was applied. The standard materials were commercially purchased calcite and coral for aragonite. Vaterite was experimentally precipitated by drop-wise addition of calcium chloride (2 M, $CaCl_2$) into sodium carbonate (2 M, Na_2CO_3) [6].

Analysis of Total Calcium Content of Gallstones

We performed analysis of total calcium content of gallstones using atomic absorption spectrophotometry as reported previously in the literature [4, 7].

Determination of GB bile pH, carbonate ion concentration, $[Ca^{++}] \times [C03^{=}]$ ion-product, saturation index for calcium carbonate (SI_$CaCO_3$) and free-ionized calcium

Gallbladder bile was aspirated anaerobically into a syringe using a 20-gauge needle. Care was taken to empty the gallbladder completely to minimize stratification effects on bile composition. All samples were immediately analyzed at 37°C for pH, partial pressure of carbon dioxide (P_{CO2}) and total CO_2 content ($[T_{CO2}]$) using a blood gas analyzer (Bayer Rapidlab 840, Diamond Diagnostics, MA, USA). In each sample, the carbonate ion concentration ($[CO3^{=}]$) was calculated from the Henderson-Hasselbalch equation. The ion-product ($[Ca^{++}] \times [C03^{=}]$) was then determined for each sample from the observed $[Ca^{++}]$ and calculated $[CO3^{=}]$ ion concentrations. The free ionized calcium concentration ($[Ca^{++}]$) was determined anaerobically at 37°C with a Ca^{++} electrode (Model SS-20 Ionalyzer; Orion Research, Inc., Cambridge, MA, USA).

Diagnostic criteria for calcium carbonate gallstones

The Evolution of the Cut-Off Value of Calcium Content

From our previous study, IAS and PM can be reliably used to determine the major compositions of gallstones [1]. When deciding the cut-off value for total calcium content (%) required diagnosing a calcium carbonate gallstone, there were 19 false positives (21.8% or 19/87 participants) diagnosed by IAS and PM when the cut-off value was set at 30%. Ten false positives (12.8% or 10/78 participants) were identified when the cut-off value was set at 40%. However, there were no false positives when the cut-off value was set at 50%. Therefore, we used 50% total calcium content as the diagnostic criteria for calcium carbonate gallstones in this study.

Ethics

The operation and sample collection procedures were explained to all patients. Informed consent was signed by each patient for both laparoscopic and open cholecystectomies. There was no formal Institutional Review Board (institutional or regional) in existence at the beginning of patient enrollment. However, the principles outlined in the Declaration of Helsinki of 1975 (revised in 1983) were followed throughout the study period.

Statistics

Chi-square tests were used for comparisons between the occurrence rates of acute cholecystitis between groups. An unpaired Student's *t*-test was used for comparisons of mean total calcium content among different gallstone composition groups. The Pearson correlation coefficient (r) was used to analyze the correlation between KUB radio-opacity and mean total calcium content (%) in gallstones with different major compositions. $P < 0.05$ was considered statistically significant.

Results

Demographics

There were no differences in gender or age between the calcium carbonate gallstone patients and the non-gallstone control patients (M/F = 53/15 vs. 8/3, $P = 0.69$; 60 ± 11 years, n = 68, vs. 62 ± 8 years; n = 11, $P = 0.57$).

KUB x-ray film radio-opacity and mean total calcium content (%) in gallstones with different major compositions

All 68 patients with calcium carbonate gallstones had calcifications present on their KUB x-ray films (Figure 4.1.1A). The mean total calcium content (%) of calcium carbonate, calcium bilirubinate and cholesterol gallstones was 75.6 ± 15.1% (n = 68), 11.8 ± 7.2% (n = 252), and 4.2 ± 4.6% (n = 161), respectively. They were significantly different from each other ($P < 0.0001$, unpaired Student's *t*-test between each two groups, Figure 4.1.1B).

Cystic Duct Obstruction

The cystic ducts were all obstructed. Twenty out of 68 patients (29.4%) had associated chronic, partial cystic duct obstructions caused by polypoid lesions at or near the GB neck region, and the remaining 70.6% obstructions were caused by stones. Twelve patients (17.6%) had acute cystic duct obstructions causing acute cholecystitis. Four out of 68 patients (5.9%) had intermittent cystic duct obstructions by the second compositions stones in the core region of calcium carbonate gallstones or in separate gallstones. The remaining 32 patients (47.1%) had calcium carbonate gallstones associated only with intermittent, partial cystic duct obstruction.

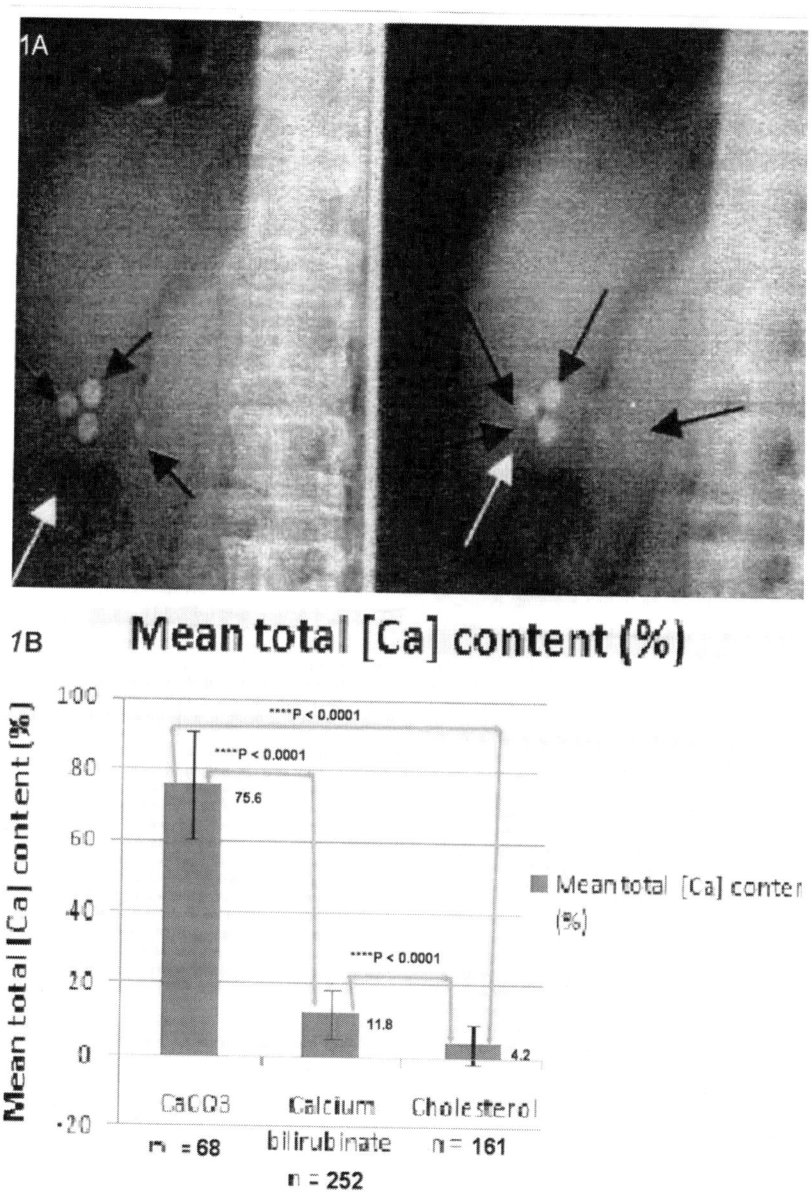

Figure 4.1.1. KUB film radio-opacity and stone total calcium content in patients with gallstones. In A black and white arrows indicate calcified gallstones. B compares the mean total calcium content in gallstones with different major compositions. [Ca]: calcium; ****: < 0.0001; upright or upside down "T" line: one standard deviation. KUB: kidney-ureter-bladder.

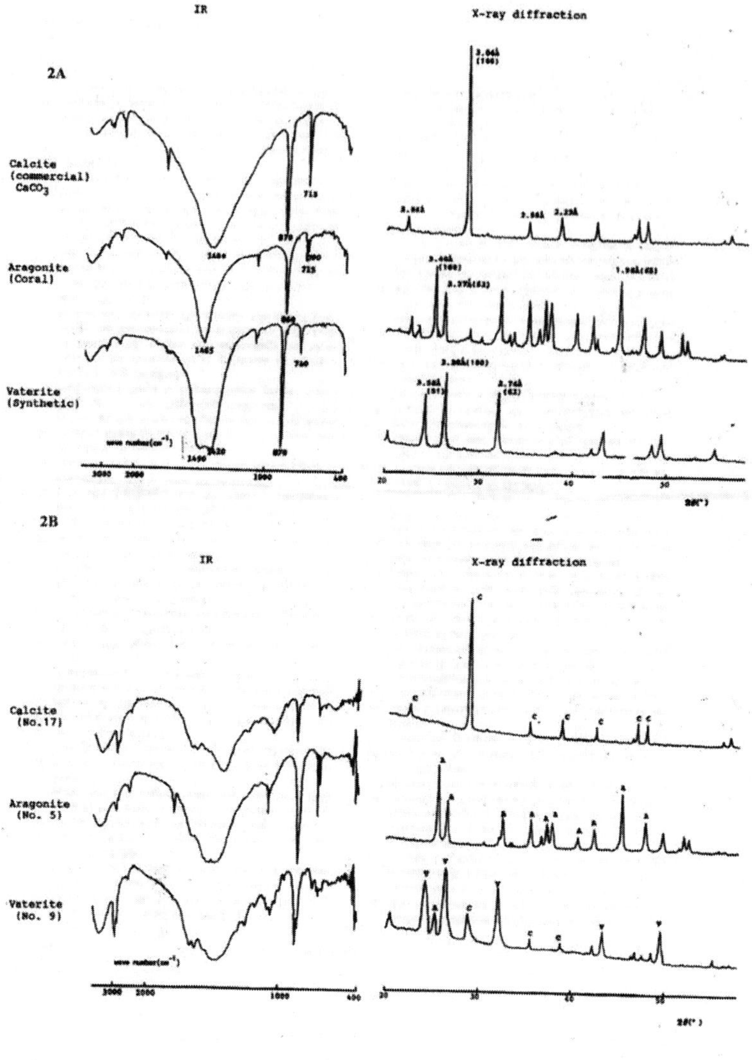

Figure 4.1.2. Infrared absorption spectroscopy, X-ray diffractometry of standard and sample calcite, aragonite and vaterite. 1a. Standard calcium carbonate. 1b. Sample of calcium carbonate gallstones (No. 17 = calcite, No. 5 = aragonite and No. 9 = vaterite).

Chronic Low-Grade Inflammation of GB Wall with/without Acute Exacerbation

All 68 patients (100%) were shown to have chronic low-grade inflammation of the GB wall at some time during the evaluation period. Among them, 12 had an acute exacerbation. In the early (clinical) stage of acute cholecystitis, which corresponds to mild (grade I) severity according to the Tokyo guidelines, [9, 10] no acute inflammatory leukocyte infiltration is observed. However, chronic inflammatory reactions are present, including subserosal fibrous tissue and lymphocyte, plasma cell, and macrophage infiltration beneath the columnar epithelium and Rokitansky-Aschoff sinus in the muscular layer, as revealed by pathological examinations. Early (clinical) stage acute cholecystitis was observed in 41.7% of patients with acute exacerbations (5/12). In the second (pathological) stage, which corresponds to moderate severity (grade II) according to the Tokyo guidelines, pathological responses of acute immunoreactive and inflammatory processes appear in the gallbladder. These include leukocyte infiltration throughout the tissues, local flattening and denuded mucosal folds, and tissue edema. This stage was observed in 41.7% of patients with acute exacerbations (5/12). If the condition goes untreated or is unresponsive to treatment, the late (complicated) stage ensues, which corresponds to severe (grade III) organ dysfunction according to the Tokyo guidelines. In this stage, aside from the pathological findings of acute immunoreactive and inflammatory responses, local gallbladder wall necrosis (gangrene), abscesses and/or perforations occur. Organ dysfunctions results thereafter. This stage was observed in 16.6% of acute exacerbations (2/12). The chronicity of gallbladder infection and inflammation are thought to be the cause of limy bile and calcium carbonate gallstone production. Chemically, the total content by weight of calcium carbonate ranged from 50.7 % to 98.5 %, averaging 75.6%. Crystallographically, calcium carbonate has three different polymorphic crystalline forms: calcite, aragonite and vaterite. Each isoform has its own characteristic absorption bands in IAS and unique d-spacings in its X-ray diffraction pattern (Figure 4.1.2, Table 4.1.1).

Table 4.1.1. Characteristic IR wave numbers, X-ray diffraction d-spacings and polarizing microscopy crystal forms of three polymorphs of calcium carbonate

$CaCO_3$ Polymorphs	R (cm^{-1})	X-diffraction d-spacings	PM
Calcite	1410 – 1450 Broad 870 715	3.04Å (100)	Irregularly isothermic layers of crystal plate with colors (red, pink, blue)
Aragonite	1410 – 1450 860 715, 700	3.40Å (100)	Serrated pieces of crystal lattice with yellow, green colors
Vaterite	1410 – 1450 860 740	3.58 Å(51) 3.30 (100)	Concentric round spheres, isolated or duplex or in clusters

$CaCO_3$: calcium carbonate, IR: infrared wave numbers, PM: polarizing microscopy.

Table 4.1.2. Comparisons of mean GB bile pH, free calcium ion concentration, carbonate anion concentration and SI_$CaCO_3^{=}$ between the calcium carbonate gallstone and NGS control patients (excluding 3 HCC and 2 GBC patients)

Stone groups / GB bile mean	$CaCO_3$ gallstone Mean ± S.D. (n = 33)	NGS control Mean ± S.D. (n = 6)	*P* - value
pH	7.87 ± 0.54	6.78 ± 0.36	< 0.0001****
free calcium ion concentration (mmol/l)	3.15 ± 0.51	1.82 ± 0.20	< 0.0001****
carbonate anion concentration (mmol/l)	0.29 ± 0.05	0.003 ± 0.0008	< 0.0001****
SI_$CaCO_3$	24.4 ± 0.64	0.14 ± 0.05	< 0.0001****

GB: gallbladder, SI_$CaCO_3$: saturation index for calcium carbonate, NGS: non-gallstone, $CaCO_3$: calcium carbonate, ****: $P < 0.0001$ by unpaired Student's *t*- test, HCC: hepatocellular carcinoma, GBC: gallbladder cancer.

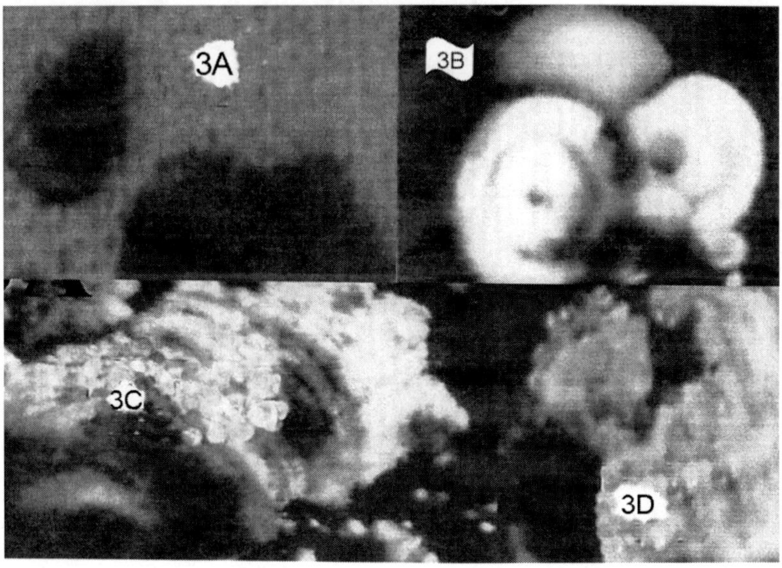

Figure 4.1.3. Gross appearance and crystallographic structures of calcium carbonate gallstone polymorphs. 3A Note mulberry or sea-urchin-like appearance. 3B Serrated pieces of crystal lattice with yellow, green colors in aragonite polymorph. 3C Irregularly isothermic layers of crystal plate with colors (red, pink and blue) in calcite polymorph. 3D Concentric round spheres, isolated, in duplex or in clusters in vaterite polymorph.

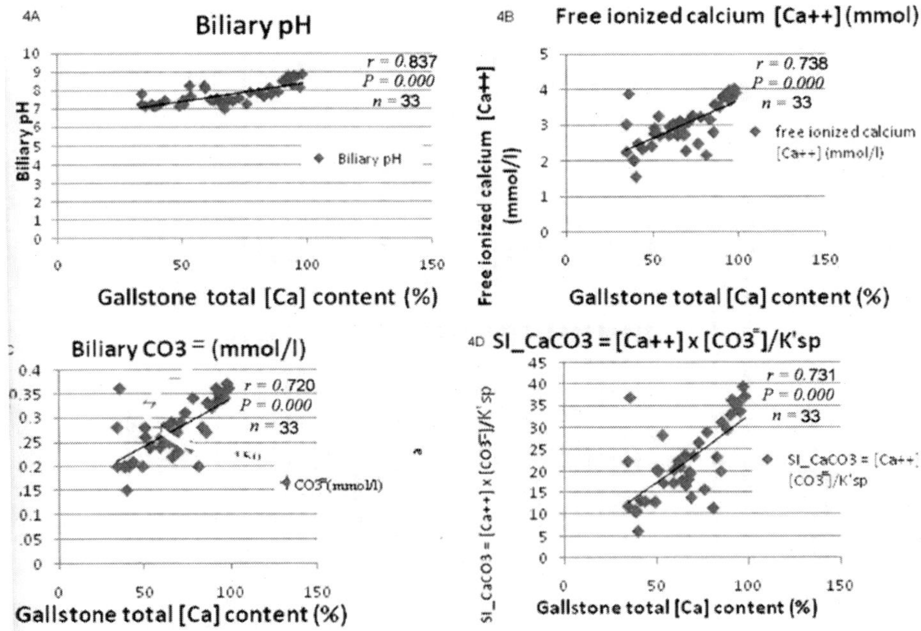

Figure 4.1.4. Correlation between total calcium content of calcium carbonate gallstones and gallbladder bile profiles. Total calcium content of calcium carbonate gallstones is positively correlated with gallbladder bile (2A) pH; (2B) free ionized calcium ion concentration; (2C) carbonate anion concentration and (2D) saturation index for calcium carbonate (SI_CaCO$_3$). (SI_CaCO$_3$) equals [Ca^{++}] x [$CO_3^{=}$] / K'sp (= 3.78 x 10^{-8}). r = Pearson correlation coefficient, *P*: probability of chance alone, n: number of patients.

Under polarizing microscopy, calcium carbonate is the most brilliant crystalline form of all gallstones (Figure 4.1.3, Table 4.1.1). In 23 cases, all three crystalline forms were detected. In comparison with NGS control patients, we found that the mean GB bile pH, free calcium ion concentration, carbonate anion concentration and SI_$CaCO_3^=$ level were significantly elevated in the calcium carbonate gallstone patients (Table 4.1.2). These findings correlated with the total calcium content (%) of the gallstones (Figure 4.1.4A – D).

Discussion

Since Churchman first described this syndrome in 1911, more than 300 cases of limy bile have been reported. [11, 12] Calcium carbonate gallstones and limy bile are characterized by the presence of radio-opaque liquid or solid calcium carbonate within the gallbladder. Limy bile may vary in consistency from a viscous liquid to a paste or solid. Saito reported cases where radio-opaque material filled the gallbladder [4]. The gallbladder and bile duct in his study were filled with radiopaque material, readily noted on plain radiographs. [13, 14] Definitive diagnosis of limy bile syndrome (LBS) is made when these characteristic findings of LBS are visualized on a plain radiograph of the abdomen. In a typical case, the gallbladder and/or the common bile duct are visualized as if contrast medium were used. On plain radiograph of the abdomen in the standing position, calcification accompanied by a hemi-oval niveau formation overlapping the gallbladder can be seen on occasion. For precise examination, including determination of the cause of LBS, ultrasonography and computed tomography should be performed [14].

In our series, all 68 patients had calcified stones in the right upper quadrant of their KUB films (Figure 4.11A). Twenty-three cases were associated with clinical findings of limy bile with radio-opacity in the shape of a gallbladder. They tended to have higher total calcium content: 73.3% to 96.1% vs. 75.6% on average. Clinically, all 68 patients with calcium carbonate gallstones had calcifications visualized on their KUB films (100%, Figure 4.1.1A).

High calcium content precludes dissolution therapy as an effective treatment modality for calcium-containing cholesterol and calcium carbonate gallstones, leaving surgery as the only effective treatment option [14, 15].

The clinical relevance of our data is that the pathogenic rules governing gallstone precipitations in patients with calcium carbonate gallstones also apply to calcium-containing cholesterol gallstones. The presence of calcium on the surface and inner layers of cholesterol gallstones precludes viable treatment by dissolution therapy, leaving cholecystectomy as the only effective management modality. LBS is frequently accompanied by lithiasis in the neck of the gallbladder, in the cystic duct and/or in the common bile duct. Complications including obstructive jaundice, acute pancreatitis, gallbladder cancer and cholangiocarcinoma were found but at a low frequency. Importantly, the diagnosis cholelithiasis and bile duct cancer can easily be missed when limy bile disease is present. Observation without treatment is, therefore, not ideal. Because endoscopic treatment does not require general anesthesia, is less invasive and requires only a short period of hospitalization, this treatment can be applied to patients with liver or kidney disorders as well as in elderly patients. Thus, endoscopic percutaneous balloon dilatation (EPBD) seems to be the best method for the treatment of limy bile disease in the common bile duct. Endoscopic therapy is an excellent method for the treatment of LBS and will likely become widely used in the future [16].

Many theories on the etiology of calcium carbonate gallstones, arising from both clinical and experimental data, have been proposed. [5] Okamura [13] reviewed the Japanese literature and found that cystic duct obstruction was present in 93% of cases whereas both Moreaux [17] and our series reported a 100% obstruction rate of the cystic duct. Generally, these were stone-related obstructions, and rarely, they were carcinoma-related. [7]

Ahronsson et al. claimed that bilirubin was degraded by infection into colorless substances, [15] and Flint postulated that chronic cholecystitis is the cause of calcium carbonate precipitation [18]

By now, most authors agree that biliary obstruction alone is the initiating factor of limy bile disease. The exact mechanism of disease remains unknown. However, successive obstruction and stasis, increased mucus secretion, pH changes, and calcium carbonate precipitation have been suggested to explain the formation of limy bile. [19]

Colorless bile, sometimes referred to as white bile, can also be found outside the gallbladder, but this should not be mistaken for limy bile. In an experimental model, it was demonstrated that when the pressure in the biliary tree rises, the gallbladder functions as a release valve for decompressing the biliary tree, and the bile becomes concentrated in the gallbladder. If the gallbladder is excluded, the bile is back-washed into the liver and leaks into the portal spaces. Normal bile is then replaced with colorless, ductular secretions of the gallbladder. This colorless bile is also found in patients with biliary obstruction. In these patients, white bile is found throughout the extra- and intra-hepatic biliary system. In the chronically an intermittently obstructed gallbladder, local changes within the gallbladder appear to be the cause of limy bile. Alternatively, an obstructed bile duct does not have absorption capabilities; therefore, the bile is either concentrated in the gallbladder or absorbed by the liver in the case of cystic duct obstruction. [19]

Light brown cholesterol (2/68) and dark brown calcium bilirubinate (1/68) precipitations were found in the core of gallstones. Externally, the stones continued calcium carbonate. Two other patients presented with a second composition (calcium bilirubinate). The presence of the second composition provides direct evidence supporting the hypothesis that partial and intermittent obstruction of the cystic duct by stones of different compositions (cholesterol or calcium bilirubinate) may precede later events that lead to calcium carbonate precipitation.

In our series, 100% (68/68) of cases were associated with cystic duct obstruction in the GB neck region: 70.6% (48/68) by stones alone, 29.4 % (20/68) by polypoid lesions alone. No cystic duct obstruction by a carcinoma was found. Twenty-four patients had chronic, partial or intermittent cystic duct obstructions caused by polypoid lesions at or near the GB neck (20 patients) or by a cholesterol-cored stone (4 patients). Twelve were associated with acute cystic duct obstructions resulting in acute cholecystitis.

According to our data, GB bile from patients with calcium carbonate gallstones has a more alkaline pH, higher free-ionized calcium concentration, higher carbonate anion concentration and higher saturation index for calcium carbonate compared with GB bile from non-gallstone patients (all $P < 0.0001$, Table 4.1.2). These pathological changes can be predicted by the total calcium content of the patients' calcium carbonate gallstones ($r = 0.717 \sim 0.837$, all $P = 0.000$, Figure 4.1.4).

Sayers [20] reported an increase in mucin-producing epithelial cells in the gallbladders of children with calcium carbonate stones. This finding supports the hypothesis that cystic duct obstruction leads to increased gallbladder mucin production and that obstruction may play a role in the development of calcium carbonate gallstones in children. Rege and Moore, [21] in a study on canine ductular and gallbladder bile, suggested the following: (1) in canine bile, as in canine pancreatic juice, a nucleating factor is necessary for $CaCO_3$ precipitation and (2) normal gallbladder mucosal function plays an important role in reducing calcium carbonate lithogenicity in gallbladder bile. Dawes and Rege [22] reported that total calcium concentration in GB bile is positively correlated with bile salt concentration in human patients with gallstone diseases and non-biliary tract diseases controls. Dawes and Rege [22] also documented the importance of calcium precipitation in pigment gallstone formation, as more than half of the samples were saturated or supersaturated with calcium carbonate.

McWhirter [16] suggested that low-grade gallbladder inflammation was necessary for calcium deposition. In our series, all 68 patients (100%) had associated chronic low-grade inflammation of the GB wall. Similar findings were also reported in the Saito [6] and Yamaguchi [23] studies.

It has been hypothesized the obstruction of the cystic duct and infection/inflammation of the gallbladder may cause an alkaline shift in the pH of the gallbladder bile. Only when the pH is greater than 6.6 [23] will calcium carbonate precipitate. This was true in the Yamaguchi study [23], in which pH ranged from 7.0 to 8.8; in our series, the pH ranged from 6.95 to 8.88.

Calcium salt is important for pigmented gallstone formation and may serve as a nidus for cholesterol precipitation. [12] Erincu demonstrated the nucleation and epitaxial growth of crystalline cholesterol monohydrate on calcite [104] surfaces. [24]

The growth rates of individual cholesterol islands that formed on calcite substrates were determined at physiological temperatures. The energetics of various calcite (104) crystalline cholesterol monohydrate interfaces were calculated to determine the most stable structure. These simulations suggest that the interface is fully hydrated and that cholesterol hydroxyl groups are preferentially positioned above carbonate ions on the calcite surface. This combination of experimental and theoretical work provides a clearer picture of how preexisting mineral seeds might provide a viable growth template that can reduce the energetics barrier to cholesterol nucleation under some physiological conditions [22]. Alternatively, calcium carbonate can precipitate on a cholesterol nidus, as demonstrated in our patients.

Limy bile is a rare finding (0.27% in 1800 cholecystectomies). Plain abdominal X-rays mostly suggest the presence of calcium carbonate precipitates in the gallbladder, but ultrasound cannot differentiate between cholelithiasis and limy bile. Laparoscopic resection can be performed without complications in most patients. Preoperative diagnosis of this rare entity is not essential, as it does not alter treatment. [25]

Moreaux [17] reports on the surgical experiences of 16 patients with limy bile disease, and this study suggests that abdominal radiographs are sufficient to identify limy bile. The presence of this condition in the gallbladder is always associated with biliary lithiasis and obstruction of the cystic duct. The presence of limy bile in the common bile duct is due to the migration of impacted stones and calceous material deposited in the gallbladder.

From the above data, a hypothetical model was proposed: Chronic and/or intermittent cystic duct obstructions and low grade GB wall inflammation lead to GB epithelium hydrogen secretion dysfunction, resulting in lower hydrogen ion concentration and higher GB bile pH as suggested by Rege and Moore [21] Greater decomposition produces more carbonate anions secondary to decreased hydrogen ion influx according to the Henderson-Hasselbalch equation. Thus, increased calcium ion efflux into the GB lumen combined with increased carbonate anion presence increases SI_$CaCO_3$ from 1 to 22.4. Thus, in an alkaline milieu with pH 7.8 (> 6.6 threshold), calcium carbonate begins to aggregate and precipitate. The model is summarized in Figure 4.1.5.

There were limitations to this study. The roles of mucin [19] and/or nucleating factors [23] were not investigated. Additionally, the effects of bile salts in GB bile on calcium concentration were not studied. [21, 26] Future investigations on these aspects are warranted.

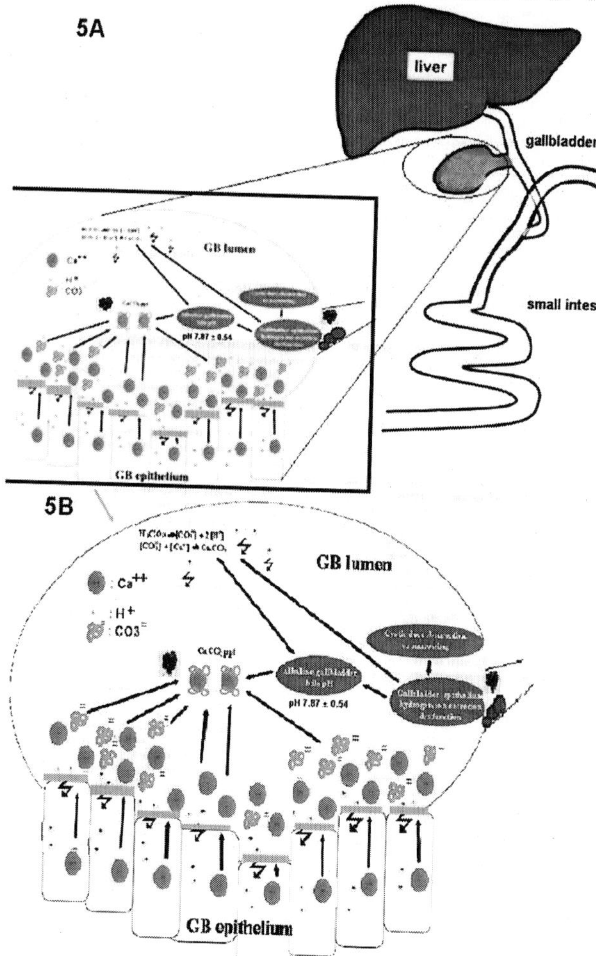

Figure 4.1.5. Schematic diagrams of hypothetical model for the pathogenesis of calcium carbonate gallstone formation. 5A demonstrates the etiologic roles of (1) cystic duct obstruction; (2) subsequent gallbladder wall low grade inflammation and epithelial dysfunction in hydrogen ion secretions leading to increased carbonate anion concentration, free calcium ion concentration, increased SI_$CaCO_3$ and alkalinization of gallbladder bile with pH above 6.6, the critical value for calcium carbonate precipitation. 3B is the magnified view of the inlet in 3A.

II. Pathogenesis of Calcium-Containing Gallstones Canine Ductular Bile, But Not Gallbladder Bile, Is Supersaturated with Calcium Carbonate [21]

Calcium precipitation in bile is a requisite event in the initiation and growth of all pigment gallstones. Calcium solubility in bile is thus of great importance. This is the first attempt to define the ion-product of $CaCO_3$ in bile in any species. If the ion-product: $[C^{++}]$ x $[CO_3^{=}1$ exceeds solubility product (K'_{sp}), the sample is supersaturated and $CaCO_3$ precipitation is thermodynamically possible. We have recently determined K' of calcite to be 3.76 X 10^{-8} mol/liter at 37^0 C and total ionic strength = 0.16 M. Gallbladder (GB) bile was obtained from 15 anesthetized dogs after 12-24-h fasts. Duct bile was obtained from three dogs (n = 12) during variable taurocholate infusion. Samples were assayed for pH, partial pressure of carbon dioxide (Pco_2), total bile salt concentration (TBS), total calcium concentration (ICaD, and free calcium ion concentration (C_a^{++}). With increasing [TBS] in both GB and duct bile, there was a linear decline in pH, a curvilinear decline in $IHCO_3^-I$ and $ICO_3^{=}j$, and linear increase in $[Ca^{++}]$ and [Cal. All ductular samples were supersaturated with $CaCO_3$, with saturation indices (SI) as high as 17.5 and a mean of 8.36±1.43 (SE). In sharp contrast, none of the GB samples were supersaturated, due to the marked decline in $[CO_2j$ upon concentration and acidification of bile. In GB bile, the SI ranged from 0.006 to 0.126, with a mean of 0.039±0.011. The gallbladder thus produced a change in the SI from a value as high as 17.5 to a value as low as 0.006 in concentrated GB bile, which is a nearly 3,000-fold change. The average change in the SI was -215-fold. Since all duct samples were supersaturated, and since the dog does not normally form gallstones, the data support our previous hypotheses that: (a) in canine bile, as in canine pancreatic juice, a nucleating factor is necessary for $CaCO_3$ precipitation; (b) bile salts are important buffers for Ca^{++} in bile; and (c) normal GB mucosal function (concentration and acidification of bile) plays an important role in reducing $CaCO_3$ lithogenicity in GB bile.

Calcium precipitation in bile is a requisite physicochemical event in the initiation and growth of all pigment gallstones. Such stones contain calcium salts of one or more readily precipitable anions in bile, which Rege and Moore [27] have recently termed "calcium-sensitive": carbonate, bilirubinate, phosphate, and long-chain fatty acids by Sutor and Wilkie. [28] Calcium solubility in bile is thus of critical importance in the formation of pigment stones. For cholesterol stones, the importance of cholesterol supersaturation in bile was clearly demonstrated by the studies of Admirand and Small. [29] More recent work has highlighted the importance of nucleation factors in the formation of cholesterol stones, since supersaturated bile occurs in individuals who do not have gallstones, [30-32] and since bile from cholesterol gallstone patients nucleates more rapidly in vitro than bile samples from subjects without gallstones for a given degree of cholesterol supersaturation by Holan, Gollish and Burnstein et al. [33-35] Precipitated calcium salts in bile are believed to serve as a nucleus for cholesterol precipitation since cholesterol stones have been found to contain pigment stone centers by Been and Wosiewitz et al. [36, 37] Therefore, Rege and Moore [27, 38] have recently advanced the hypothesis that calcium precipitation is important in the initiation of cholesterol gallstones by forming a nucleus on which cholesterol can precipitate from its supersaturated state. A similar view has been expressed by Williamson and Percy-Robb. [39] In addition to possibly having a role in the initiation of cholesterol stones, calcium precipitation may occur on the surface of such stones either spontaneously, [40] during chenodeoxycholic acid treatment, [41] or during ursodeoxycholic acid treatment. [40] Such precipitation is clinically important, as it usually precludes successful gallstone dissolution. In any given bile sample, the limiting solubility of a calcium salt is determined by the ion-product: $[Ca^{++}]$ x $[anion^{-}]$ for that salt. If this product exceeds the solubility product constant (Ksp)' of that salt, the sample is supersaturated (metastable) and calcium precipitation is thermodynamically possible. Of the four anions listed above that precipitate with calcium in bile, only the K's ofCaCO3 (calcite) has been determined under physiologic conditions. Recently, using the Ca^{++} electrode, Moore and Verine [42] have reported Ksp for calcite to be 3.76×10^{-8} mol/ liter at 37°C. Comparison of the ion-product: $[Ca^{++}]$ x $[CO_3^{=}]$ in a given bile sample at 37°C with the value of Ks allows a quantitative statement as to whether that sample is supersaturated with respect to calcite. This study is the first attempt to determine the ion-product of a calcium salt in bile in any species. We will show that canine ductular bile, but not gallbladder bile, is supersaturated with calcium carbonate. The results suggest that: (a) nucleating factor(s) are necessary for calcium precipitation in bile, and (b) normal gallbladder mucosal function (absorption and acidification) greatly reduces the $[Ca^{++}]$ x $[CO_3^{=}]$ ion product, so that gallbladder bile is normally unsaturated with calcite. Gallbladder bile was obtained from 15 mongrel dogs anesthetized with sodium pentobarbitol (25 mg/kg) after 12-24-h fasts. The period of fasting as intentionally varied to achieve variable degrees of bile concentration and acidification. Laparotomy was performed and gallbladder bile aspirated anaerobically into a syringe using a 20-gauge needle. Care was taken to empty the gallbladder completely to minimize stratification effects on bile composition. [43] 2 samples of common duct bile were also obtained from three dogs during variable infusion of sodium taurocholate (0-100 Mmol/min), obtained from Calbiochem-Behring Corp., La Jolla, CA (purity > 98%). t laparotomy, the cystic duct was ligated, and the common duct was intubated with PE-190 tubing, and ligated distally. For each rate of infusion, bile flow was allowed to stabilize until it was relatively constant. At this time, a sample of duct bile was slowly withdrawn anaerobically into a syringe. A second higher rate of taurocholate infusion was then begun and the procedure repeated. All samples were immediately analyzed at 370C for pH and partial pressure of carbon dioxide (Pco2) using a blood gas analyzer (model 13; Instrumentation Laboratory, Inc., Lexington, MA). Total CO_2 content $[TCO_2]$) was determined in triplicate with an S/Special Chem Micro O2 System (American Scientific Products, McGaw Park, IL). Total bile salt concentration was assessed by the 3-hydroxysteroid dehydrogenase method by Talalay. [44] Total calcium concentration ([Ca]) was determined by atomic absorption spectroscopy using a spectrometer (model 305B; Perkin- Elmer Corp., Instrument Div., Norwalk, CT). Free ionized calcium concentration ([Ca++]) was determined anaerobically at 370C with a Ca++ electrode (Model SS-20 Ionalyzer; Orion Research, Inc., Cambridge, A). In each sample, the bicarbonate ion concentration ($[HCO_3^{-}]$) was calculated from the Henderson-Hasselbalch equation:

$$pH = pK_1' + \log\ [HCO_3^{-}] / Pco_2 \cdot Q' \quad \text{(Eq. la)}$$

$$[HCO_3^{-}] = (Pco_2 \cdot Q') \times (10^{pH - pK1'}) \quad \text{(Eq. Ib)}$$

here $pK'_1 = 6.1$ at 37°C,(45) and Q' is the CO_2 solubility coefficient. The product: Pco2 * Q' is the concentration of dissolved CO_2. Rege have recently reported Q' to be 0.0288 mol/liter per mmHg in canine bile at 37°C; this value was used in the calculations. In each sample, the carbonate ion concentration ($[CO_3^{=}]$) was similarly calculated:

$$pH = pK'_2 + \log [HCO^-]/[CO_3^{=}] \quad \text{(Eq. 2a)}$$
$$[CO_3^{=}] = [HCO_3^- J \times (10^{pH-pK2'}) \quad \text{(Eq. 2b)}$$

here $pK'_2 = 9.8$ at 37°C (19). The ion-product: $[Ca^{++}] \times [CO_3^{=}]$ was then determined for each sample from observed electrode $[Ca^{++}]$ and calculated $[CO_3^{=}]$ concentrations. All calculations were made with a computer PC-XT; IBM Instruments, Inc., Danbury, CT); graphs were made using lotus 1-2-3 software and Hewlett-Packard Model 7470A plotter.

In the results section, pH vs. total bile salt concentration ([TBS]). As shown in Figure 1, there was an apparently linear decline in pH with increasing [TBS]. The slopes of the regressions for duct and gallbladder bile samples were not significantly different from one another (variance analysis), so the two sets of data were combined to yield the tentative regression: pH = 8.03 - 0.008 [TBS], (r = 0.97). In duct samples, with increasing taurocholate infusion and increasing [TBS], pH declined from 7.85 to 7.37. The linear decline in pH continued in gallbladder samples as bile salt con centration rose during sodium and water reabsorption. Thus, in the most concentrated gallbladder bile sample, [TBS] was 305 mM and pH was 5.86; the lowest observed pH was 5.81 at a [TBS] of 298 mM. $[HCO_3^-]$ and $[CO_3^{=}]$ vs. [TBS]. The above-mentioned decline in pH was accompanied by a curvilinear decrease in calculated bicarbonate and carbonate ion concentrations. In ductular bile, maximally observed $[HCO_3]$ was 38.6 mM, with a decline to <1 mM in concentrated gallbladder bile. Similarly, $[CO_3^{=}]$ declined from a maximal value of 0.34 mM in ductular bile to <7 X 10-8 M in concentrated and acidified gallbladder bile. This decline was - 5,000-fold. Thus, the normal concentration and acidification of bile in the canine gallbladder resulted in a striking decrease in the concentration of one component of the ion-product: $[Ca^{++}] \times [CO_3^{=}]$. This decline in $[CO_3^{=}]$ would correspondingly increase the maximal allowable $[Ca^{++}]$ concentration within the limits of calcium carbonate solubility, as dictated by K,'. [Ca] and free $[Ca^{++}]$ vs. [TBS]. In sharp contrast to the above decrease in [CO], the concentrations of total calcium and free ionized $[Ca^{++}]$ rose linearly with increasing bile salt concentration in both ductular and gallbladder bile samples. For total calcium, the combined tentative regression was: [Ca] = 2.73 + 0.026 [TBS], (r = 0.96), while for free $[Ca^{++}]$ it was: $[Ca^{++}]$ = 1. 16 + 0.0063 [TBS], (r = 0.90). The $[Ca^{++}]$- intercept of the latter regression, 1. 16 mM, is the approximate normal canine ionized calcium concentration in plasma. This suggests that free Ca^{++} ion in the proximal biliary tract is at or near electrochemical equilibrium with plasma. The slope of 0.0063 (Figure 4) for the rise in $[Ca^{++}]$ was considerably lower than the slope of0.026 (Figure 5) observed for total calcium, which indicates that free $[Ca^{++}]$ rises more slowly than [Ca] during bile concentration. Thus, in ductular samples, mean [Ca] was 3.98±0.18 mM (SE), whereas in gallbladder bile it was 9.30±0.28 mM. In contrast, mean [Ca++] rose from 1.47±0.08 mM in ductular bile to a mean of only 2.7 1±0.1 I mM in gallbladder bile. This difference between total and free Ca+4 concentrations largely reflects binding of calcium to bile salts. Thus, the ratio of mean $[Ca^{++}]$ to mean [Ca]: 2.71/9.30 = 0.291 in gallbladder bile indicates that only about 29. 1% of total calcium was present as the free ion, while 70.9% was present as bound and complexed species. Significant calcium-binding would be expected, since taurocholate is the major bile acid in canine bile, and since we have recently found affinity constants of - 151 liters/mol and 7.1 liters/mol for the binding of calcium to free and micellar taurocholate species, respectively. (27, 38) Ion product: $[Ca^{++}]$ x $[CO_3^{=}]$ The above-mentioned decline in $[CO_3^{=}]$ was much greater than the rise in free $[Ca^{++}]$, so that the ion-product: $[Ca^{++}]$ x $[CO_3^{=}]$ sharply declined with increasing bile salt concentration. The dashed line at 3.76 X 10-8 mol/liter is the value of K', for calcite at 37°C and total ionic strength 0. 16 M [17]. It can be seen that all duct bile samples were supersaturated, with ion-products that exceeded K' . The most marked degree§ of supersaturation were at the lowest bile salt concentrations. These data indicate that canine ductular bile is metastable with respect to calcium carbonate (calcite). In sharp contrast, all gallbladder bile samples were far below K', which indicates that canine gallbladder bile is normally unsaturated with respect to calcite. Saturation index. Another way of considering calcium sol- from 0.006 to 0.126, with a mean of only 0.039±0.01 Thus, the mean ion-product in gallbladder bile was only 3.9% K'_{SP} so that, on the average, gallbladder bile was unsaturated factor of ~25. These data show that normal gallbladder mucosal function, i.e., concentration and acidification of bile, produced change in the saturation index from a value as high as 17.5 in ductular bile to a value as low as 0.006 in gallbladder bile, a nearly 3,000- fold change. The average change in the saturation index ductular (8.34) to gallbladder (0.039) bile was -215-fold.

In the discussion section, these studies represent the first attempt in any species to determine whether bile is supersaturated with respect to calcium carbonate. Using the Ca^{++} ion electrode for measurement ionized calcium, and established relationships and constants calculation of free carbonate ion concentration, the ion-product: $[Ca^{++}]$ x $[CO_3^{=}]$ has been assessed in 12 samples of canine ductular bile and in 15 samples of gallbladder bile. The results show striking differences between ductular and gallbladder bile. Therefore, all ductular samples, but none of the gallbladder samples, were supersaturated with calcium carbonate. They believe these findings have important implications regarding the pathogenesis of calcium- containing gallstones. First, a metastable state has been shown to exist in ductular bile samples of the dog, a species that does not normally form gallstones. This strongly suggests that a nucleating factor is necessary for $CaCO_3$ precipitation to occur in bile. It has been previously reported a very analogous situation in canine pancreatic juice,(47) in which both basal and stimulated samples were consistently supersaturated with respect to calcite, yet the dog is not known to form pancreatic stones. Pancreatic stones have been reported only in humans and cattle by Sarles and Verine, [48, 49] and are composed largely or entirely of calcite in both species by Perinet, Mallet-Guy and Perrin et al. [50-52] The presence of supersaturated juice, but no stones, strongly suggests that for a pancreatic stone to develop, a nidus for CaCO3 precipitation is necessary. Verine and Lafont [53] have demonstrated the presence of protein in pancreatic stones from humans and cattle, and Sarles [48] has suggested that such a protein "plug" forms a nidus for $CaCO_3$ precipitation in human pancreatic calcific disease. The present studies thus indicate that there are strong analogies between bile and pancreatic juice in the dog; both fluids are supersaturated with $CaCO_3$, yet neither gallstones nor pancreatic stones have been reported in this species. These findings suggest that a nucleating factor, presumably mucus and/or protein, is required for $CaCO_3$ precipitation in bile, similar to the "protein plug" theory of Sarles for $CaC0_3$ precipitation in pancreatic juice. Any measure that reduces the free Ca^{++} concentration (activity) in bile will reduce the likelihood of pigment gallstone formation. The second implication of these studies is that bile salts are the major buffers for free Ca^{++} in bile, in conformity with our previous hypothesis in studies of calcium-binding to taurocholate by Moore et al. [38] This is indicated by the finding that, on the average, only about 29% of the total calcium in gallbladder bile was present as free Ca^{++}ion; the remainder was present as bound or complexed species. At given total calcium, this buffer action would tend to reduce free Ca^{++}, and thus serve to reduce the $[Ca^{++}]$ $[CO_3^{=}]$ ion product, thereby reducing the likelihood of $CaCO_3$ precipitation in bile. The third implication of the present study relates to gallbladder mucosal function, and the protection that this provides against calcium precipitation in bile. Therefore, it was seen that all ductular samples were supersaturated with $CaCO_3$, whereas none of the gallbladder bile samples were supersaturated. This reduction in lithogenicity of gallbladder bile occurred in the face of increasing $[C_a^{++}]$, and was due to a marked reduction in free carbonate ion concentration. They now will consider the mechanisms by which $[CO_3^{=}]$ may be so dramatically reduced in gallbladder bile. The reduction in free$[CO_3^{=}]$ is due primarily to two factors: (a) reduction in total carbonate (totalCO_2 in all forms) in gallbladder bile, and (b) reduction in the relative proportion of $[CO_3^{=}]$ as pH declines. In the past, it has been generally held that the reduction in total carbonate in gallbladder bile that occurs during the concentrating process is due to bicarbonate ion reabsorption. Recently, nevertheless, in studies reported elsewhere (Rege., and. Moore, manuscript submitted for publication), they have shown that in the dog, there is substantial ion secretion by gallbladder mucosa. This presumably represents a Na^+/H^+ exchange in the epithelial cell, similar to that recently described in Necturus gallbladder in vitro by Weinman and Reuss [28]. Acidification by H^+ secretion would result in a greater pH decline, at given luminal bicarbonate, than would occur by simple bicarbonate absorption alone, due to an increase in the denominator of the Henderson-Hasselbalch equation (increase in CO_2 from luminal bicarbonate neutralization). As a result of this pH decline, the proportion of total CO_2 present as carbonate ion would be substantially lower. These considerations regarding gallbladder mucosal function may be summarized as follows: upon delivery of ductular bile to the gallbladder, the mucosa absorbs Na' and water, while secreting H' ion. The latter reacts with luminal bicarbonate to produce CO_2 and water. As a result of bicarbonate neutralization and CO_2 production, there is a decline in pH and total $C0_2$, with dramatic decline in the concentration of free $[CO_3^{=}]$ ion. The decrease in $[CO_3^{=}]$ is so substantial that gallbladder bile remains very unsaturated with respect to $CaCO_3$, despite a rise in free $[Ca^{++}]$ during the concentrating process. In addition, upon removal of water by mucosal function (Na^+ absorption), the total bile salt concentration increases, with a corresponding increase in calcium-binding capacity, so that free $[Ca^{++}]$ remains relatively low in the face of increasing total calcium. Resulting [COT] and $[Ca^{++}]$ are thus sufficiently low to produce an ion product that is well below K'_{sp} for calcite. Note that assessment of $CaCO_3$ solubility is strongly dependent on the constants used in the calculations: pK'_1, pK'_2, and K'_{sp}. For the first two of these, we have used values given by Edsall and Wyman [19], who have noted that these are probably accurate to within 0.1 pH unit [29]. For K',, we have used the value 3.76 X 10-8 mol/liter, recently obtained with the Ca^{++} electrode [16]; this value is similar to that of Hastings, Murray, and Sendroy [30] who, in 1926, obtained a K', of 3.98×10^{-8} mol/liter (37°C, total ionic strength $[\mu] = 0.15$ M), and is almost identical to the results of Broman and Hastings [31] who, in 1937, obtained a calcite K' value of 3.72 X 10-8 mol/liter. All of the above Ksp values were obtained at a total ionic strength of 0.15 or 0.16 M, which is the approximate ionic strength of ductular bile. As bile undergoes concentration by the gallbladder, the total ionic strength increases, so that in fully concentrated bile the sodium concentration may exceed 300 mM. As it has been noted previously [1], the term "total ionic strength" has no clearly defined meaning in such samples, because bile salt anions aggregate to form micelles and the activities of Na^+ and K^+, [54] and also Ca^{++} [38] are suppressed by virtue of binding to the micelle. In gallbladder bile, it is therefore likely that K' varies somewhat from sample to sample, so that the saturation indices for gallbladder samples should be viewed as approximate estimations. Since gallbladder samples were unsaturated by a factor of ~25, minor variations in KSP due to ionic strength effects would not diminish the striking differences between ductular and gallbladder bile, and would not alter the conclusion that gallbladder bile is unsaturated with respect to calcite. Also note that three different polymorphs of $CaCO_3$ have been identified in human gallstones: calcite, aragonite, and vaterite [36, 55].

Vaterite is rarely found elsewhere in nature, and the physicochemical significance of the various polymorphs in gallstone disease is not known. Insofar as relative solubility of the various polymorphs is concerned, Broman and Hastings [31] found aragonite to be somewhat more soluble than calcite; we know of no studies of vaterite solubility under physiologic conditions. Should future studies show that vaterite is less soluble than calcite, then resulting saturation indices would be higher than those depicted. On the other hand, if vaterite is more soluble than calcite, then Ksp for calcite will determine $CaCO_3$ solubility, since limiting solubility is determined by the least soluble species present. The relative solubilities of aragonite and vaterite are worthy of future investigation.

We believe these studies have provided new insights into some of the factors that may lead to calcium precipitation and gallstone formation. The results support our previous hypothesis (I) that in canine bile, as in canine pancreatic juice, a nucleating factor is necessary for $CaCO_3$ precipitation. In addition, it is proposed that normal gallbladder mucosal function plays an important role in reducing calcium carbonate lithogenicity in gallbladder bile. Similar studies are now needed in human.

III. Limy Bile Syndrome [12]

Milk of calcium bile or limy bile is a rare disorder in which the gall bladder is filled with a thick, paste-like, radiopaque material. Seven patients with limy bile syndrome were treated in our department from 1980 to 2003. There were five women and two men, and their age ranged from 30 to 64 years.

A retrospective analysis of clinical symptoms, diagnostic work-up, treatment approach and operative findings was performed. All patients presented with intermittent right upper abdominal quadrant pain. Three of the seven patients (42.85%) presented with complications like acute cholecystitis (two of seven patients) and obstructive jaundice (one of seven patients). Diagnosis was based on clinical findings, plain abdominal X-rays, ultrasonography and computed tomography scanning. Surgery was the treatment of choice and cholecystectomy alone or in combination with common bile duct exploration and drainage (if needed) was performed.

Conclusion

The clinical aspect of the disease is similar to that of biliary lithiasis and the diagnosis is easily made by the characteristic spontaneous opacification of the gall bladder on plain abdominal X-rays. Complications such as acute cholecystitis, pancreatitis or obstructive jaundice can also be present. Although some cases of conservative pharmaceutical treatment as well as cases of spontaneous disappearance of limy bile have been reported, surgical treatment remains the treatment of choice.

Limy bile is a rare disorder in which the gall bladder, and rarely the common bile duct, are filled with a thick paste-like radiopaque material by Hatzigcorgiadis et al. [11, 56] This is almost entirely composed of calcium carbonate by weight Komblum and Phemister et al. [5, 57, 58] and the precipitation of these inorganic calcium salts results in spontaneous opacification of the gall bladder on plain abdominal X-rays. The aim of the present study was the retrospective analysis of clinical symptoms and signs, diagnostic work-up and the treatment approach of patients with limy bile referred to their department.

In the methods section, in a retrospective analysis of patients who underwent cholecystectomy in Konstantino et al.'s department from 1980 to 2003, seven patients were found to have a radiopaque gall bladder in plain abdominal X-rays, suggesting limy bile. There were five women and two men, and their age ranged from 30 to 64 years. No patient had other abnormal calcifications. Serum calcium levels and urinary calcium output, measured in all patients, were consistently normal. Two of these patients were operated on early after their admission due to acute cholecystitis, while the rest underwent elective surgery. In six patients limy bile was limited to the gall bladder while in one it was present in both the gall bladder and common bile duct. All patients were operated on under general anaesthesia, through a right subcostal incision and cholecystectomy was performed along with common bile duct exploration when indicated. A review of data on all patients treated is presented in Table 1.

In the results section, all patients presented with intermittent right upper abdominal quadrant pain, lasting from 3 months to 7 years. Three of the 7 patients (42.85%) presented with complications like acute cholecystitis (two of seven patients) and obstructive jaundice (one of seven patients). Patients with acute cholecystitis presented with fever and right upper abdominal quadrant tenderness on physical examination. Abdominal tenderness and jaundice were the main physical findings in the patient with limy bile extending to the common bile duct while laboratory studies revealed a total bilirubin level of 4.4 mg/dL with direct bilirubin at 3 mg/dL, and increased levels of liver function tests (serum glutamate oxaloacetate 170 IU/l, serum glutamate pyruvate transaminase 300 IU/l, alkaline phosphatase 166 IU/L). Laboratory data were within normal limits in all other patients but the two with acute cholecystitis who presented with leukocytosis. There were no severe associated diseases in any patient. Spontaneous opacification of the gall bladder on plain abdominal X-rays (Figure 1) was revealed in all patients. In one patient, the cystic duct was also opacified, while opacification of the common bile duct, with the characteristic 'exclamation sign', was revealed in another patient. Ultrasonography showed hyperechogenic material in the gall bladder's lumen associated with lithiasis in all patients and with dilation of extra- and intrahepatic bile ducts in one patient. Computed tomography (CT) scanning, performed in two patients, revealed the presence of high density material in the gall bladder. The two patients with acute cholecystitis were operated on during the first 24 h after their admission, while the rest underwent elective surgery. All patients underwent cholecystectomy. The gallbladder was macroscopically normal or had minimal changes in all patients, with a slightly thick wall in patients with acute cholecystitis, and moderately distended in the patient with jaundice. It was filled with a white, thick, paste-like material in all patients. An impacted stone was found in the cystic duct of one patient. Intraoperative cholangiography and common bile duct exploration through cystic duct remnant was performed in the patient with limy bile extending to the common bile duct and two clots of limy bile were extracted. All patients recovered uneventfully. Biochemical analysis of the paste-like material revealed the presence of calcium carbonate but no quantitative analysis was performed in any specimen.

In the discussion section, churchman first described limy bile in 1911. [59] Volkmann, [60] in 1926, called this disorder 'kalkmilchgalle' or milk of calcium bile. The term limy bile was introduced in 1933 by Knutsson [61] to denote the condition in which calcium, usually in the form of carbonate, is precipitated in the gall bladder, rendering it radiopaque. Limy bile syndrome is a rare disorder compared to the prevalence of biliary lithiasis. It is characterized by: the presence of a thick, paste-like, radiopaque material in the gall bladder and/or common bile duct lumen; its clinical aspect similar to that of biliary lithiasis, and spontaneous opacification of the gall bladder and/or common bile duct on plain abdominal X-rays, which is due to calcium carbonate precipitation by Cohen, Nomura, Marquis and Morehouse et al. [62-65] Prevalence of the syndrome ranges between 0.1 and 1.7% of patients operated on for biliary lithiasis by Katsuda, Mouchet, Love and Treyve et al. [66-69] it is more common in women (men : women ratio = 1:3) by Moreaux and Roux, [17]and all ages are affected by Grand and Amand et al. [70, 71] (from the age of 3 years) but more commonly after the age of 40 years reported by LeGnissel and Schwartz et al. [14, 67, 72, 73] Concomitant biliary lithiasis was present in all patients in our series and in 60–81% of patients in other series by Delgotte et al. [17, 74] Constant association of limy bile with biliary lithiasis must be emphasized. Presence of limy bile in the common bile duct is rare – only a few cases have been reported [17, 56, 65, 74] (one in our series) – and it always occurs in patients with limy bile in the gall bladder, and can be attributed to migration of small impacted stones from the cystic duct or the neck of the gall bladder, followed by passage of the calcareous material from the gall bladder to the common bile duct. 6 Formation of limy bile in the gall bladder is not well understood, although it is generally agreed that some form of obstruction in the cystic duct or gall bladder neck and the resultant bile stasis are necessary. 1,6 Under these circumstances precipitation of calcium carbonate, which is normally present in bile, is the end result of local changes in the gall bladder, but the exact mechanism and the time required for these biochemical changes are not fully elucidated. [17] Chronic inflammatory changes of the gall bladder, which are often observed, seem to be not specific and probably secondary by Knutsson and Cohen et al. [17, 61, 62]. The clinical aspect of the syndrome is similar to that of biliary lithiasis. Presence of limy bile in the gall bladder can be an incidental finding on plain abdominal X-rays of patients with no symptoms at all. Biliary symptoms are, however, present in most patients with limy bile syndrome by Delgotte et al. [14, 67, 72-74] Complications such as acute cholecystitis, pancreatitis or obstructive jaundice can also be present. Symptoms and complications do not seem to be the result of limy bile, but of the associated calculous biliary tract disease by Delgotte et al. [17, 74]. In our series three of seven patients presented one of the above-mentioned complications (acute cholecystitis two of seven, obstructive jaundice one of seven patients). Plain abdominal X-rays are crucial in diagnosis. Characteristic findings are the presence of radiopaque material in the gall bladder, the cystic duct and/or the common bile duct and the exclamation mark sign, which is present when limy bile and gallstones coexist in the common bile duct by Cohen, Nokuda, Marquis and Chun et al. [62-64, 75] Limy bile may resemble a normally opacified gall bladder following oral cholecystography. It must though be determined whether the patient received cholecystographic contrast medium before definitive diagnosis of limy bile is established. Ultrasonography is much less specific [76, 77] and in most cases simply reveals concomitant biliary lithiasis. Routine use of plain abdominal X-rays on admission for all patients presenting with right upper abdominal quadrant pain is the rule in our department, and the rarity of the syndrome cannot be attributed to the routine use of ultrasonography in the last decade. Interestingly, six of the seven patients were diagnosed before the laparoscopic era while the more recently presented was not considered a candidate for laparoscopic cholecystectomy because of a previous operation in the upper abdomen. Differential diagnosis from a porcelain gall bladder, in which extensive calcification of the gall bladder wall is present, is also necessary. Ultrasonography and abdominal CT are considered highly specific in differentiating porcelain gall bladder from other calcifying pathologies like limy bile syndrome. In such cases, complete or partial calcification of the gall bladder wall is easily differentiated from radiopaque material filling the gall bladder. This differential diagnosis is essential as porcelain gall bladder is considered to be a premalignant condition. Although some cases of conservative pharmaceutical treatment [78-80] as well as cases of spontaneous disappearance of limy bile have been reported, [64, 66, 74, 78] surgical treatment remains the treatment of choice. Cholecystectomy, intraoperative cholangiography and common bile duct exploration when necessary seems justified in patients with specific biliary symptoms. In nonsymptomatic patients, however, or in patients with spontaneous disappearance of limy bile, surgical treatment is not recommended unless biliary lithiasis coexists.

IV. Gallbladder Mucin Production and Calcium Carbonate Gallstones in Children [20]

In contrast to adults, calcium carbonate gallstones are relatively common in children. Their pathogenesis is poorly understood. Cystic duct obstruction promotes calcium carbonate formation in bile and increases gallbladder mucin production. Sayers et al. tested the hypothesis that mucin producing epithelial cells would be increased in gallbladders of children with calcium carbonate gallstones. Archival gallbladder specimens from 20 consecutive children who had undergone elective cholecystectomy for cholelithiasis were examined. In each case, gallstone composition was determined by Fourier transform infrared microspectroscopy. Gallbladder specimens from six children who had undergone cholecystectomy for conditions other than cholelithiasis during the same period were used as controls. Multiple sections were examined in a blinded fashion and scored semiquantitatively for mucin production using two stains (alcian blue and periodic acid-Schiff). Increased mucin staining was observed in 50% or more epithelial cells in five gallbladder specimens from seven children with calcium carbonate stones, compared to 5 of 13 with other stone types ($P = 0.17$) and none of the control gallbladders ($P = 0.02$). Gallbladders containing calcium carbonate stones were significantly more likely than those containing other stone types or controls to contain epithelial cells with the greatest mucin content (P = 0.03).

Gallbladders containing calcium carbonate stones were also more likely to show the ulcer-associated cell lineage. These results demonstrate an increase in mucin producing epithelial cells in gallbladders from children containing calcium carbonate stones. This supports the hypothesis that cystic duct obstruction leading to increased gallbladder mucin production may play a role in the development of calcium carbonate gallstones in children.

Studies in Western children have shown an increase in the prevalence of gallstones during the last three decades [81-83]. Traditionally, three types of gallstones have been recognized. Cholesterol stones develop from cholesterol supersaturation of bile; they account for 70–90% of gallstones in Western adults and also occur in overweight adolescent girls. Black pigment stones represent the commonest type of gallstone in children. They are formed from the supersaturation of bile with calcium bilirubinate, the calcium salt of unconjugated bilirubin. Black pigment stones are typically found in hemolytic disorders and also develop in association with parenteral nutrition by Takiff and O'Brien et al. [84, 85] Brown pigment stones are rare and form in presence of biliary stasis and bacterial infection. They occur more often in the bile ducts than the gallbladder and are composed of calcium bilirubinate and calcium salts of fatty acids. [86] In 2003, we reported a detailed composition analysis of a consecutive series of pediatric gallstones from the United Kingdom. [87] The stones were analyzed using Fourier transform infrared microspectroscopy, a highly accurate method of determining stone composition. The relative proportions of each major stone component were assessed: cholesterol, protein and calcium salts of bilirubin, fatty acids, carbonate and hydroxyapatite. Of the 20 children, 10 had black pigment stones, 2 had cholesterol stones and one had brown pigment stones. Remarkably, 7 (35%) children were found to have calcium carbonate stones, composed of 90% or more of calcium carbonate polymorphs. Prior to this study, calcium carbonate stones were considered very rare in both adults and children. Their occurrence in children had been confined to isolated case reports by Beauregard and Wu et al. [88, 89] The pathogenesis of calcium carbonate gallstones is not understood. One possible factor contributing to a higher prevalence of calcium carbonate stones in children could be cystic duct obstruction, since this promotes calcium carbonate formation in bile. [90] Cystic duct obstruction is also known to cause markedly increased gallbladder mucin production by Harvey et al. [91] Gallbladder mucin is rich in calcium carbonate. [92] Our hypothesis would be supported if it could be shown that mucin producing cells in the gallbladder mucosa of children with calcium carbonate gallstones were increased in comparison to children with other gallstone types. We therefore investigated gallbladder histology in children whose gallstone composition had been previously established.

In the patients and methods section, cholecystectomy specimens Archival gallbladder specimens from a series of 20 consecutive children who had undergone elective cholecystectomy for cholelithiasis between June 1997 and January 2002 were examined. The chemical composition of the gallstones in each of these patients had been previously determined by Fourier transform infrared microspectroscopy [7]. Archival gallbladder specimens from children who had undergone cholecystectomy for conditions other than cholelithiasis during the same period were used as controls. The study was approved by institutional and research ethical committees. Histochemistry Two sections, each of 4 *l*m thickness, were cut from each specimen of formalin fixed paraffin embedded tissue and stained separately with two mucin stains, alcian blue and periodic acid-Schiff. For the former, tissue sections were immersed in alcian blue reagent (1 g alcian blue in 0.1 M hydrochloric acid) for 15 min, washed in water, and immersed in 1% aqueous neutral red solution for 1 min, before being dehydrated with 100% alcohol, cleared in xylene and mounted. For the latter, tissue sections were immersed in 1% periodic acid solution, washed in water, immersed in Schiff's reagent for 5 min, washed in water for 10 min, and immersed in Harris's haematoxylin for 2 min, before being dehydrated in 100% alcohol, cleared in xylene and mounted. Microscopy Stained sections were examined using light microscopy by a histopathologist (CS) blinded to the chemical composition of the gallstones and to the clinical details on the histopathology request form. Epithelial cells from representative sections of each gallbladder were scored according to their mucin content. A scale of 0 to + + + was employed, with zero representing no staining, + representing weak staining in the apical cytoplasm, + + representing moderate staining in the apical half of the cytoplasm, and + + + representing strong staining throughout the cytoplasm. The presence of goblet cells, indicative of intestinal metaplasia, was also noted. Ten representative high power fields were examined in each case, and the percentage (and thus density) of cells within each category of the staining scale determined. In 14 cases, sections from the fundus, body and neck of the gallbladder were examined; in the remaining six cases the exact site of origin of the paraffin embedded tissue could not be confirmed with certainty. Statistics Fisher's exact test was used to compare categorical variables, taking $P < 0.05$ as statistical significance.

In the results section, the study group consisted of 20 consecutive cholecystectomy specimens from children (11 boys, 9 girls) with a median age of 8 (0.3–13.9) years. Control gallbladders were from six children (three boys and girls) with a median age of 7.9 (0.3–12.3) years; this group included five children undergoing cholecystectomy at the time of choledochal cyst excision and one child who had a prophylactic cholecystectomy whilst undergoing biliopancreatic diversion for familial lipoprotein lipase deficiency. Mucin content of gallbladder epithelial cells In ten of the study group cases the majority of epithelial cells scored + for mucin. In nine cases, the majority scored + + and in one case, the majority scored + + +. Epithelial cell mucin stained positive with periodic acid-Schiff suggesting relatively neutral mucin. Goblet cells were identified in four gallbladder specimens and their mucin content was positive with alcian blue suggesting acidic mucin. Analysis of the control group showed that in all six cases, the majority of epithelial cells scored + for mucin. Goblet cells were identified in only one specimen. Ulcer-associated cell lineage In nine of the study group cases, focal glandular structures were seen budding from the base of mucosal folds. These consisted of cuboidal cells with small, round, basal nuclei and pale cytoplasm. The latter stained particularly strongly with periodic acid- Schiff and less so with alcian blue. In one case, an adjacent duct-like structure was seen near the mucosal surface. These morphological features were suggestive of the ulcer-associated cell lineage (UACL). (93) Correlation with gallstone type Mucin staining + + or + + + was observed in 50% or more epithelial cells in five gallbladder specimens from seven children with calcium carbonate stones, compared to 5 of 13 with other stone types ($P = 0.17$) and none of the control gallbladders ($P = 0.02$). Of the ten gallbladders demonstrating + + + mucin containing cells, six were from patients with calcium carbonate stones; only one of the control gallbladders showed epithelial cells with + + + mucin content. Of the nine gallbladders with UACL features, five were from children with calcium carbonate stones.

In the discussion section, the gallbladder is conventionally regarded as an absorptive organ but the gallbladder mucosa also secretes water, electrolytes and mucin into the lumen reported by Klinkspoor et al. [94] This fluid is rich in bicarbonate by Glickman et al. [95] Calcium ions also enter the gallbladder lumen when mucus is secreted, because the intracellular mucin storage granules contain high concentrations of calcium by Taylor et al. [92]. If the cystic duct is obstructed, gallbladder bicarbonate and mucin secretion are stimulated and gallbladder bile becomes rich in calcium carbonate. [58] Mucins themselves may also influence calcium carbonate precipitation. In one study, mucin purified from T-tube bile of a patient with intrahepatic stones was more highly sulfated than control mucin from a patient with no biliary tract disease, and it also had a significantly greater ability to cause aggregation of finely divided calcium carbonate. [96] Gallbladder mucin also increases acid buffering capacity, which encourages calcium carbonate precipitation by Shiffman et al. [97] In contrast to the our pediatric series of gallstones where calcium carbonate stones accounted for 7 of 20 gallstone samples, [87] only 2 of 50 adults undergoing cholecystectomy for cholelithiasis at our institution had this type of gallstone (unpublished data). The reason for this markedly higher prevalence of calcium carbonate stones in our pediatric patients is unknown. The results of our study demonstrate a statistically significant increase in mucin producing epithelial cells in gallbladders from children containing calcium carbonate stones compared to controls.

In addition, there was a non-significant statistical trend toward an increase in mucin producing cells in gallbladders from patients with calcium carbonate stones compared to other stone types. This supports Sayers et al.'s hypothesis that cystic duct obstruction leading to increased gallbladder mucin production may play a role in the development of calcium carbonate stones in children. Children may have a greater tendency to cystic duct obstruction because of the relatively small size of their cystic duct. Mucin is a high-molecular-weight glycoprotein that is synthesized, stored, and secreted by epithelial mucosal cells. Its production is under the control of many different genes (MUC genes). A biological role for mucin has been previously suggested in experimental and human cholesterol gallstone formation and mucin hypersecretion has been documented in several animal models of gallstone formation by Bar Dayan et al. [98] Thus, various factors controlling gallbladder mucin production might influence the tendency to calcium carbonate gallstone formation.

Our study also found evidence of the ulcer-associated cell lineage in cholecystectomy specimens from children with gallstones. UACL has been observed in relation to chronic gastrointestinal ulceration, particularly adjacent to small bowel ulceration in Crohn's disease by Wright et al. [99, 100] It has been suggested that this may represent a form of gastrointestinal 'repair kit by Hanby et al. [101] The appearance of such glands has long been termed 'pyloric metaplasia', owing to their morphological similarity to pyloric glands by Lee et al, [102] but 'ulcer-associated cell lineage' is now considered a more appropriate description, in recognition of the unique morphological and functional characteristics of these glands. [100, 103] 'Pyloric metaplasia' of the gallbladder mucosa is well recognized in association with chronic calculous cholecystitis. Ulcer-associated cell lineage in gallbladder mucosa (PAS stain).

Glandular structures composed of cuboidal cells are present at the base of the mucosal folds. Their cytoplasm stains strongly for mucin. This is in contrast with the columnar epithelial cells on the luminal surface. Gallbladder epithelial mucin staining and type of gallstone cholecystitis [104, 105] but the characteristic morphological appearance of the ulcer-associated cell lineage has not been previously described at this site.

V. Observations on Some Causes of Gall Stone Formation. The Relation of the Reaction of the Bile to Experimental Cholelitiasis

In previous papers it has been shown that there exists a well-defined tendency for calculi to form out of the sterile liver bile of dogs, irrespective of whether or not these animals are losing the secretion; [106] and that after hepatic injury of various sorts potential centers for lithiasis are frequently abundant therein by Rous et al. [107] Why, then, are gall stones almost never encountered in autopsies on dogs dying from ordinary causes? Scientists have suggested an answer to this question insofar as it concerns the ducts. There are several evident safeguards against stone formation within them,-their motility, the cleansing and possibly antagonistic action of the secretion they themselves elaborate, and the flushing out effected by an intermittently quickened bile stream. But how is one to explain the absence of calculi from the gall bladder, a viscus which, according to the latest evidence, empties itself but poorly, and in which the bile often undergoes great concentrations and must frequently be held for many hours together. Nearly half of the score or more of normal canine gall bladders that we have examined contained an abundant debris consisting of shreddy mucous particles and lakes of long desquamated epithelium not infrequently stained black as result of secondary changes in pigment during the course of their sojourn in the organ. Once actual quartz sand was present,- small granules resisting aqua regia, likewise not infrequently recovered from the biliary system of other domestic animals, [108] into which they were presumably forced from the intestine by the muscular contractions of the gut. Yet never have gall stones been present. In view of the marked tendency for calcium carbonate to come down out of liver bile on standing, and for it to deposit within old organic debris, it seems certain that the normal gall bladder must either effect some change in the secretion in the direction of safety, or else add some preventative against deposition. Both possibilities are within reason, since the *vesica fellea is* known to alter markedly the fluid coming to it.

Influence of the Gall Bladder on the Bile Reaction

The solubility of calcium carbonate, the substance most abundant in the gall stones that we have induced experimentally in dogs, is greatly affected by the reaction of the fluid in which it is contained. Lichtwitzs has touched upon the possible influence of the bile reaction on gall stone formation in his discussion of the puzzling absence of calcium bilirubinate from normal human bile. Naunyn before him had tentatively advanced the view that a special reaction may be necessary for the formation of the substance. Following the line of thought suggested by our own work, and by such speculative reasoning, we have tested the reaction of bladder bile of the dog and have compared it with that of the secretion as derived from the hepatic tissue. To our surprise bladder bile proved frankly acid to litmus in a large proportion of instances, whereas liver bile was nearly always somewhat alkaline, and usually markedly so. The literature showed that the difference had already been noticed by Okada [109] for the dog, and by Neilson and Meyer [110] for the rabbit. Curiously enough, it has failed to attract attention in its possible bearing on gall stone formation.

Okada used the capillary electrometer. He ascertained that the pH of the gall bladder bile of dogs ranged from 5.43 to 6.97. His animals almost without exception had been fasting; but the data he obtained in other species supported the view that bladder specimens may be alkaline, acid, or neutral, with a tendency for them to be relatively acid after fasting. Liver bile, procured through a fistula of Schwann, was, by contrast, always alkaline, with a range in pH of 7.54 to 8.15. Fasting was without an evident influence upon such specimens. Those exposed to air rapidly became more alkaline. Neilson and Meyer made use of a calorimetric method and studied rabbit bile especially, but some other biles also. They corroborated Okada's findings and traced the change in pH on exposure to air to a loss of CO_2. They showed further that base-forming diets notably increase the average titrable alkalinity of rabbit bile, whence they inferred that this alkalinity is due to the presence of carbonates. We have employed the potentiometer. The readings were made in duplicate at 37°C. Exposure of the specimens to air was avoided by withdrawing them from the collecting balloons, or from the gall bladder, directly into Luer syringes cleansed of alkali by long previous use and boiled in water for present purposes. The determinations were made as soon as possible after the bile had been procured, though tests showed that even several hours in the syringe did not notably alter the pH. Day-to-day pH determinations were made on the liver bile of twelve dogs studied with special reference to the bile sediment. The observations in some instances extended over many weeks. In addition, the total calcium content of the bile was determined as routine by ashing, precipitation with sodium oxalate, and titration with potassium permanganate. The results of the analyses will form the topic of a separate communication. They will be considered here only in so far as they bear directly on the problem under discussion. The liver bile regularly proved alkaline, often more strongly so than Okada found. The pH ranged from 7.07 to 8.55 and tended to approximate 8.20 ordinarily. But Okada's specimens, unlike ours, had been subjected to gall bladder influence, owing to the circumstance that the organ formed a link in the fistula system. On the other hand some carbonate precipitation had occurred in our specimens during their period of sojourn in the collecting balloons. This should have rendered the bile less alkaline, if anything, owing to the fact that calcium carbonate represents the union of a strong base with a weak acid. The precipitate was present in proportionate amount in the samples tested. Fasting is attended by a great diminution in the amount of bile secreted, and in a marked and in some instances closely reciprocal increase in the concentration of certain of its constituents. [111] According to Okada, the reaction undergoes no change. But the contrary that the bile regularly becomes less alkaline during a fast, and, as this progresses, may become approximately neutral to litmus, though the pH has never in our experience quite reached 7.00 (Figure 4.5.1). The gall bladder bile of a number of normal dogs was procured by operation under ether. As in the case of liver biles, the individual differences in reaction were greater than those noted by Okada,- which would naturally follow from the larger and more various material at our disposal. The gall bladder specimens obtained a few hours after a meal were either neutral to litmus or alkaline-not infrequently as alkaline as some liver biles,--whereas those procured after 48 hours of fasting, were as a rule markedly acid and reddened litmus promptly. Specimens of this latter sort were heavily pigmented and syrupy, appearing greatly concentrated. It has long been supposed on good evidence that during intervals between meals bile accumulates in the gall baldder and is concentrated and stored there, to be more or less gradually voided and replaced with new when the digestion of a meal takes place.

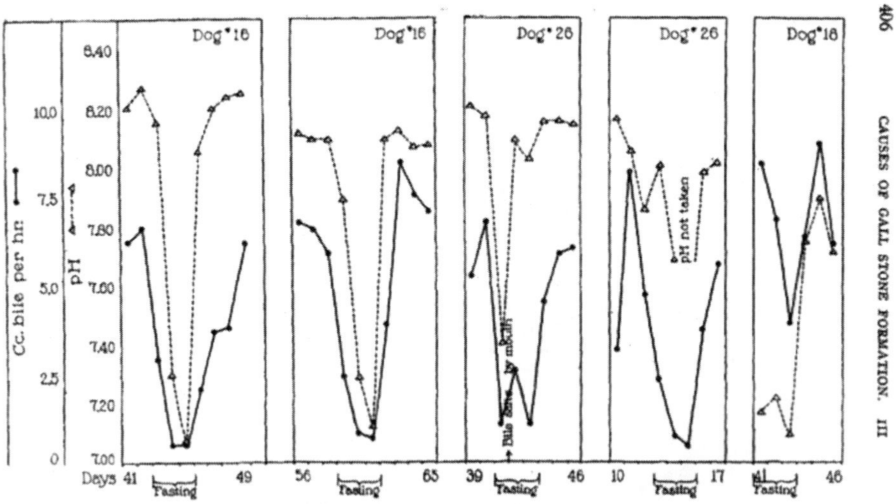

All biles sterile except that of Dog 18.

TEXT-FIG. 1. Influence of fasting on the amount and pH of liver bile.

Figure 4.5.1. All biles sterile except Dog 18. The influence of fasting on the amount and pH of liver biles.

Recent observations which indicate that the viscus empties itself imperfectly do not invalidate this view. Fresh support for it is to be found in our observations. In normal dogs recently fed, the reaction of the gall bladder contents approximated that of liver bile, whereas after fasting it was found acid, and concentrated and thickened, all to a degree never encountered in liver bile, as procured from fistulas. That the prevailing alkalinity of liver bile is not due to the loss of secretion entailed by the fistula may be safely inferred from the alkaline character of the gall bladder contents of full fed normal animals. The alteration that takes place in the reaction of bile within the gall bladder may conceivably be the result of chemical changes occurring in a labile secretion as result of its prolonged retention at body heat, or on the other hand, of some influence exerted by the organ of retention. That the latter is the true explanation may be inferred from the fact that liver bile collected into a balloon and kept warm remains highly alkaline, as further from the demonstrated activity of the gall bladder influence the bile in other ways, and from Neilson and Meyer's s observation that in gall bladders so injured by infection as to lose the function just referred to, the pH of the bile remains that of the secretion as derived from the liver.

Influence of the Bile Reaction on Carbonate Precipitates

Granting, then, that the gall bladder acts to render the bile acid, it has remained to demonstrate an influence of changes in the reaction of dog bile upon carbonate precipitation. This has been sufficiently accomplished by a series of simple experiments with bile that contained such a precipitate. They need be but briefly described. Several like portions of a single specimen of dog bile, each with its share of crystalline carbonate, as obtained from the collecting balloon, were distributed in 50 cc. Pyrex centrifuge tubes previously rinsed with distilled water. Some were rendered neutral to litmus, and others made faintly acid thereto, while still others were kept as controls. The acids employed for the purpose were N/10 hydrochloric acid, concentrated lactic acid, and 3 per cent acetic acid. The specimens treated with hydrochloric acid became opalescent owing to the development of a finely divided mucous precipitate, but the others appeared unchanged.

All were now brought to the same bulk by the addition of distilled water, and either centrifuged at once or allowed to stand overnight at room temperature before so doing. The experiment was several times repeated. The controls regularly yielded the sediment of carbonate originally present, whereas in the portions made neutral or acid it was completely or partially dissolved. Some of the original specimens contained pigmented nuclei, potential centers for lithiasis, of the sort heretofore described as well as carbonate crystals. These nuclei dissolved, but somewhat less rapidly than the associated carbonate crystals. Several unsuccessful attempts were made to determine a precipitation of calcium carbonate out of liver bile by exhausting it of free carbonic acid. For the purpose, the secretion was taken from the collecting balloon into large centrifuge tubes filled with CO_2 gas, deprived by centrifugation of the sediment previously formed, separated into portions under CO_2, and some of these portions placed *in vacuo* for several hours, with the container tilted so that a large surface of fluid was exposed. No carbonate came out, nor did it in the controls. Evidently the precipitation of the salt occurring in the balloon had reduced the bile content of it far below the saturation point. Efforts to dissolve a carbonate sediment by bubbling CO2 through the bile were likewise unsuccessful, probably because the period of a few hours allotted to the tests was too short. The greatest change accomplished was a dubious rounding of the crystal edges. The results have an interest in connection with the not infrequent presence of carbonate calculi within glass bulb connections interpolated in the course of the common duct of animals otherwise normal, which connections must have been flushed at intervals with more or less acid bile from the gall bladder. The persistence of the calculi may be laid to the transitory nature of this flushing. The bulbs when removed from the animals always contained alkaline bile. It would seem from these experiments, crude though they are, that no other explanation is needed for the lack of carbonate deposition in the normal gall bladder than the changes in reaction of the bile effected by this viscus. Further observations upon the changes occurring in the liver bile during a fast, and on those in the bile that assembles and distends the gall bladder after obstruction of the common duct clearly indicate that the reaction of the secretion undergoes an alteration in the direction of safety when there might otherwise be danger of carbonate precipitation.

The Calcium Concentration and Reaction of the Bile As Affected by Fasting

On the withdrawal of food from the intubated dog for 2 or 3 days, the bile output usually lessens greatly, and may diminish to less than one-tenth of the ordinary amount. Such alterations are accompanied by a reciprocal increase in the concentration of bilirubin, and the total output from day to day remains the same. There is a marked but less considerable increase in the calcium per cc. And *pari passu* with this increase and the pronounced slowing of the bile stream, changes both that, other things being equal, would favor precipitation within the duct system, there occurs a change in the reaction of the bile such as would tend to rule out this possibility. The pH falls from an average of approximately 8.20 to close to 7.00, that is to say to approximately the neutral point for litmus (Text-figures 4.5.1 and 4.5.2).

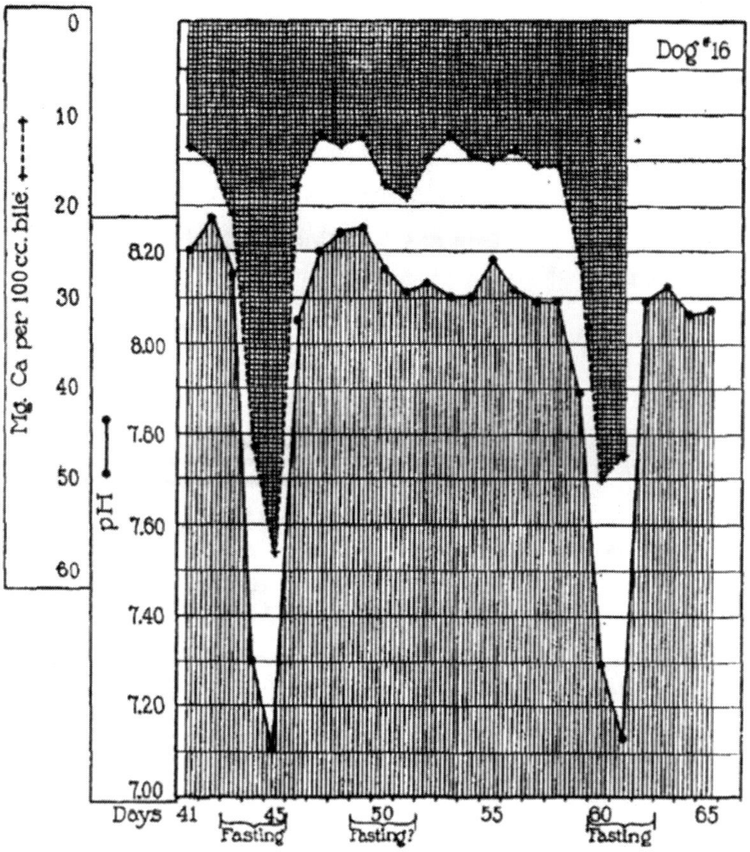

Figure 4.5.2 Calcium concentration and pH of liver bile. by a reciprocal increase in the concentration of bilirubin, and the total output from day to day remains the same. There is a marked but less considerable increase in the calcium per cc. (Text-figure 2) and *pari passu* with this increase and the pronounced slowing of the bile stream.

The precipitate found in balloon specimens collected under these circumstances is often far less than the ordinary, and never greater despite the high concentration of the bile.

The Calcium Concentration and Reaction of Stasis Bile. When the common duct of a previously normal animal is obstructed When the common duct of a previously normal animal is obstructed very great concentration of the bile pent in the bladder may come about through. the action of this viscus [12]. Yet, as is well known, stones fail to form out of the dark, thick fluid. We have, in seven instances of experimentally induced stasis, ascertained the reaction of the bladder bile and determined its bilirubin and calcium content. Obstruction was produced by tying and cutting the common duct in every instance save one in which it followed the clotting of blood within a glass tube which had been interpolated in the duct. Asepsis was maintained during the operations and the eventual stasis fluid regularly proved sterile on culture. It was taken into syringes under the precautions already described. For comparison with it the gall bladder content was removed at the initial laparotomy through a rubber catheter run up into the viscus by way of a slit made in the common duct below the point at which this was to be ligated. The dogs had purposely been fed full a few hours before operation. Thereafter they as a rule ate fitfully, if sometimes well. From the table it will be seen that the period of obstruction ranged from 2 to 6 days. The eventual bladder contents showed, in comparison with that originally procured, a pigment concentration which was sometimes nothing less than startling. In the case of Dog, there was 18 times as much pigment per cc. in the stasis specimen as in the normal sample originally had, and in Dog 6, 53 times as much. Part of this increase is attributable to the influence of operation on the character of the bile but most of it is undoubtedly due to the concentrating activity of the *vesica fellea*. The change in calcium concentration was, relatively speaking, negligible, though in four out of five instances there was a well-defined increase, once to double the initial amount. No calcium precipitate was ever found. The pH of the initial specimens has been either alkaline or neutral, whereas that of the stasis bile was acid, sometimes notably so. The changes in reaction which occur in normal bladder bile, in the liver bile of fasting animals, and in stasis bile take place at times when the calcium content of the bile is increased. That they are not an indirect result of such increases is sufficiently shown by the lack of correspondence between the two under conditions of stasis. If changes in bile reaction effected by the gall bladder act as the normal preventative of carbonate lithiasis, when these changes are suppressed stones should form. We have been spared the labor of experiments on the point through the existence in the literature of observations which suffice to illustrate it and which are the more telling because recorded in another connection. Meyer, Neilson, and Feusier13 have noted that in rabbits with a typhoid infection of the gall bladder, stones consisting of calcium carbonate regularly develop when the animal survives for a considerable period (100 days). They attribute the calculi, as have others in the past, to the inflammation set up by the infection, and they believe that all carbonate stones are traceable to infection, a view rendered untenable by our work.1 In a separate paper, Neilson and Meyer have dealt exhaustively with the reaction of normal and pathological bile but in no reference to stone formation. They state that the liver bile of the rabbit is regularly alkaline, having a pH of 7.6 to 7.9, whereas that from normal gall bladders may be acid, neutral, or alkaline, the pH ranging between 5.7 and 7.7, mu as in the dog. The bladder biles of typhoid carrier rabbits were, by contrast alkaline with the pH never less than 7.00 and on the average approximating that of normal liver bile. They conclude that "the gall bladder of a 'carrier' animal has apparently lost its concentrating function and therefore fails to change the reaction of its content." They mention that some of the carrier biles they tested contained carbonate sediment. In brief, these observations dearly show that gall bladders which have been damaged by the typhoid bacillus fail to alter the character, and in special the pH, of the bile coming to them from the liver. When this abnormal state of affairs endures for some time a carbonate lithiasis inevitably develops. That there is a relationship of cause and effect between the bladder shortcomings and the development of stones cannot be definitely affirmed. Yet the findings bring support by the method of difference to the conception,-based initially on evidence through the method of agreement,-that the formation of carbonate stones in the gall bladder of the dog and rabbit is prevented under normal conditions by changes in the reaction of the bile that the organ effects.

The Reaction of the Bile in Its Relation to Human Cholelithiasis. Stones formed predominantly of calcium carbonate are rare in man. Human calculi are of such varied character that a single factor can scarcely be the prime agent in the genesis of all. Yet the question is worth asking whether the reaction of the bile, or to speak more concretely, the failure of a pathologically damaged gall bladder to alter the reaction of the bile, may not have a share in determining human lithiasis. In a preceding paper2 we have described spheroliths of calcium carbonate occurring in the sterile bile from human gall bladders containing calculi, and serving as centers for a formation of secondary stones. It has been interesting to compare the reaction of biles containing such spheroliths with that of specimens in which they were not present. Nine samples of bile in all have been tested, which were removed from the gall bladder at operation, and also subsequent fistula specimens from four of the cases. The derivation and general characters of the material have been described in the paper just referred to. We are indebted for the specimens to Doctor Allen Whipple of the College of Physicians and Surgeons of Columbia University. The bladder biles were aspirated direct from the organ into Luer syringes previously submitted to boiling water; and the drainage specimens were collected, under oil occasionally, in Pyrex centrifuge tubes. The patients had received no food on the day of operation. While care was exercised to prevent exposure of the bladder contents to air, in most instances this was not wholly prevented. Frog or rabbit bile becomes more alkaline on contact with air, and some alteration in the same direction may be expected in the human instance. When the amount of bile was sufficient its reaction was determined in duplicate with the potentiometer; but frequently reliance had to be placed on litmus. In two out of four instances of cholelithiasis with mild chronic cholecystitis the bladder bile had a pH of 7.00 and of 6.98, respectively and in one of the others,--the sole one of them with an infected bile -it was neutral to litmus, and in the fourth alkaline. The bile from a peculiarly shaped but otherwise normal gall bladder had a pH of 6.72; that from a case with dubious cholecystitis in the absence of infection a pH of 7.28; while in an instance of mild chronic inflammation with infection, the pH was 7.06. The sterile white bile associated with a carcinoma of the head of the pancreas that had metastasized to the gall bladder wall was markedly acid, having a pH of 6.29; whereas another instance of a growth localized as yet to the pancreas but producing intermittent biliary obstruction the tarry specimen proved alkaline to litmus, possibly as result of the presence of blood intermixed with it when procured. There must have been little, if any, impairment of the concentrating activity of the bladder in this last case.

All of the fistula specimens were highly alkaline, their pH averaging 8.00. But they were collected during the adjustment period after obstruction, while the patient was still jaundiced, and hence must be regarded as abnormal.' Also there had been a relatively great exposure-of them to air. The reaction of human bile has received much notice in the past, though usually of a perfunctory character. The secretion is stated to be either alkaline or neutral to litmus. Little distinction has been made between gall bladder and duct specimens and some authors do not mention the indicator that they employed. Neilso and Meyer have cited the literature. They alone made pH determinations, on fistula specimens from a single patient. They found that the pH from day to day approximated 8.00. They do not mention precautions to prevent exposure of the material to air. An immediate conclusion which follows upon the inspection of our scanty data together with the prior ones of Neilson and Meyer is that many more cases must be studied, and under conditions better controlled, before certainty will be reached as concerns the effect of the gall bladder upon the reaction of the bile. But the available data show at least that the gall bladder bile of man is in some instances neutral or slightly acid to litmus, whereas liver bile tends to be alkaline. And the findings as a whole support the supposition that the secretion is alkaline as it comes from the liver, but that it undergoes an alteration toward the acid side during its sojourn in the *vesica fellea,* just as in the rabbit and the dog.

Changes in Reaction Determining Precipitation from Human Bile. Is the solubility of the substances out of which human stones form affected by slight changes in the bile reaction? Some simple experiments have been made on the point.

Experiment .--Into each of five small test-tubes, there was put 1 cc. of a medium brown bile with pH of 7.00 from a gall bladder containing "old" cholesterol stones. The fluid was sterile but slightly cloudy, because of the distribution through it of fine, myelin-like bodies, as the microscope showed. No sediment came down from it on centrifugation. To four of the tubes were added respectively 1, 2, 3, and 4 drops of N/10 potassium hydrate in water. All were now allowed to stand overnight at room temperature and again centrifuged. From the tube to which nothing had been added and from that containing 1 drop of potassium hydrate there was recovered a copious, light brown sediment of yelin-like material which dissolved almost completely in acetone and proved on test to be mainly cholesterol. The supernatant bile was alkaline to litmus in both instances. Acidification of it with HCl failed to cause the sediment to go into solution again. In the tubes containing 2 to 4 drops of hydroxide, no precipitation had occurred.

Experiment 2.-A bile, dark brown, thin, and faintly cloudy, from a case of chronic cholecystitis, was rid of slight mucous sediment by centrifugation and is distributed in center portions in each of four small test-tubes. The fluid had been sterile, with a pH of 7.06. To one portion a drop of 1 per cent lactic acid added, to others, 1 and 2 drops of potassium hydrate, respectively, while a fourth s kept as such. All were allowed to stand at room temperature for 3 hours and then centrifuged. The acid specimen yielded no sediment, whereas that ept as such gave a slight one of mucus and myelin bodies (cholesterol), while hose containing potassium hydrate yielded a well marked one of the same arterials.

Experiment 3.-A sterile, medium brown, clear, and slightly syrupy bilerom a case of dubious cholecystitis was centrifuged to rid it of a few cells which t contained; and 1 cc. specimens were placed in each of three test-tubes. The initial pH of the fluid was 7.28. To one tube a drop of 1 per cent lactic acid was added, to another a drop of N/10 potassium hydrate, while the third was left as such. After 1 hours at room temperature all were centrifuged, sedimentation noted, and they were let stand overnight and centrifuged again. No further sediment had come down during the interval. In the tube receiving alkali there had been present, after the initial hour and a half, a considerable deposit of cholesterol in myelin form, and in the tube let be as such, a slight sediment of the same material, whereas in that containing acid no deposition whatever occurred. Another experiment similar to that just described, carried out with a ropy, lack bile, failed of result in the way of sediment, as did one with a thin, lightly pigmented, and presumably highly dilute, fistula specimen secreted during the adjustment period after relief from obstruction. Our finding, that small quantities of base or acid will determine or prevent a precipitation of cholesterol from human bile, might perhaps have been predicted from the known complexity of the secretion and, in special, from that of the relationships whereby cholesterol is maintained in its distribution through the fluid. Yet the results do not pose in significance for this reason. Human bile is a well buffered fluid; and the quantity of hydrate or acid added in our tests cannot have greatly altered the reaction. Nilson and Meyer neutralized some rabbit biles with concentrated acetic acid or N/10 HC1 and found that there occurred only a temporary change in the hydrogen ion concentration which in some instances returned to the initial figure within 24 hours. Others before us have noted that cholesterol frequently falls out of human specimens that have stood for a few hours *in vitro*. An explanation for the phenomenon may be found in alkali derived from the glassware; and another in a presumptive loss of carbon dioxide on exposure of the bile to air. Whatever the cause for the deposition, it has, in our experience, proved preventable through the addition to the bile of a trace of acid. On the other hand, bile rendered acid to litmus may have no effect to dissolve cholesterol deposit that has once formed. Certainly it had none in the single test made in three instances of cholelithiasis there was present in the gall bladder a quantity of bile sand in addition to urge stones. Fragments of the older stones together with cholesterol plates made up the bulk of the sand in two of the cases; but there were present as well, in all, minute concretions, spheroliths which consisted of calcium carbonate in impure form. These have been described in detail in a previous communication. 2 They were beautifully concentric in structure, and on the surface of some of them a deposition of cholesterol, or of pigmented amorphous material, or of both had taken place, while still others were situated deep within larger stones. Their interest in the resent connection lies in their association with heavily pigmented, thick bile, one that is to say which had undergone alterations within the gall bladder. For it may be recalled that in the case of the dog and rabbit carbonate precipitation tends to take place from the unchanged liver bile on standing; and we have referred the absence of precipitation within the gall bladder to the activities of this viscus o prevent it by altering the bile. There can be no doubt that in the human instances now under discussion one of these activities, namely hat through which concentration of the bile is effected, had still been retained in considerable part by the pathologically altered bladder; hile that the ability to alter the reaction of the secretion had not been wholly lost seems probable from the fact that one specimen containing spheroliths was neutral to litmus and another had a pH of 6.98. The third bile was faintly alkaline to litmus. The circumstances under which the spheroliths originally formed re of course unknown. We have already drawn attention to the fact that carbonate concretions may not readily redissolve in bile,-this hile discussing their presence upon the walls of glass tubes interpolated in the common duct of dogs and intermittently flushed with formal bladder bile. It is possible as accounting both for their origin and survival in our human cases that there was a pathological increase in the bile content of calcium; or that the concentration of the secretion effected by the gall bladder was of an abnormal sort, preventing solution of the spheroliths despite favorable changes in the bile reaction, or that these changes themselves were never sufficiently great to accomplish this. Speculation upon the point is idle. But the findings themselves serve to forecast a difficulty which may be expected in attempts to correlate the reaction of human bile with the presence of stones.

In the **discussion** section, the problem of cholelithiasis presents two major facets to the pathologist, why stones begin, and why they grow. In a previous paper we have considered some aspects of that first mentioned and have shown that in the dog, at least, potential opportunities for stones to begin are offered in many sorts of liver disturbance. Out of the bile elaborated under such pathological conditions there come down "showers" of little concretions, nuclei which can serve as centers of stone formation, and which frequently did so under the abnormal circumstances of our experiments. Potential nuclei of other sorts, organic debris in special, must pass along the biliary channels at some time or other in the life of many individuals. In the present communication we have been concerned with why stones grow, or, to put the problem in a form more accessible to attack, why, given the recurring opportunities just mentioned for stones to arise they remain rare, relatively speaking. The question is an old one, if stressed anew by our observations. For the statement has often been made, with a query appended, that gall stones seldom form on the sediment so frequently contained in the gall bladder; and the fact has repeatedly been noticed that although foreign bodies frequently serve as the nuclei of gall stones, their presence in the biliary tract is not of itself sufficient to cause lithiasis.'[4] The experiments and observations here recounted afford an explanation for the occurrence of calcium carbonate stones in laboratory animals which is more than merely rational being probably the real one. A study along similar lines of the reaction of the bile in its possible relation to the development of calculi consisting of calcium bilirubinate would appear to be highly desirable, because of the important r6le conceded to the substance in human stones. But the indications are that this may prove difficult. For the physical chemistry of bilirubinate precipitation is a complicated matter; while furthermore the methods at present available do not always enable one to identify the substance with certainty in the test-tube. It is deposited from the bile of the dog only on special occasions and then in small amount.' The existing literature on stones of the guinea pig and rabbit suggests that in these species as well it is seldom formed in quantity. According to the thesis supported by our work, carbonate stones develop in intubated dogs and in typhoid carrier rabbits as the result of a tendency for the salt to be deposited out of the normal bile of both species. In healthy animals of the sorts mentioned this tendency is counteracted in the gall bladder by a change that the organ effects in the reaction of the bile, as result of which carbonate remains in solution despite the great diminution its fluid vehicle undergoes. When the gall bladder function is so impaired that it fails to effect this change and the reaction of the bile remains what it was when first derived from the hepatic tissue, carbonate lithiasis may automatically ensue. Does this explanation of the occurrence of a certain type of calculi under controlled conditions in some laboratory animals bring with it any implications as regards the causes for human cholelithiasis? Needless to say, a single factor can scarcely be expected to account for all the diverse categories of human stones. Yet the fact is worth recalling that calcium carbonate is no uncommon constituent of these stones, if seldom a principal one. As already mentioned, we have recovered calcium spheroliths from human gall bladders in which they were serving as centers for a secondary formation of gall stones. The suggestion that calcium bilirubinate may be precipitated from human bile at a certain reaction only was made years ago.' And the test-tube findings of the present work sufficiently prove that a precipitation of cholesterol out of the bladder bile of man can be determined or prevented *in vitro* by slight additions of base or acid which would tend to effect alterations in the bile reaction such as there is reason to suppose may be decisive within the organism. These are suggestive facts. Our purpose is not to emphasize them but to outline, irrespective of them, an attitude toward the problem of human cholelithiasis which may perhaps have advantages besides novelty. It has become old habit to ask, why do stones form? But might not the question better be, why are they ever absent? May not a gall bladder or duct functionally impaired through infection or by other means (recurring stasis? become *particeps criminis* to stone formation as result of its sins of omission? Faulty evacuation of the bile channels has long been deemed a contributary element in lithiasis. But may not a failure on the part of the gall bladder to modify the bile committed to it be sometimes the decisive factor? To test the hypothesis in its bearing on the human case will require a large material. Quite possibly the normal gall bladder effects other changes in the bile besides those of reaction, that are inimical to stone formation, serving in this way to offset the favoring influences of concentration and retention. But much remains to be learnt in relation to the influences of the bile reaction. It is needful to ascertain first of all whether, as our findings seem to indicate, the normal gall bladder of man effects changes in the reaction of its content comparable with the changes occurring in the dog and rabbit. In these days of "prophylactic" ablation, data on the point will not be difficult to procure. But to determinewhether stones form when the gall bladder fails to alter the reaction of the bile may prove an arduous task. A few of the difficulties have already been touched upon in connection with the figures on the pH of human biles containing carbonate spheroliths. The problem was simpler in the case of typhoid carrier rabbits, because of the limiting conditions and the type of calculus encountered. But in patients coming to operation, the manifestations of physiological principles are only too often overlaid by phenomena irrelevant to them, for example those of infection. That the human gall bladder, though containing stones, may retain part at least of its ability to concentrate the bile is certain. Our findings suggest that the ability to alter the bile reaction may likewise not be totally lost under these circumstances. Fitz [112] has concluded as the result of a series of observations upon operative material that bladder bile from gall stone patients tends to be less pigmented, of lower specific gravity, and less rich in nitrogen than that from cases of cholecystitis only. The finding might perhaps be taken to suggest, in line with our hypothesis, that a failure of the bile reservoir to modify the secretion coming to it from the liver is concerned in the development of stones. But the need of the moment is for data. Conjectures only can be made as to the means whereby alterations in the reaction of the bile come about in the *vesica fellea* of the dog and rabbit. It is reasonable to suppose that the same processes of osmosis and diffusion may be responsible which bring about a reduction in the bulk of the secretion. Were this the case, one would expect to find an impairment of the concentrating ability constantly associated with a greater or less failure to alter the bile reaction,-unless indeed the permeability of the bladder wall for some substances may be altered without affecting that for others.

Summary

As previous papers from our laboratory have shown, there exists a well-defined tendency for calcium carbonate to come out of solution in the normal liver bile of the dog, and for it to be deposited on certain nuclei not infrequent in the secretion under pathological circumstances. Gall stones that had arisen in this fashion were a frequent occurrence in the intubated animals we studied. The present paper is concerned with the reasons for the absence of such stones from dogs with an intact biliary tract. The solubility of calcium carbonate is known to be markedly affected by the reaction of the fluid in which it is contained. The normal liver bile, out of which it tends to precipitate, is alkaline, with an average pH of 8.20 but in the gall bladder where conditions might otherwise seem especially favorable to precipitation, the secretion undergoes a change toward the acid side, becoming on long sojourn there, strongly acid to litmus (pH 5.18 to 6.00). From bile as thus altered, no carbonate precipitation takes place, even when it becomes greatly concentrated as in fasting animals or after obstruction of the common duct. Furthermore, carbonate which has precipitated out of liver bile on standing dissolves again in it when the fluid is rendered slightly acid *in vitro,* or, in some cases merely neutral to litmus. There are several obvious reasons for the absence of carbonate stones from the normal ducts under ordinary conditions,-notably the motility of these latter, the flushing that they undergo from an intermittently quickened bile stream, and the cleansing and possibly antagonistic action of the secretion elaborated by the duct mucosa. In the fasting animal, one at least of these influences is almost done away with the rate of bile flow is so greatly cut down; while furthermore the calcium concentration of the secretion undergoes a considerable increase. But *pari passu* with these changes there occurs one in the bile reaction, a diminution in alkalinity so great that the pH often approximates that of the neutral point for litmus. That this change is not a direct consequence of the increase in calcium, may be inferred from the findings with stasis bile, the calcium content and reaction of which were observed to vary independently, if in general in the same direction. These adjustments within the organism, some of which may be thought to exhibit an element of the purposeful, when considered with the test-tube experiments, strongly suggest that the reaction of the bile plays a critical part in determining the occurrence of carbonate stones, as furthermore that their absence from the normal gall bladder is a consequence of the changes in the bile reaction there occurring. The changes come about through a functional activity of the bladder. This being the case, one might suppose that the failure to act would be followed by a formation of carbonate stones. There is sufficient evidence available in the literature to indicate that this happens, in rabbits at least.

VI. The Epitaxial Growth of Cholesterol Crystals From Bile Solutions on Calcite Substrates [25]

Epitaxial relationships between the surfaces of inorganic and bioorganic crystals can be an important factor in crystal nucleation and growth processes in a variety of biological environments. Crystalline cholesterol monohydrate (ChM), a constituent of both gallstone and atherosclerotic plaques, is often found in association with assorted mineral phases. Using in situ atomic force microscopy (AFM) and well-characterized model bile solutions, the nucleation and epitaxial growth of ChM on calcite (101h4) surfaces in real-time is demonstrated. The growth rates of individual cholesterol islands formed on calcite substrates were determined at physiological temperatures. Evidence of Ostwald's ripening was also observed under these experimental conditions. The energetics of various (101h4) calcite/(001) ChM interfaces were calculated to determine the most stable interfacial structure. These simulations suggest that the interface is fully hydrated and that cholesterol hydroxyl groups are preferentially positioned above carbonate ions in the calcite surface. This combination of experimental and theoretical work provides a clearer picture of how preexisting mineral seeds might provide a viable growth template that can reduce the energetic barrier to cholesterol nucleation under some physiological conditions.

The deposition of cholesterol crystals in vivo is an undesirable crystallization process that is implicated in a variety of human diseases including the formation of gallstones and atherosclerotic plaques. Although the detailed step-by-step formation of these entities is not yet fully understood, the nucleation of cholesterol crystals is regarded as an important first step in the formation of these pathogenic deposits. Free cholesterol has extremely low solubility in pure aqueous solutions (-3 ~ 10.8 mol/L, at 30 °C), [113] and only slightly higher solubility in dilute bile salt solutions (~(1-3) x 10^{-3} mol/L, at 35 °C) by Corradini et al. [114] Nevertheless, the presence of phospholipids (usually phosphatidylcholine) or other detergents drastically increases the solubility of cholesterol by enabling it to form vesicles or mixed micelle solutions (~7 g/L at 37 °C) by Small. [115] Previous studies using cryo-transmission electron microscopy by Konikoff and Kaplun et al, [116, 117], light microscopy, [118] and synchrotron X-ray diffraction(119) have been used to characterize the evolution of vesicular microstructures in well-characterized model bile and gallbladder bile solutions. In these bile systems, the aggregation and fusion of cholesterol-rich vesicles is generally thought to facilitate nucleation. Interestingly, a number of clinical studies have demonstrated Somewhat less attention has been paid to the potential effects of insoluble species that may also exist under physiological conditions and influence cholesterol crystallization. Compositional analyses of human gallstones have established the presence of a number of calcium carbonate and calcium phosphate phases by Malet, Nagpal and Bogren et al. [120-122] Although the primary component of most human gallstones is cholesterol (~80 wt %), the calcium carbonate (~15 wt %) and calcium phosphate (~3 wt %) content can also be quite significant. [122] These mineral phases are often found in the central nidius of the stone as well as radially distributed in the successive outer rings reported by van den Bert et al. [123] Heterogeneous nucleation is generally considered to be energetically more favorable than homogeneous nucleation, and the presence of an epitaxial surface can reduce the nucleation barrier such that crystal growth can occur in solutions that have otherwise not met supersaturation conditions. Epitaxial is defined as the growth of one crystal on the substrate of another, such that there is at least one preferred orientation and a near geometrical fit between the contacting surface lattices. That these mineral phases frequently coexist with cholesterol deposits suggests a synergistic influence of one crystalline phase on the other may be an important factor in nucleation and growth under physiological conditions.

Crystalline cholesterol deposited under physiological conditions is typically in the form of cholesterol monohydrate (ChM) by Craven et al. [124] ChM crystals grown from bile solutions or from aqueous alcohol solutions consistently develop a similar platelike morphology in which the largest face is (001) by Abendan et al. [125] The plates are usually bounded by smaller [100], (011), and (010) side faces, and often exhibit a small (01h1) notch. The deposition of metastable crystalline intermediates including anhydrous cholesterol by Shieh et al. [126] and/or polymorphs of unknown structure by Konikoff et al. [127] may also precede ChM formation under some conditions. Previously in their laboratory, the geometric lattice-matching program EpiCalc [128] was used as a systematic screening tool to identify which of the low index faces of anhydrous cholesterol and ChM are epitaxially matched with the naturally abundant faces of calcium carbonate (calcite, vaterite, aragonite) and calcium phosphate (hydroxyapatite, brushite). [129] For molecular crystal systems, which often contain many molecules per unit cell, simple geometric matching can be performed in a reasonable amount of time and has been shown in many cases to give predictions similar to those of the more rigorous potential energy calculations. [130, 131] Our geometric screening protocol predicted 186 coincident epitaxial relationships between the surfaces of these cholesterol and mineral phases, [132] of which were between various combinations of calcite and ChM surfaces. By far, the best geometric lattice match was found between the largest (001) plate-face of ChM and the natural (101h4) cleavage face of calcite when the two surfaces are rotated by an azimuthal angle of 39°. In the present study, we demonstrate experimentally the nucleation and epitaxial growth of ChM from model bile solutions on calcite (101h4) using in situ atomic force microscopy (AFM) under physiological temperature. The time-resolved data generated in this AFM study confirm the earlier EpiCalc predictions. As geometric matching alone does not provide any information about the molecular structure of the interface or its energetics, we have also undertaken more rigorous molecular simulations of the cholesterol-calcite interface. These calculations involve optimizing slabs of cholesterol with different terminations on the calcite basal plane, which yield not only the most stable interface but also information on the intermolecular interactions that direct the precise positioning of the contacting crystal surfaces. This dual approach affords a more detailed nanoscale understanding of how mineral seeds may have a profound effect on cholesterol crystallization in vivo.

Experimental Section

Materials. High purity cholesterol (Aldrich, 99+%) and sodium taurocholate (**TC**) (Sigma, 97%) were used without further purification. Egg yolk phosphatidyl choline (**PC**) in chloroform solution (20 mg/ mL) was purchased from Avanti Polar-Lipids (Alabaster, AL). Calcite was purchased from the Smithsonian Museum of Natural History (Washington, DC). Water was purified by passage through two Barnstead deionizing cartridges followed by distillation. All glassware was cleaned with an alcohol-alkali solution (ethanol:KOH 1:1 vol), acid washed (1 M HNO3) and thoroughly rinsed with deionized distilled water, wrapped in aluminum foil, and oven dried before use.

Model Bile Solution. Model bile solutions mimicking human gallbladder bile were prepared according to the system developed by Konikoff et al. [133] Stock solutions of 99+% cholesterol (in methanol), PC (in chloroform), and TC (in methanol) were mixed in a molar ratio of 18:37:120 and subsequently dried under nitrogen and low vacuum for 18 h to form a lipid film. Resuspension of the film in an aqueous solution containing 0.15 M NaCl and 0.003 M sodium azide (an antimicrobial agent) and heating to 56 °C for 1 h yielded a concentrated lipid solution (90 g/dL). The solution was diluted with additional 0.15 M NaCl to yield a total lipid concentration of 10 g/dL and was maintained at 37 °C in a water bath for a period of 21 days. The turbidity of the solution appeared to increase over days 1-10, then slowly decreased over time until day 21, at which time a white precipitate containing ChM crystals had completely separated from the clear yellowish supernatant. Small aliquots of the clear supernatant were removed with a disposable Pasteur pipet, transferred onto a glass microscope slide, and examined under polarized optical microscopy. Aliquots free of visible particulates were removed from the solution and used in AFM experiments without any further processing.

Cholesterol Monohydrate Crystal Growth. Cholesterol monohydrate crystals were grown both from model bile solutions as described above and from the slow evaporation of supersaturated aqueous acetone or 95% ethanol solutions. Optical micrographs obtained on an Olympus BX50 microscope of bile-grown and conventional solvent-grown ChM crystals reveal that they are identical morphologically. Single ChM crystals selected for AFM imaging studies were those that appeared to have the smoothest surfaces under optical microscopy.

Substrate Preparation. Calcite has a natural cleavage plane along (101h4). Fresh (101h4) surfaces of calcite were cleaved immediately prior that cholesterol supersaturation is not the sole prerequisite for to AFM experiments. Contact-mode imaging of freshly cleaved calcite surfaces reveals well-defined and oriented facets, which are easily distinguishable from the surface topography of cholesterol monohydrate crystals.

Atomic Force Microscopy (AFM). All real-time cholesterol growth studies were performed on a Nanoscope IIIa atomic force microscope (Digital Instruments, Santa Barbara, CA) equipped with Nanoscope III 4.43r8 software, an E-scanner (17.4 ím2 max. area), and

Si3N4 tips with a force constant of 0.12 N/m. The AFM is also equipped with a temperature stage (DI Metrology Group Heater Controller, model HS-1), which allows for heating from room temperature to 50 °C. A custom-built fluid reservoir was designed to precondition the temperature of the bile solution before it enters the 30 ίL glass fluid cell. The fluid was introduced with a 10 mL Hamilton syringe (model 81620); a syringe pump (KD Scientific 200) was used to regulate the flow rate (between 0.5 and 4 mL/h) through the fluid cell.

Calcite and cholesterol crystal samples were mounted to a metallic sample puck with double sided tape or with a mixture of 5 min epoxy/5 min epoxy hardener (Devcon, ITW Brands). Except in control experiments calcite samples were usually oriented such that the *X*-scan axis is parallel to one of the crystal edges. AFM images of calcite (101h4) surfaces exposed to aqueous solutions at 37 °C with pH's similar to those of the model bile solutions used did not show any appreciable changes over a period of several hours. Both contact- and tapping mode techniques were used to image cholesterol and calcite crystals in air and in fluid (model bile solution or pure water) at room temperature and at 37°C. We note that contact-mode imaging of cholesterol crystals in air often results in tip-induced etching, although contact imaging in solution and/or tapping-mode imaging can usually be performed without evidence of sample surface damage.

Computation and Molecular Simulation. The crystal structure of ChM was taken from the work of Craven [124] and the Cerius [132] molecular modeling package31 was used to add the hydrogen atoms. Visual inspection showed that the added hydrogen atoms were not in the correct orientation to form a hydrogen bonded network in the middle of the cholesterol/water bilayer. Thus, the hydrogen atoms were subjected to 1000 ps of molecular dynamics at 750 K, followed by 250 ps at 298 K after which they were minimized. The time step used was 1 fs. These calculations utilized the CVFF force field [134] within the Discover molecular simulation program by Disco Ver. (135) The van der Waals interactions were cut off after 12 Å, and the electrostatic contribution to the lattice energy was evaluated using the Ewald sum. Each water molecule in the minimized structure was found to form three hydrogen bonds, two with hydroxyl groups on cholesterol molecules and the third with a neighboring water molecule. A CIF file containing the minimized hydrogen coordinates is available as Supporting Information. This model was then fully minimized using the CVFF, CFF91 by Maple et al. [136] and ESFF [137] force fields using the same treatment of the long-range potentials in Discover. The vacuum growth morphology of ChM was derived by calculating the unrelaxed attachment energy (*E*att) of a growth slice of thickness *dhkl* to the 15 faces with the largest interplanar spacings by Gay et al. [138]. The calculations were done using the latest version of GULP by Gale et al., [139] which can simulate surfaces with two-dimensional periodic boundary conditions. This code utilizes a two-region approach, where the top layers of the surface are placed in region I and it is possible for these ions to be relaxed. The ions in region II are kept fixed and represent the potential of the bulk on region I. The CVFF force field was used in these simulations with identical treatment of the long-range interactions as for the Discover simulations above. Note that ChM crystallizes in a non-centrosymmetric space group and thus the face (*hkl*) is crystallographically distinct to (*h*h *k*h *l*h). However, the unrelaxed attachment energies of these two faces are identical as the growth slices are the same (they are just attached to opposite sides of the crystal), and the sum of the attachment energy and the slice energy is the crystal energy. [140].

To determine the possible surface terminations for face (*hkl*), the surface cell is cleaved in the *z* direction. To ensure that complete molecules result from this procedure, the position of each molecule is represented by its centroid. Starting at the origin and moving the cleavage plane by translating it in *z*, a different surface termination will occur when the slice moves from between two neighboring centroids to the next pair of centroids. Thus, in general, the number of possible surface terminations is equal to the number of centroids, unless symmetry is present. In cholesterol, there are 16 molecules (8 cholesterol and 8 water) and no symmetry, so each face has 16 different possible surface terminations. The attachment energies of all 16 were calculated, and the smallest in absolute value was retained because the morphological importance of a face is inversely proportional to the absolute value of the attachment energy. Finally, the calculated morphology is displayed via a Wulff plot by Wulff. [141].

The energetics of the cholesterol/calcite interactions were determined and subsequently used to provide a nanoscale description of the cholesterol/calcite interface. The interatomic potentials for calcite were taken from our previous work by Rohl et al, [142] and the calcite to cholesterol potentials were taken from the ESFF force field. Next, a 2 x 2 supercell of the (101h4) calcite cleavage plane with three layers in region II and three layers in region I was constructed. A growth slice of the (001) surface of cholesterol is rotated by 39° and placed in region I above the calcite surface. The growth slice is first kept rigid and allowed to translate in *x*, *y*, and *z* with respect to the fixed calcite surface, until the minimum *E*att calcite/cholesterol) (*E*calcite+cholesterol - *E*calcite - *E*cholesterol)/8 energy is found. All of the region I ions are then allowed to relax to their minimum energy positions. To try and ensure that the global minimum was found, each growth slice is started from four different starting positions. The first configuration is manually placed at a reasonable position above the surface. This is then translated half a lattice translation of the 1 _ 1 (101h4) calcite surface cell, first along **a**, then along **b**, and finally along both. Although the (001) growth slice has 16 possible terminations, only 4 of these produce a flat surface, which we have termed hydrophobic, hydrophilic, half water layer, and full water layer. These slices are more stable than the remaining 12 corrugated surfaces and thus are the only ones considered in the interfacial calculations. To assess which configuration is the most favorable, the attachment energy of the cholesterol layer to the calcite was calculated. The attachment energy is defined by: where the first term on the right is the minimum energy of the system containing the cholesterol slab on the calcite surface, the second term is the energy of the calcite surface minimized without the cholesterol slab present, and the final term is the energy of the cholesterol slab minimized in the absence of the calcite surface. As there are 8 cholesterol molecules in the slab, the total energy is divided by 8 to yield the attachment energy per molecule. The relaxed attachment energy can also be calculated for the cholesterol slab and a cholesterol surface by repeating the above calculations but replacing the calcite surface with the (001) surface of cholesterol with one layer in region I, and one layer in region II. The GDIS program (http://gdis.sf.net) was used to do all the manipulations required to construct the various interfaces, and the optimizations of these configurations were done using GULP by Gale et al. (139) ChM crystal deposition by Whiting et al. [29, 143]. Some patients with high cholesterol levels that meet the supersaturation conditions do not develop gallstones, while others who do not meet the prerequisite saturation levels can exhibit cholesterol deposits. This clinical evidence suggests that the presence of nucleating or antinucleating agents may also play a fundamental role in the cholesterol nucleation and/or growth processes under biological conditions. Although it is not known exactly which molecules might regulate cholesterol crystallization in vivo, a number of studies have examined the effect of soluble species such as mucin by Levy et al, [144] proteins, [145, 146] phospholipids Lafont and

Rapaport et al, [147, 148] monoclonal antibodies, [149] and metal ions by Toor and Moore et al. [150, 151] on the cholesterol nucleation and growth rates.

In **results and discussion** section, their experimental epitaxy studies utilize model bile solutions and freshly cleaved calcite surfaces. The model bile used in this work was based on a system developed by Konikoff et al., [116, 133] which has previously been shown via cryo-TEM studies to contain micellar aggregates that are similar to those present in human gallbladder bile solutions. The bile is prepared by mixing three key reagents - cholesterol, phosphatidylcholine, and sodium taurocholate - in an 18:37:120 molar ratio. When a 10 g/dL lipid solution of this composition is maintained at 37 °C, for the initial first 10 days immediately following the solution preparation, the bile solution shows a noticeable increase in turbidity. After that time, the turbidity appears to decrease, and on or about day 21, a white precipitate containing ChM crystals separates from the clear yellowish supernatant. The ChM crystals deposited from this solution are clear plates and are typically 0.10 mm in their largest dimension (Figure 4.6.1).

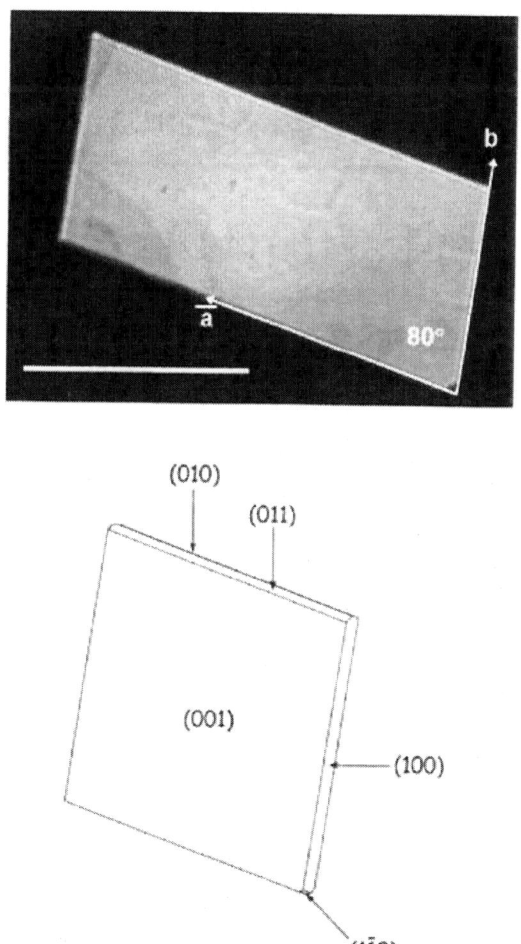

Figure 4.6.1. (top) ChM plates grown from model bile solution, scale bar) 0.05 mm. (bottom) Theoretical ChM morphology.

The acute angle observed between [100] and (010) side faces typically measures 80 (0.7°, which is consistent with the expected complement to the known crystallographic angle ç) 100.8°. ChM crystals grown from bile solution are morphologically identical to those grown from conventional aqueous alcohol solutions. The calculated theoretical morphology is also a rhombic plate, with the largest (001) face bounded by smaller side [100] and (010) faces with a (011) chamfering face and a very small (11h0) facet. While the calculated major faces are consistent with the experimental growth morphology, the small (011) and (11h0) faces are not always observed experimentally, although (11h0) is clearly visible in the experimental morphology in Figure 4.6.1. The EpiCalc screening procedure utilized in previous work predicted the best epitaxial match to be between calcite (101h4) and ChM (001). Frincu et al. thus focused our initial experimental studies on calcite (101h4) substrates. Calcite has a natural cleavage plane along (101h4); this surface is charge neutral, with an even number of carbonate and calcium groups. Using in situ atomic force microscopy, changes to the calcite surface upon introduction of model bile solutions could be examined in real time.

AFM images were collected continuously over a time frame of about 2-3 h, although some experiments involved imaging over longer time periods. Experiments were performed under both dynamic- and static-mode conditions (i.e., with or without flow). The series of images in Figure 4.6.2 depict typical changes resulting from the introduction and continuous flow (2 mL/h) of mature 30-day old model bile solution over the calcite (101h4) surface. Image A is that of calcite in pure aqueous solution. Soon after the bile solution is introduced to the fluid cell, a number of cholesterol islands appear on the surface. Images B (13 min), C (68 min), and D (126 min) are representative images selected from a larger series to illustrate changes to the surface over time. They note that for approximately the first 5-10 min immediately following bile introduction, AFM properties of bile and pure water are sufficiently different that the AFM detector must be realigned once the solutions are exchanged. Only images collected after the initial 10 min blackout period are used for analysis of the cholesterol growth process. There is substantial evidence to suggest that these islands formed on the calcite surface are ChM. The angle made between the side faces of any individual island measures ~80° throughout the series. None of the other known cholesterol crystal phases, including anhydrous cholesterol, [152] are known to exhibit this angle. Cross-sectional analyses of the island surfaces also reveal molecular-scale steps that have minimum heights of ~34 Å, a value that matches the expected heights for cholesterol bilayers in ChM. AFM images of the earliest islands observed may suggest a morphology that resembles half-pyramids more so than the characteristic plate shape expected of ChM. However, the skewed aspect ratio of the islands is due at least in part to the very different horizontal and vertical scales used in presenting these AFM images. After several hours of growth, when the islands are significantly larger, the scale of the AFM images obtained more clearly resembles the plate shape morphology indicative of macroscopic ChM crystals (Figure 4.6.3). Figure 4.6.3 depicts the theoretical match based on geometric considerations between a 2 x 1 supercell of calcite (101h4) substrate (with $a1$ = 4.989 Å, $a2$ = 8.095 Å, a = 90°) and a ChM (001) overlayer (with $b1$ = 12.39 Å, $b2$ = 12.41 Å, β = 100.8°) at an azimuthal rotation angle θ = 39°. [129]. In our in situ AFM studies, the calcite substrate is typically positioned such that one of the macroscopic edge faces is parallel to the *X*-scan direction. On the basis of the calcite substrate orientation and the lattice-matching predictions, one would expect the (010) edge of ChM islands nucleated and/or grown on these substrates to lie nearly parallel to the *X*-scan direction. Indeed, in every experiment, we find this to be the case. All cholesterol islands observed are aligned relative to one another and to the substrate at the 39° angle predicted by the lattice-matching protocol. The common orientation of islands is indicated in Figures 4.6.2c and 4.6.3 to show the influence of the underlying epitaxial substrate.

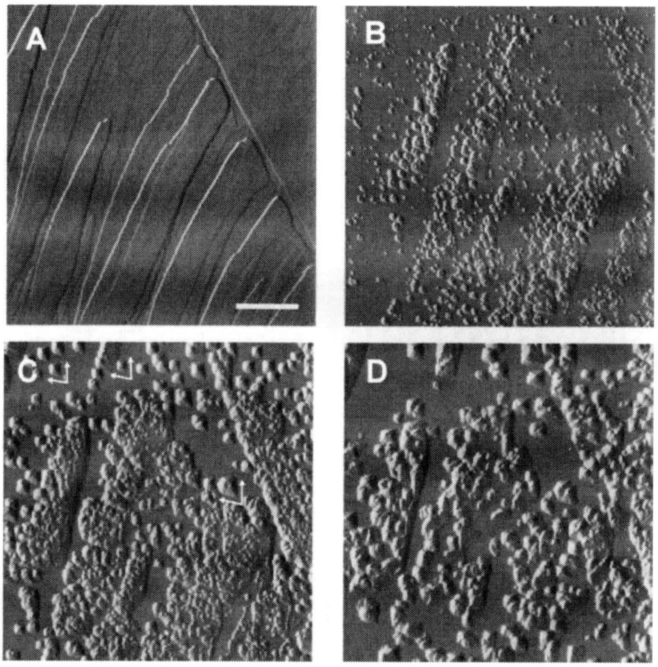

Figure 4.6.2. Selected sequential deflection-mode AFM images of the calcite (101h4) surface before and after exposure to flowing model bile solution. Temperature) 37 °C, pH) 5.4. Image A is a contact-mode image of calcite in water before the introduction of bile solution. Bile solution is introduced to the fluid cell and continuously flowed over the surface at 2 mL/h. Images B, C, and D were obtained 12, 68, and 126 min after initial bile introduction, respectively (scale bar) 2 ím).

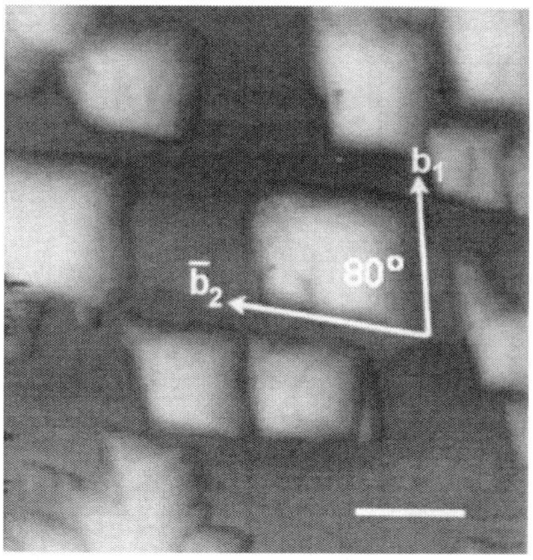

Figure 4.6.3. (top) Schematic of the best coincident epitaxial match between calcite (101h4) and **ChM** (001) surfaces predicted by geometric lattice matching. The calcite lattice is oriented the same as that in all AFM images presented. (bottom) Tapping-mode AFM images taken after 53 min of growth show platelike **ChM** island morphologies similar to macroscopic crystals. Overlayer cell vectors are indicated (scale bar) 1 ím, *z*-scale) 800 nm).

Tracking Individual Island Growth

Surface growth rates can be obtained by different methods. The first method, which yields average growth rates, is based on changes in the surface roughness (*R*a) over time, a value that can be readily calculated using standard DI software. Frames A-D in Figure 4.6.1 have increasing roughness values ranging from R_a) 0.438 nm (A) for pure calcite, to R_a) 1.633 nm (B), 4.790 nm (C), and 6.621 nm (D) at times after bile is introduced. This type of quick measurement provides at least a qualitative estimate of the growth. A more detailed analysis of individual islands over sequential images is required to determine relative and absolute growth rates as well as any apparent growth anisotropy. The height, width, and volume of eight individual islands were extracted from sequential AFM images obtained over a 2 h growth experiment. Those islands selected for growth measurements are identified in Figure 4.6.4 with white circles. Islands 1-3 appear in the lower left side of the images, while islands 4-8 are in the top central part of the images. Typical islands first observed on the calcite surface are approximately 2500 Å wide by 250 Å high, giving them a cross-sectional volume of 1.6 x 109 Å3. Using molecular volume estimates based on one-eighth of the ChM unit cell volume (5128.193 Å3) reported by Craven,(124) this corresponds to ~2.4 x 106 molecules of cholesterol per island. The growth rate of individual islands can be quite variable (Figure 4.6.5a). For the eight islands examined, the average growth rate over the course of the experiment ranges between 3 x 105 and 1.4 x 106 molecules/min. Careful tracking of a single island's size over time reveals that the growth rate of any given island is also not uniform over the duration of the experiment; rather, an island can grow much faster or slower than the average at different times. The variability of an island's absolute growth rate may be due to a variety of factors. A ChM island that resides in an area with a relatively high density of islands might be expected to grow at a slower rate than one in a less dense area, if the growth rate is at all limited by local competition for nutrients. Other factors such as sudden increases in a particular island's surface defect density by Shieh et al,(153) the coalescence of multiple islands, and/or local concentration gradients in solution might also contribute to spontaneous changes in the observed growth rates. In a few cases, sudden growth rate changes of islands 1-8 seem to be correlated with other events on the surface. For example, the growth of island 1 increases significantly between T = 87 min and T =107 min, while island 2 appears to actually decrease in size over the same time frame. While there is no direct evidence that cholesterol molecules from islands 1 and 2 were exchanged, the islands' close proximity and the timing of the sudden growth rate changes suggest at least qualitatively that local changes in growth rates may be related.

The growth is also highly anisotropic, as evidenced by the changing relative and absolute aspect ratios (horizontal vs. vertical growth) of individual islands. In general, growth parallel to the calcite surface occurs much faster than growth normal to it, which is what one would expect on the basis of the platelike morphology of ChM. Interestingly, the aspect ratios of islands 1-8 all decrease over the course of the experiment (Figure 4.6.5b). While islands start off with a broad distribution of aspect ratios, after 2 h of growth, most of the islands have attained aspect ratios of ~5:1 (width:height). In the absence of a substrate, the aspect ratio may be quite different, as macroscopic ChM crystals tend to have aspect ratios of ~15:1. While there is clear evidence for island growth in both the horizontal and the vertical directions, it can be easy to miss some of the other more subtle changes in the surface topography.

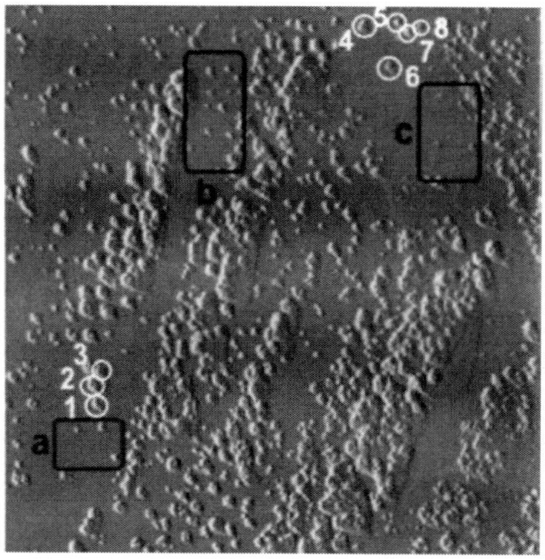

Figure 4.6.4. Islands 1-8 circled in white were found to grow both horizontally and vertically over the course of several hours. Black rectangles a-c identify areas where small islands disappeared over the same period of time in which others grow, presumably due to Ostwald's ripening.

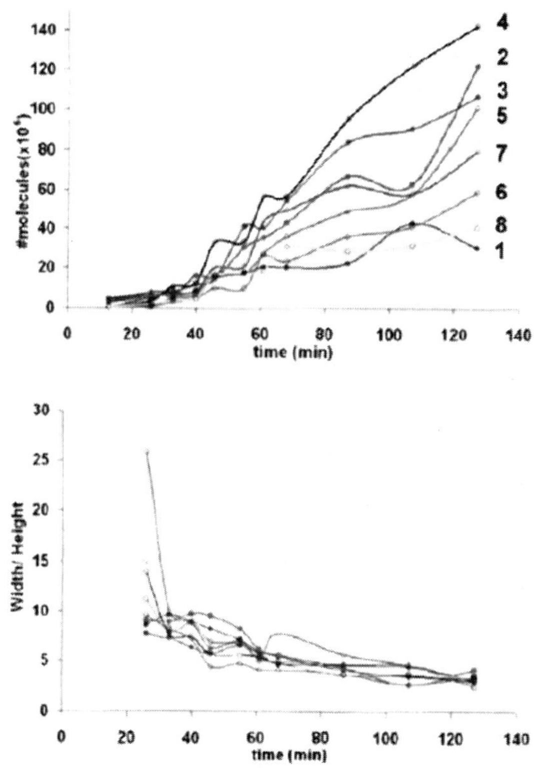

Figure 4.6.5. (top) Estimated number of molecules in individual **ChM** islands1-8 plotted as a function of time. (bottom) The aspect ratio of islands 1-8 during growth plotted as a function of time. Numbers 1-8 correspond to the islands identified in Figure 4/6.4. Reprinted (adapted) with permission from (Complete Reference Citation). Copyright (2004) American Chemical Society.

In nearly every set of cholesterol growth images collected, careful analysis revealed some evidence for disappearing islands concomitant with the growth of a large majority of islands. Those islands that disappear tend to be among the smallest ones observed (relative to the other islands present on the surface). Three regions marked with black rectangles in Figure 4.6.4 identify areas that contain some of the smallest (3 x 108 Å^3) cholesterol islands seen in our AFM bile studies on calcite. Some of the islands in these regions were observed to disappear at different times in the image sequence. For example, islands in box disappear after the topograph collected at T = 107 min. In boxes b and c, some of the islands disappear between T = 33-40 min, while others continue to reside in those areas for even longer periods of time. All are gone in the image collected at T = 127 min. We surmise that this complex growth and dissolution behavior is clear evidence for an Ostwald ripening process. From a kinetic standpoint, the formation of many small islands is favored because they nucleate more easily. Nevertheless, because molecules on the surface of these islands are energetically less stable than those in the interior, larger islands with a smaller surface/volume ratio represent a lower energy state. Thus, in this spontaneous ripening process, small islands can serve as nutrients for the growth of larger islands so that a lower total energy state can be attained. While it can be argued that disappearing islands might also be due to image artifacts, surface ripening was observed in both contact- and tapping-mode imaging with about equal frequency, suggesting that tip-induced shear forces are not a major contributor to this effect. Similarly, rotation of the substrate and/or changing the image scanning direction had no discernible effect.

Molecular Simulation of the Calcite/Cholesterol Interface

Although EpiCalc can determine which facets of ChM are likely to grow on calcite substrates and their required orientation, these calculations only take into account geometric factors. Such calculations offer no information about the chemistry of the interface. More rigorous molecular simulations are required if one is to determine which of the possible ChM (001) surface terminations are most energetically favorable to bind to the calcite surface. Such calculations also provide a means to assess which calcite-cholesterol interactions direct the precise positioning of the facet, a factor that is critical for determining the position of the supercell's origin. There are two previous molecular modeling studies of the solid-state structures of cholesterol and its derivatives. In the first, Liang and co-workers [154] simulated the condensed phase structures of anhydrous cholesterol and cholesteryl acetate using the CVFF class I force field as well as the CFF91 class II force field. They found that for the structures minimized with the latter force field, all cell vectors and volumes were reproduced to within 2.4% of experimental values and that employing molecular dynamics averaged structures resulted in an even better description. Limited comparisons with the class I force field showed no major differences. Ma et al. [155] used the MM3 class II force field to examine the solid-state structure of cholesteryl acetate and found that the cell vectors and volume were reproduced to within 0.7% as compared to 1.1% for CVFF and 2.1% for CFF91. The results of our crystal structure optimizations are summarized in Table 4.6.1. The magnitude of the changes in lattice parameters is larger than that previously reported for cholesteryl acetate, with a maximum deviation of 2.6% in the cell lengths (ESFF) and larger changes in the angles, particularly R (4.2% for ESFF).

Table 4.6.1. Comparison of Experimental and Optimized Cell Parameters Using Three Different Force Fields

	expt22	CVFF	CFF91	ESFF
a	12.390	12.510	12.558	12.472
b	12.410	12.112	12.193	12.092
			34.595	
c	34.959	34.959	88.51 1	34.570
			00.21	88. 0
α	88.47	R 91.90	102.44	100.10
β	98.10	100.93	5090.3	101.53
	100.80		-0.74	5029.3
γ	5128.2	101.24		-1.93
cell volume		5100.3		
deviation (%)		-0.54		

What is most surprising is that all three force fields produce very similar cells, with the *a* and *c* axes larger than the experimental structure and the *b* axis smaller. The angles all show similar trends. Visualization of the calculated structures reveals why the calculations deviate from the experimental results. The water-water and water-hydroxyl interactions are stronger in the calculations than in the experimental structure. The water interaction potentials were derived for liquid water, but the layer of water in the middle of the bilayers is not as polarized as liquid water. None of the potentials studied allow for variations in polarizability as a function of environment; thus all of the force fields overbind the water molecules, leading to the differences between the calculated and experimental cells. The CVFF and CFF91 potentials fare better than the ESFF force field. They have utilized the CVFF force field in the surface simulations rather than CFF91, as it is much simpler and thus less computationally demanding. The unrelaxed attachment energies of the 15 cholesterol faces with the highest interplanar *d* spacings were calculated. The (001) face was found to have a much smaller attachment energy (-0.0669 eV/mol) than all of the other faces. There is a group comprising the (100), (010), (011), and [101] faces which have attachment energies between -0.28 and -0.31 eV/mol, but all of the remaining faces have absolute energies greater than 0.38 eV/mol. (156) It has been shown that under a given set of solution conditions, the largest plate face of ChM may be either hydrophilic with surfaces terminated with 3-hydroxyl groups or hydrophobic exposing the tail groups [125] (Figure 4.6.6). The results from docking a cholesterol monohydrate layer with varying surface terminations onto the basal plane of calcite are compared to the values calculated for attaching the same cholesterol monohydrate layer to a ChM surface in Table 4.6.2. Based on calculations, it appears that more energy is liberated when the cholesterol slice (with any termination) is added to the basal surface of a calcite crystal than when the same slice is added to the (001) surface of a ChM crystal. This is perhaps not surprising because the cholesterol slices all have a dipole moment that will interact more strongly with the highly ionic calcite surface than with the organic cholesterol surface. The final optimized configurations for the four different slabs are reproduced in Figure 4.6.7. Magnified images of the various cholesterol-calcite interfaces are shown in Figure 4.5.8. The surface termination of the slab that interacts least strongly with the calcite basal surface is the hydrophobic one.

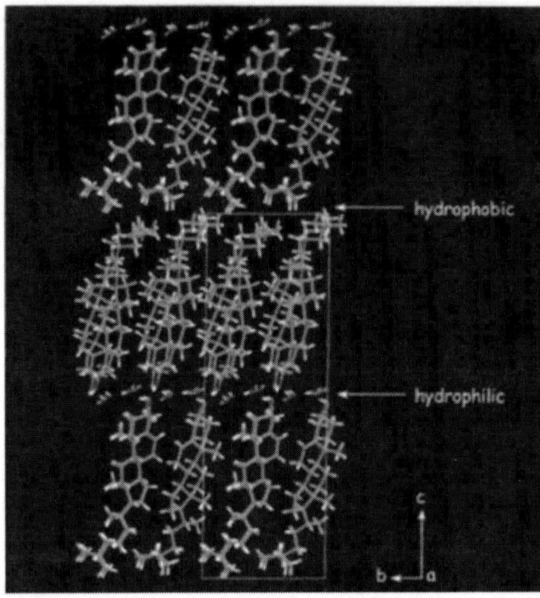

Figure 4.6.6. Schematic of hydrophilic versus hydrophobic ChM surfaces.

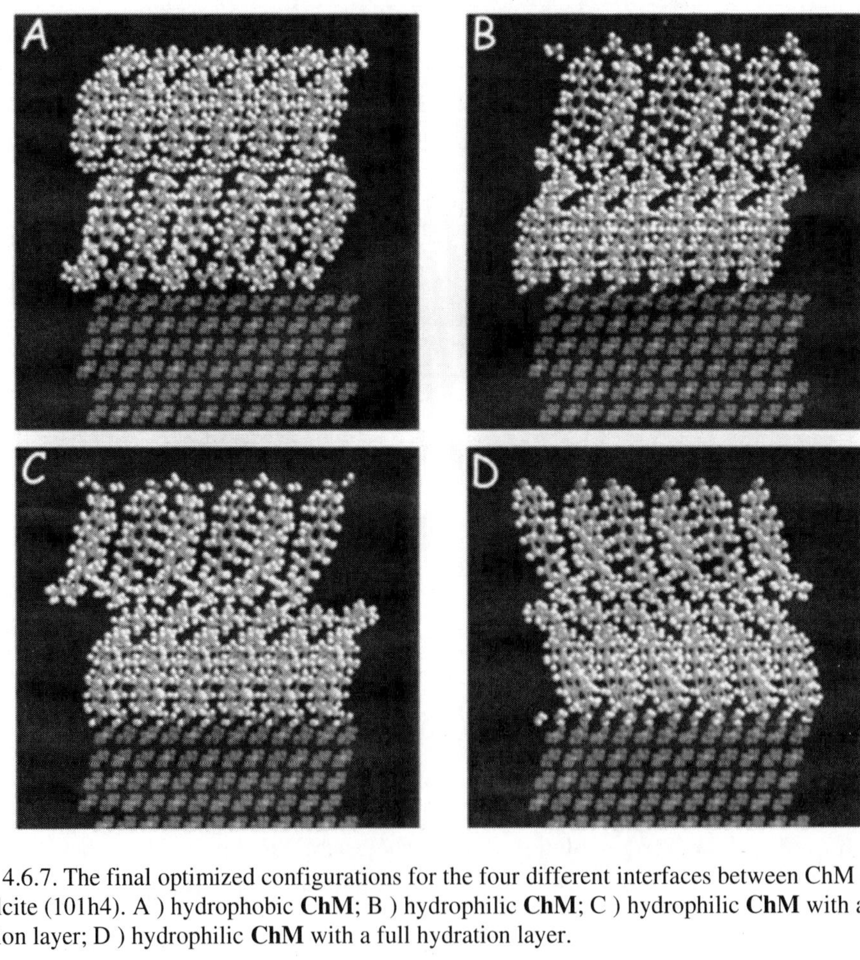

Figure 4.6.7. The final optimized configurations for the four different interfaces between ChM (001) and calcite (101h4). A) hydrophobic **ChM**; B) hydrophilic **ChM**; C) hydrophilic **ChM** with a half hydration layer; D) hydrophilic **ChM** with a full hydration layer.

Table 4.6.2. Attachment Energies of Cholesterol (001) Growth Slices with Four Different Terminations to Calcite and Cholesterol Surfaces

	(calcitechol) *E*att (eV/mol)	(cholchol) *E*att (eV/mol)
hydrophobic	-0.1	-0.12
6hydrophili3	c -0.4	-0.28
hydrophilic + half water	-0.75	
hydrophilic + full water	-0.84 -	-0.35

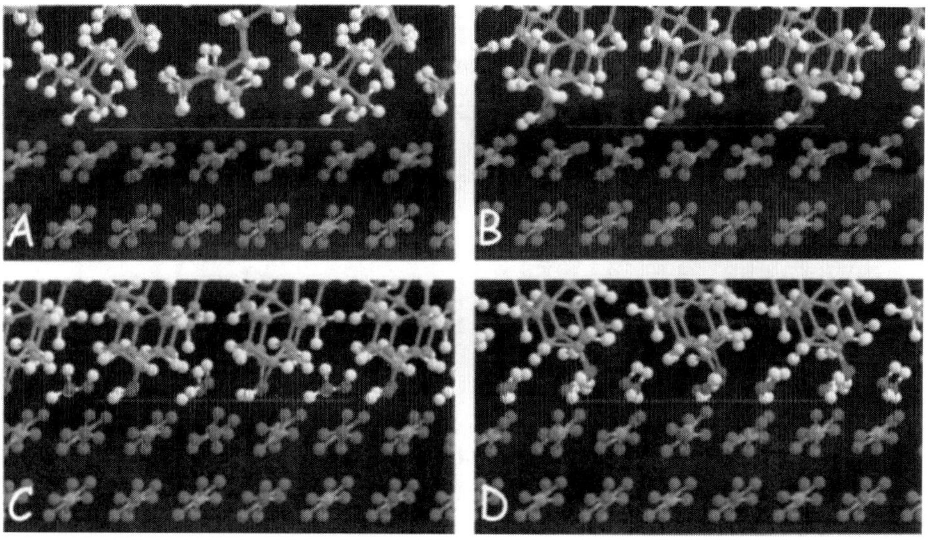

Figure 4.6.8. View of the optimized interfaces for the **ChM** (001) docked onto calcite (101h4). A) hydrophobic **ChM**; B) hydrophilic **ChM**; C) hydrophilic **ChM** with a half hydration layer; D) hydrophilic **ChM** with a full hydration layer.

This is also the surface termination with the smallest difference in attachment energies between adding to a calcite crystal or a ChM crystal. This illustrates that the interactions between a hydrophobic surface and an ionic crystal are weak. As we move from the slab with a hydrophilic termination, to a half water layer termination, and finally from a slab with a full layer of water termination, there is an increase in the energy liberated upon attachment. The hydrophilic terminated surface shows directional bonding with the calcite surface, in which the hydroxyl groups of the cholesterol molecules hydrogen bond to half of the surface carbonate anions (Figures 4.6.7 and 4.6.8B). The four unique H···O (O···O) distances are 1.500 (2.451), 1.504 (2.405), 1.540 (2.474), and 1.767 (2.462) Å with associated O-H···O angles of 148.2°, 158.0°, 154.8°, and 125.0°, respectively. Three of the four cholesterol molecules hydrogen bond very strongly to the surface, but the fourth one is unable to because even though the (001) face of cholesterol lattice matches the calcite basal plane well, there is still some residual lattice misfit. When half a layer of water is present at the interface, a similar hydrogen bonding arrangement is observed between the hydroxyl groups of the cholesterol molecule and the surface carbonate anions. The water molecules are located in rows between the cholesterol hydroxyl groups (Figures 4.6.7 and 4.6.8C), which allow the hydroxyl groups of the cholesterol to get closer to the carbonate groups. The H···O (O···O) distances are now 1.460 (2.421), 1.469 (2.376), 1.524 (2.412), and 1.528 (2.471) Å with O-

H···O angles of 159.4°, 148.6°, 146.1°, and 156.6°, respectively. The water molecules also hydrogen bond to a single carbonate group with distances of 1.510 (2.506), 1.521 (2.465), 1.524 (2.516), and 1.655 (2.541) Å and associated angles of 170.1°, 154.5°, 169.1°, and 146.2°, respectively. The second hydrogen atom on each water molecule projects into the hydrophobic areas above the hydroxyl groups of the cholesterol molecules. Thus, the water has improved the interaction energy between contacting surfaces, in essence acting as a screen between the calcite surface and the hydrophobic parts of the cholesterol molecule. The presence of a whole layer of water allows the hydroxyl groups of cholesterol to approach the carbonate ions of calcite still further (Figures 4.6.7 and 4.6.8D). The HâââO (OâââO) distances are now 1.411 (2.399), 1.414 (2.404), 1.507 (2.461), and 1.518 (2.464) Å with associated angles of 169.6°, 170.8°, 160.4°, and 158.5°, respectively. The additional water molecules are positioned in the same rows as the hydroxyl groups, with each water molecule lying between two cholesterol molecule.

Conclusion

There are presumably a variety of different mechanisms by which cholesterol nucleation can occur in complex biological solutions. In the present work, they have focused our attention solely on the potential influence that insoluble calcite seeds might play in the crystallization of cholesterol monohydrate. Using in situ AFM, they have demonstrated experimentally that the (101h4) calcite surface can serve to catalyze the precipitation of cholesterol monohydrate from bile solutions under physiologic temperature conditions. Analysis of sequential images reveals that the evolution of these surface-bound ChM islands over time is a complex balance of individual island growth and Ostwald's ripening. However, the strong orientation and directional growth of all ChM islands provide unambiguous evidence that epitaxial matching at the calcite/cholesterol interface is an important factor. While the orientation observed matches the values predicted in an earlier geometric lattice-matching study, the more rigorous molecular simulations of the (101h4) calcite/ (001) ChM interfaces provide significantly greater insight into the energetics of that interface. Both geometric and chemical interactions influence the alignment of ions and molecules at the boundary of these two different crystalline materials. Perhaps not surprisingly, the presence of interfacial water molecules plays a key role in mediating the repulsive interactions associated with bringing ionic and neutral surfaces together. The dual theoretical and experimental approaches adopted in this study bring them closer to a molecular-scale understanding of at least one viable means by which the energetic barrier to cholesterol nucleation can be reduced under some physiological conditions.

References

[1] Yu, J., Pan, H., Huang, S., Huang, N., Yao, C., Hsiao, K., and Wu, C. 2012. Calcium content of different compositions gallstones and pathogenesis of calcium carbonate gallstones. *Asian Journal of Surgery* (In Press).

[2] Kim, I., Myung, S., Lee, S., Lee, S., and MH.., K. 2003;. Classification and nomenclature of gallstones. *Yonsci Medical Journal* 44:10.

[3] Huang, S., Su, C., Wu, L., Chang, T., Wu, C., Lee, C., and Lui, W. 1989. Polarizing microscopy versus infrared absorption spectrcscopy in gallstone analysis. *Asian J Surg* 12:6.

[4] Wei, T. 1982. Quantitative determination of chemical composition of gallstones by infrared absorption spectrophotometry. *J Formosan Med Assoc* 81:13.

[5] Saito, K., Hatafuka, T., and Kanno, S., et al.. 1979. Review of five cases of limy bile – particular ly on radiological, chemical and crystallographic studies. *Gastroenterologia Japonica* 14:6.

[6] Stinton, L.M., Myers, R.P., and Shaffer, E.A. 2010. Epidemiology of gallstones. *Gastroenterol Clin North Am* 39:157-169, vii.

[7] Saito, K., Omor, i.H., Kanno, S., Hirata, Y., Okada, T., Mori, S., and Nakadate, K. 1986. Chemical and crystallographic studies on 33 cases of calcium carbonate gallstones (so-called limy bile). *Gastroenterologia Japonica* 21:5.

[8] Davies, T. 1963. The determination of calcite: aragonite ratio in mollusc shells by the x-ray diffraction. *Mineralogical magazine* 33:5.

[9] Saito, K., Omor, i.H., Kanno, S., Hirata, Y., Okada, T., Mori, S., Nakadate, K., Miura, F., Takada, T., Kawarada, Y., et al. 2007. Flowcharts for the diagnosis and treatment of acute cholangitis and cholecystitis: Tokyo Guidelines. *J Hepatobiliary Pancreat Surg* 14:8.

[10] Huang, S.M., Yao, C.C., Pan, H., Hsiao, K.M., Yu, J.K., Lai, T.J., and Huang, S.D. 2010. Pathophysiological significance of gallbladder volume changes in gallstone diseases. *World J Gastroenterol* 16:4341-4347.

[11] Naryshkin, S., Trotman, B.W., and Raffensperger, E.C. 1987. Milk of calcium bile. Evidence that gallbladder stasis is a key factor. *Dig Dis Sci* 32:1051-1055.

[12] Ballas, K.D., Alatsakis, M.B., Rafailidis, S.F., Psarras, K., and Sakadamis, A.K. 2005. Limy bile syndrome: review of seven cases. *ANZ J Surg* 75:787-789.

[13] Okamura, N. 1974. On limy bile. *The Journal of the Japanese Practical Surgeon Society* 35:7.

[14] Sava, G., Millot, P., Becmeur, F., Vaxman, F., and Grenier, J.F. 1988. [Limy bile syndrome. Study of a case with double localization in the gallbladder and common bile duct]. *Gastroenterol Clin Biol* 12:156-159.

[15] Ahronsohn, H. 1936. Pathogenesis of white bile. *Arch Surg* 32:25.

[16] McWhirter, R. 1935. Cholecystography: Its present clinical value. *Br J Surg* 23:33.

[17] Moreaux, J., and Roux, J.M. 1994. Limy bile. A surgical experience in 16 patients. *Gastroenterol Clin Biol* 18:550-555.

[18] Flint, E.R. 1937. Obstructions of the Common Bile Duct. *Br Med J* 2:253-256.

[19] Onghena, T., De Waele, J.J., Vereecken, L., and Van Loon, C. 2001. Limy bile and laparoscopic cholecystectomy. *Acta Chir Belg* 101:31-34.

[20] Sayers, C., Wyatt, J., Soloway, R.D., Taylor, D.R., and Stringer, M.D. 2007. Gallbladder mucin production and calcium carbonate gallstones in children. *Pediatr Surg Int* 23:219-223.

[21] Rege, R.V., and Moore, E.W. 1986. Pathogenesis of calcium-containing gallstones. Canine ductular bile, but not gallbladder bile, is supersaturated with calcium carbonate. *J Clin Invest* 77:21-26.

[22] Dawes, L.G., and Rege, R.V. 1990. Calcium and calcium binding in human gallstone disease. *Arch Surg* 125:1606-1609.

[23] Yamaguchi, S. 1974. On limy bile. *Operation* 28:7.

[24] Itoh, H. 2003. Management of limy bile syndrome: no therapy, laparotomy or endoscopic treatment? *Intern Med* 42:1-2.

[25] Frincu, M.C., Fleming, S.D., Rohl, A.L., and Swift, J.A. 2004. The epitaxial growth of cholesterol crystals from bile solutions on calcite substrates. *J Am Chem Soc* 126:7915-7924.

[26] Knyrim, K., and Vakil, N. 1990. The effects of synthetic human secretin on calcium carbonate solubility in human bile. *Gastroenterology* 99:1445-1451.

[27] Moore, E.W. 1984. The role of calcium in the pathogenesis of gallstones: Ca++ electrode studies of model bile salt solutions and other biologic systems. With an hypothesis on structural requirements for Ca++ binding to proteins and bile acids. *Hepatology* 4:228S-243S.

[28] Sutor, D.J., and Wilkie, L.I. 1977. Calcium in bile and calcium salts in gallstones. *Clin Chim Acta* 79:119-127.

[29] Admirand, W.H., and Small, D.M. 1968. The physicochemical basis of cholesterol gallstone formation in man. *J Clin Invest* 47:1043-1052.

[30] Holzbach, R.T., Marsh, M., Olszewski, M., and Holan, K. 1973. Cholesterol solubility in bile. Evidence that supersaturated bile is frequent in healthy man. *J Clin Invest* 52:1467-1479.

[31] Carey, M.C., and Small, D.M. 1978. The physical chemistry of cholesterol solubility in bile. Relationship to gallstone formation and dissolution in man. *J Clin Invest* 61:998-1026.

[32] Hofmann, A.F., Grundy, S.M., Lachin, J.M., Lan, S.P., Baum, R.A., Hanson, R.F., Hersh, T., Hightower, N.C., Jr., Marks, J.W., Mekhjian, H., et al. 1982. Pretreatment biliary lipid composition in white patients with radiolucent gallstones in the National Cooperative Gallstone Study. *Gastroenterology* 83:738-752.

[33] Holan, K.R., Holzbach, R.T., Hermann, R.E., Cooperman, A.M., and Claffey, W.J. 1979. Nucleation time: a key factor in the pathogenesis of cholesterol gallstone disease. *Gastroenterology* 77:611-617.

[34] Gollish, S.H., Burnstein, M.J., Ilson, R.G., Petrunka, C.N., and Strasberg, S.M. 1983. Nucleation of cholesterol monohydrate crystals from hepatic and gall-bladder bile of patients with cholesterol gall stones. *Gut* 24:836-844.

[35] Burnstein, M.J., Ilson, R.G., Petrunka, C.N., Taylor, R.D., and Strasberg, S.M. 1983. Evidence for a potent nucleating factor in the gallbladder bile of patients with cholesterol gallstones. *Gastroenterology* 85:801-807.

[36] Been, J.M., Bills, P.M., and Lewis, D. 1979. Microstructure of gallstones. *Gastroenterology* 76:548-555.

[37] Wosiewitz, U. 1980. Limy bile and radiopaque, calcified gallstones: a combined analytical, radiographic, and micromorphologic investigation. *Pathol Res Pract* 167:273-286.

[38] Moore, E.W., Celic, L., and Ostrow, J.D. 1982. Interactions between ionized calcium and sodium taurocholate: bile salts are important buffers for prevention of calcium-containing gallstones. *Gastroenterology* 83:1079-1089.

[39] Williamson, B.W., and Percy-Robb, I.W. 1980. Contribution of biliary lipids to calcium binding in bile. *Gastroenterology* 78:696-702.
[40] Bateson, M., Bouchier, I., Trash, D., Maudgal, D., and Northfield, T. 1981. Calcification of radiolucent gall stone during treatment with ursodeoxycholic acid. *Br Med J (Clin Res Ed)* 283:2.
[41] Schoenfield, L.J., and Lachin, J.M. 1981. Chenodiol (chenodeoxycholic acid) for dissolution of gallstones: the National Cooperative Gallstone Study. A controlled trial of efficacy and safety. *Ann Intern Med* 95:257-282.
[42] Moore, E.W., and Verine, H.J. 1985. Pathogenesis of pancreatic and biliary CaCO3 lithiasis: the solubility product (K'sp) of calcite determined with the Ca++ electrode. *J Lab Clin Med* 106:611-618.
[43] Tera, H. . 1960. Stratification of human gallbladder bile in vivo. *Acla Chir. Scand.* 256 (Suppl.):85.
[44] Talalay, P. 1960. Enzymatic analysis of steroid hormones. *Meth. Biochem. Anal* 8:25.
[45] Edsall, J., and Wyman, J. 1958. *Biophysical Chemistry*. New York.: Academic Press, Inc.
[46] Rege, R., and Moore, E. 1984. Pathogenesis of CaCO3-containing gallstones: I. The solubility coefficient (Q') of CO2 in canine bile. *Hepatology (Baltimore).* 4.
[47] Moore, E., and Zimmerman, M. 1982. Pancreatic ionized and total calcium secretion: a test of the thermodynamic model for pancreatic lithogenicity. *Gastroenterology* 82.
[48] Sarles, H. 1974. Chronic calcifying pancreatitis--chronic alcoholic pancreatitis. *Gastroenterology* 66:604-616.
[49] Verine, H.J. 1973. Reserches sur la lithogenese pancreatique: apports de la pathologie comparee et de la pathologie experimentale. Lyon, France.: Lyon, No. 8, Universite de.
[50] Perinet, G., Verine, H., and Lafont, R. 1972. Etude thermique de calculs pancreatiques humains et bovins. *Seances Acad. Sci.* 274D:3.
[51] Mallet-Guy, P., Perrin, M., and A, T. 1969. Etude radiocristallographique de calculs pancreatiques humains. *C. R. Seances Soc. Biol.* 163:4.
[52] Perrin, M., Thozet, A., and HJ.., V. 1969. . Etude radiocristallographique de calculs pancreatiques bovins. *C. R. Seances Soc. Biol.* 163:3.
[53] Verine, H., and H, L. Existence d'une matrice proteique dans les calculs pancreatiques de vertebres superieurs comparaison avec les matrices proteiques a calcite des mollusques. *Haliotis* 2:5.
[54] Moore, E., and Dietschy, J. 1964. . Na and K activity coefficients in bile and bile salt solutions determined with glass electrodes. *Am. J. Physiol* 3:8.
[55] Bogren, H., and Larsson, K. 1963. Crystalline components of biliary caluli. . *Scand. J. Clin. Lab. Invest* 15:6.
[56] Hatzigeorgiadis, A., Mavroudis, N., Alatsakis, M., and C., S. 1990. Milk of calcium bile. *Hellenic. Med.* 56:4.
[57] Kornblum, K., and Hall, W. 1935. The roentgenologic significance of 'milk of calcium' bile. *Am. J. Roentgenol* 33:13.
[58] Phemister, D., Rewbridge, A., and Rudstill, H. 1931. Calcium carbonate gallstones and calcification of the gall bladder following cystic duct obstruction. *Ann. Surg* 94:24.
[59] Churchman, J. 1911;. Acute cholecystitis with large amount of calcium soap in gall bladder. *ull. Johns Hopkins. Hosp.* 22:2.
[60] Volkmann, J. 1926. Uber kalkmilchgalle. *Munchen. Med. Wochen.* 73:2.

[61] Knutsson, F. 1933. On limy bile. *Acta Radiol* 14:10.

[62] Cohen, O.H. 1955. Limy ductus choledochus. *Radiology* 65:78-80.

[63] Nomura, F., Suzuki, Y., Suzuki, K., Yamamoto, K., Ohshima, H., Nakayama, T., Yokosuka, O., Ohnishi, K., Saisho, H., Ohhara, K., et al. 1984. Spontaneous disappearance of limy bile: report of a case with review of the literature. *Am J Gastroenterol* 79:884-888.

[64] Marquis, J.R., and Densler, J. 1970. The disappearing limy bile syndrome. *Radiology* 94:311-312.

[65] Morehouse, H.T., Roush, G., Deshmukh, S., and Baker, S. 1984. Milk of calcium in the common bile duct. *J Comput Assist Tomogr* 8:177-179.

[66] Katsuda, H., Ueda, K., and Kawashima, H.e.a. 1979. On limy bile. *Wakayama Med. Rep* 22:8.

[67] Mouchet, A., Marquand, J., M., G., ;, 22, and :. 1968. Le syndrome de la bile calcique, a propos de deux observations de vesicule a contenu calcique. *Ann. Chir.* 22:7.

[68] Love, M. 1982. Sonographic features of milk of calcium bile. . *J.Ultrasound Med* 1:3.

[69] Treyve, D. 1981. *Lithiase vesiculaire calcique chez l'.* Paris: nfant, a propos de deux cas (These Medecine). 18 pp.

[70] Grand, A., Bismuth, V., Bourgeois, R., and Julien, M. 1966;. Syndrome de la bile calcique. A propos de deux observations. *Press Med* 74:6.

[71] Arnaud, J., Aprahamian, M., Eloy, R., Daly, R., Graff, P., Adloff, M., and Electrol., J.R. 1978. Le syndrome de la bile calcique. A propos de deux observations. 59:4.

[72] LeGenissel, M., LeComte, P., Benejam, Y., Vedel, J., and Commadre, F. 1967. Observations de bile calcique. *Arch. Fr. Mal. App. Dig.* 56:2.

[73] Schwartz, A., and Feuchwanger, M. 1961. Radiographic demonstration of spontaneous disappearance of limy bile. *Gastroenterology* 40:4.

[74] Delgoffe, C., Regent, D., Chaulieu, C., and Treheux, A. 1981. [Ultrasonographic appearance of gallbladder calcification: a case report (author's transl)]. *J Radiol* 62:669-672.

[75] Chun, G.H., Deutsch, A.L., and Scheible, W. 1982. Sonographic findings in milk of calcium bile. *Gastrointest Radiol* 7:371-373.

[76] Bergeret, A., Caroli, J., and Lagarenne, P. 1947. Ictere par migration de la bile calcaire dans le choledoque. .*Arch. Fr. Mal. App. Dig* 36:6.

[77] Walter, H. 1949. [Not Available]. *Acta Gastroenterol Belg* 12:112-118; Disc , 135.

[78] Warmoes, F. 1939. Calculs et boues biliaires calcifiees. *J. Belg. Gastroenterol.* 7:5.

[79] Coupris, L., Varlet, F., Duverne, C., Laumonier, F., and Alliot, G. 1985. Le syndrome de la bile calcique chez. *l'enfant. Chir. Pediatr.* 26:7.

[80] Holden, W.S., and Turner, M.J. 1972. Disappearing limy bile. *Clin Radiol* 23:500-507.

[81] Bailey, P.V., Connors, R.H., Tracy, T.F., Jr., Sotelo-Avila, C., Lewis, J.E., and Weber, T.R. 1989. Changing spectrum of cholelithiasis and cholecystitis in infants and children. *Am J Surg* 158:585-588.

[82] Waldhausen, J.H., and Benjamin, D.R. 1999. Cholecystectomy is becoming an increasingly common operation in children. *Am J Surg* 177:364-367.

[83] Miltenburg, D.M., Schaffer, R., 3rd, Breslin, T., and Brandt, M.L. 2000. Changing indications for pediatric cholecystectomy. *Pediatrics* 105:1250-1253.

[84] Takiff, H., and Fonkalsrud, E.W. 1984. Gallbladder disease in childhood. *Am J Dis Child* 138:565-568.

[85] O'Brien, C., Berman, J., Fleming, C., Malet, P., and RD, S. 1986. Total parenteral nutrition gallstones contain more calcium bilirubinate than sickle cell gallstones. *Gastroenterol* 90.

[86] Soloway, R., Kemmer, M., Wu, J., ., I.e., and , pp 2000. *Pigment gallstones.* New York: Marcel Dekker Inc. 18 pp.

[87] Stringer, M.D., Taylor, D.R., and Soloway, R.D. 2003. Gallstone composition: are children different? *J Pediatr* 142:435-440.

[88] Beauregard, W.G., and Ferguson, W.T. 1980. Milk of calcium cholecystitis. *J Pediatr* 96:876-877.

[89] Wu, S.S., Casas, A.T., Abraham, S.K., Billmire, D.F., Smergel, E.M., and de Chadarevian, J.P. 2001. Milk of calcium cholelithiasis in children. *J Pediatr Surg* 36:644-647.

[90] Phemister, D.B., Aronsohn, H.G., and Pepinsky, R. 1939. Variation in the Cholesterol, Bile Pigment and Calcium Salts Contents of Gallstones Formed in Gallbladder and in Bile Ducts with the Degree of Associated Obstruction. *Ann Surg* 109:161-186.

[91] Harvey, P.R., Rupar, C.A., Gallinger, S., Petrunka, C.N., and Strasberg, S.M. 1986. Quantitative and qualitative comparison of gall bladder mucus glycoprotein from patients with and without gall stones. *Gut* 27:374-381.

[92] Taylor, D.R., Crowther, R.S., Cozart, J.C., Sharrock, P., Wu, J., and Soloway, R.D. 1995. Calcium carbonate in cholesterol gallstones: polymorphism, distribution, and hypotheses about pathogenesis. *Hepatology* 22:488-496.

[93] Jass, J.R., and Walsh, M.D. 2001. Altered mucin expression in the gastrointestinal tract: a review. *J Cell Mol Med* 5:327-351.

[94] Klinkspoor, J., Lee, S., I.e., and , pp 2000. *Gallbladder mucosal funtion.* New York: Marcel Dekker Inc. 18 pp.

[95] Glickerman, D.J., Kim, M.H., Malik, R., and Lee, S.P. 1997. The gallbladder also secretes. *Dig Dis Sci* 42:489-491.

[96] Nagashima, H., Masubuchi, M., and Yosizawa, Z. 1974. Sulfated glycoproteins capable of coagulating calcium carbonate isolated from pathological human bile. *J Biochem* 75:779-786.

[97] Shiffman, M.L., Sugerman, H.J., and Moore, E.W. 1990. Human gallbladder mucosal function. Effect of concentration and acidification of bile on cholesterol and calcium solubility. *Gastroenterology* 99:1452-1459.

[98] Bar Dayan, Y., Vilkin, A., and Niv, Y. 2004. Gallbladder mucin plays a role in gallstone formation. *Eur J Intern Med* 15:411-414.

[99] Wright, N.A., Pike, C., and Elia, G. 1990. Induction of a novel epidermal growth factor-secreting cell lineage by mucosal ulceration in human gastrointestinal stem cells. *Nature* 343:82-85.

[100] Wright, N.A., Poulsom, R., Stamp, G.W., Hall, P.A., Jeffery, R.E., Longcroft, J.M., Rio, M.C., Tomasetto, C., and Chambon, P. 1990. Epidermal growth factor (EGF/URO) induces expression of regulatory peptides in damaged human gastrointestinal tissues. *J Pathol* 162:279-284.

[101] Hanby, A.M., and Wright, N.A. 1993. The ulcer-associated cell lineage: the gastrointestinal repair kit? *J Pathol* 171:3-4.

[102] Lee, F.D. 1964. Pyloric Metaplasia in the Small Intestine. *J Pathol Bacteriol* 87:267-277.

[103] Roberts, I.S., and Stoddart, R.W. 1993. Ulcer-associated cell lineage ('pyloric metaplasia') in Crohn's disease: a lectin histochemical study. *J Pathol* 171:13-19.

[104] Rosai, J.I. 2004. *Gallbladder and extrahepatic bile ducts*. Edinburgh: Elsevier.

[105] Adsay, N. 2004. *Gallbladder, extrahepatic biliary tree, and ampulla*: Lippincott Williams and Wilkins. 3 pp.

[106] Rous, P., McMaster, P., and Drury, D. 1924. Tendency For Calculi To Form Out Of The Sterile Liver Bile Of Dogs *J. Exp. Med.*

[107] Rous, P., Drury, D., and McMaster, P. 1924. After hepatic injury of various sorts potential centers for lithiasis are frequently abundant. *J. Exp. Med.*

[108] Kitt, T. 1906. *Lehrbuch path.* Stuttgart: Haustiere.

[109] Okada, S. 1915. Liver bile was nearly always somewhat alkaline. *J. Physiol.* 16.

[110] Neilson, N., and Meyer, K. 1921. The literature showed that the differenc. *J. Infect. Dis.*

[111] Nervi, F., Marinovic, I., Rigotti, A., and Ulloa, N. 1988. Regulation of biliary cholesterol secretion. Functional relationship between the canalicular and sinusoidal cholesterol secretory pathways in the rat. *J Clin Invest* 82:1818-1825.

[112] Lichtwitz, L. 1914,. Ergebn. *inn. Med.*

[113] Saad, H.Y., and Higuchi, W.I. 1965. Water solubility of cholesterol. *J Pharm Sci* 54:1205-1206.

[114] Corradini, S.G., Elisei, W., Giovannelli, L., Ripani, C., Della Guardia, P., Corsi, A., Cantafora, A., Capocaccia, L., Ziparo, V., Stipa, V., et al. 2000. Impaired human gallbladder lipid absorption in cholesterol gallstone disease and its effect on cholesterol solubility in bile. *Gastroenterology* 118:912-920.

[115] Small, D.M. 2003. Role of ABC transporters in secretion of cholesterol from liver into bile. *Proc Natl Acad Sci USA* 100:4-6.

[116] Konikoff, F.M., Danino, D., Weihs, D., Rubin, M., and Talmon, Y. 2000. Microstructural evolution of lipid aggregates in nucleating model and human biles visualized by cryogenic transmission electron microscopy. *Hepatology* 31:261-268.

[117] Kaplun, A., Talmon, Y., Konikoff, F.M., Rubin, M., Eitan, A., Tadmor, M., and Lichtenberg, D. 1994. Direct visualization of lipid aggregates in native human bile by light- and cryo-transmission electron-microscopy. *FEBS Lett* 340:78-82.

[118] Wang, D.Q., and Carey, M.C. 1996. Characterization of crystallization pathways during cholesterol precipitation from human gallbladder biles: identical pathways to corresponding model biles with three predominating sequences. *J Lipid Res* 37:2539-2549.

[119] Somjen, G.J., Lipka, G., Schulthess, G., Koch, M.H., Wachtel, E., Gilat, T., and Hauser, H. 1995. Behavior of cholesterol and spin-labeled cholestane in model bile systems studied by electron spin resonance and synchrotron x-ray. *Biophys J* 68:2342-2349.

[120] Malet, P.F., Dabezies, M.A., Huang, G.H., Long, W.B., Gadacz, T.R., and Soloway, R.D. 1988. Quantitative infrared spectroscopy of common bile duct gallstones. *Gastroenterology* 94:1217-1221.

[121] Nagpal, K., Ghori, T., and Ali, S. 1982. A number of calcium carbonate and calcium phosphate phases. *Curr. Sci* 51:2.

[122] Bogren, H.G., Mutvei, H., and Renberg, G. 1995. Scanning electron microscope studies of human gallstones after plasma etching. *Ultrastruct Pathol* 19:447-453.

[123] van den Berg, A.A., van Buul, J.D., Tytgat, G.N., Groen, A.K., and Ostrow, J.D. 1998. Mucins and calcium phosphate precipitates additively stimulate cholesterol crystallization. *J Lipid Res* 39:1744-1751.

[124] Craven, B.M. 1976. Crystal structure of cholesterol monohydrate. *Nature* 260:727-729.

[125] Abendan, R., and Swift, J. 2002. ChM crystals grown from bile solutions or from aqueous alcohol solutions consistently develop a similar platelike morphology *Langmuir* 18:7.

[126] Shieh, H.S., Hoard, L.G., and Nordman, C.E. 1977. Crystal structure of anhydrous cholesterol. *Nature* 267:287-289.

[127] Konikoff, F.M., Chung, D.S., Donovan, J.M., Small, D.M., and Carey, M.C. 1992. Filamentous, helical, and tubular microstructures during cholesterol crystallization from bile. Evidence that cholesterol does not nucleate classic monohydrate plates. *J Clin Invest* 90:1155-1160.

[128] Hillier, A., and Ward, M. 1996,. The geometric lattice-matching program EpiCalc was used as a systematic screening tool. *Phys. ReV. B* 54:15.

[129] Frincu, M., Sharpe, R., and Swift, J. 2004. Identify which of the low index faces of anhydrous cholesterol and ChM are epitaxially matched with the naturally abundant faces of calcium carbonate (calcite, vaterite, aragonite) and calcium phosphate (hydroxyapatite, brushite). *Cryst. Growth Des* 4:4.

[130] Hooks, D., and Ward, M. 2001. Predictions similar to those of the more rigorous potential energy calculations *AdV. Mater* 13.

[131] Last, J., Hooks, D., Hillier, A., and Ward, M. 1999. Predictions similar to those of the more rigorous. *J. Phys. Chem* 103:11.

[132] Cerius. 1999. *Cerius2.*

[133] Konikoff, F.M., Laufer, H., Messer, G., and Gilat, T. 1997. Monitoring cholesterol crystallization from lithogenic model bile by time-lapse density gradient ultracentrifugation. *J Hepatol* 26:703-710.

[134] Dauber-Osguthorpe, P., Roberts, V., Osguthorpe, D., Wolff, J., Genest, M., and Hagler, A. 1988. The CVFF force field. *Proteins: Struct., Func. Genet.* 4:17.

[135] .DiscoVer. 1999. *DiscoVer, 99.*

[136] Maple, J.R., Dinur, U., and Hagler, A.T. 1988. Derivation of force fields for molecular mechanics and dynamics from ab initio energy surfaces. *Proc Natl Acad Sci U S A* 85:5350-5354.

[137] Shi, S., Yan, L., Yang, Y., Fisher-Shaulsky, J., and Thacher, T. 2003. This model was then fully minimized using ESFF35 force fields. *J. Comput. Chem* 24:18.

[138] Gay, D., and Rohl, A. 1995,. Growth slice of thickness. *J. Chem. Soc., Faraday Trans* 91:12.

[139] Gale, J., and Rohl, A. . 2003. The calculations were done using the latest version of GULP. *Mol. Simul* 29:51.

[140] Hartman, P., and ennema, P. 1980. The sum of the attachment energy and the slice energy is the crystal energy *Cryst. Growth* 49:12.

[141] Wulff, G. 1901. The calculated morphology is displayed via a Wulff plot. *Krystallogr* 34:82.

[142] Rohl, A., Wright, K., and Gale, J. 2003. The interatomic potentials for calcite were taken *Am. Mineral* 88:5.

[143] Whiting, M.J., and Watts, J.M. 1985. Cholesterol gallstone pathogenesis: a study of potential nucleating agents for cholesterol crystal formation in bile. *Clin Sci (Lond)* 68:589-596.

[144] Levy, P.F., Smith, B.F., and LaMont, J.T. 1984. Human gallbladder mucin accelerates nucleation of cholesterol in artificial bile. *Gastroenterology* 87:270-275.

[145] Harvey, P., Upadhya, G., and Strasberg, S. 1992,. The effect of soluble species such as proteins *J. Biol. Chem.* 266:8.

[146] Kibe, A., Holzbach, R.T., LaRusso, N.F., and Mao, S.J. 1984. Inhibition of cholesterol crystal formation by apolipoproteins in supersaturated model bile. *Science* 225:514-516.

[147] Lafont, S., Rapaport, H., Somjen, G., Renault, A., Howes, P., Kjaer, K., Als-Nielsen, J., Leiserowitz, L., and Lahav, M. 1998,. The effect of soluble species such as phospholipids. *J. Phys. Chem* 102:5.

[148] Rapaport, H., Kuzmenko, I., Lafont, S., Kjaer, K., Howes, P.-., Nielsen, J., Lahav, M., and Leiserowitz, L. 2001,. Effect of soluble species such as phospholipids Biophys. *Biophys. J.*:18.

[149] Perl-Treves, D., Kessler, N., Izhaky, D., and Addadi, L. 1996. Monoclonal antibody recognition of cholesterol monohydrate crystal faces. *Chem Biol* 3:567-577.

[150] Toor, E.W., Evans, D.F., and Cussler, E.L. 1978. Cholesterol monohydrate growth in model bile solutions. *Proc Natl Acad Sci U S A* 75:6230-6234.

[151] Moore, E.W. 1990. Biliary calcium and gallstone formation. *Hepatology* 12:206S-214S; discussion 214S-218S.

[152] Shieh, H., Hoard, L., and Nordman, C. 1981. None of the other known cholesterol crystal phases, including anhydrous cholesterol are known to exhibit this angle. *Acta Crystallogr* B37:6.

[153] Burton, W., Cabrera, N., Frank, F., and Sudden increases in a particular island's surface defect density. 1951. *Proc. R. Soc. London, Ser. A* 243:42.

[154] Liang, C., Yan, L., Hill, J., Ewig, C., Stouch, T., and Hagler, A. 1995. Simulated the condensed phase structures of anhydrous cholesterol. *J. Comput. Chem* 16:15.

[155] Ma, B., Lii, J., Chen, K., and Allinger, N. 1997,. Use the MM3 class II force field to examine the solid-state structure of cholesteryl acetate *J. Am. Chem. Soc* 119:4.

[156] Frincu, M. (hh kh lh)) Eatt: (10-1)) -0.3892 eV/mol; (100)) -0.2818 eV/mol; (010), = -0.3071 eV/mol; (01-1) = -0.3566 eV/mol; (011) = -0.2940 eV/ mol; (10-2) = -0.4855 eV/mol; (101) = -0.2915 eV/mol, (01-2) = -0.4995 eV/mol; (012) = -0.3971 eV/mol; (-111) = -0.4741 eV/mol; (1-10) = -0.4581 eV/mol; (10-3) = -0.5542 eV/mol; (102) = -0.4108.

Chapter V

Reactive Oxygen Species, Melatonin, Methionine, Ezetimibe and Gallstones

I. Potential Gallstone Disease (GD)-Preventing Drugs [1]

Among the GD-preventing drugs, ezetimibe is noteworthy as advocated by Ahmed. [2] This agent prevents the formation of cholesterol stones in mice by reducing cholesterol absorption (by 35% in the animals on a lithogenic diet and by 90% in the controls) and bile cholesterol saturation index (by 60% on a lithogenic diet), intensifying bile flow, and enhancing the secretion of bile salts (by 60%), phospholipids (by 44%) and glutathione (by 100%), which is associated with the slightly increased expression of bile acid carriers. According to the preliminary data, the major effect of ezetimibe in man is to lower cholesterol absorption reported by Zuniga et al. [3].

The drug is also effective in resorbing cholesterol stones by producing excess unsaturated micelles. Furthermore, it increases the time of cholesterol crystallization in patients by Wang et al. [4] The long-term use of magnesium preparations has been demonstrated to prevent the occurrence of clinical forms of GD. Magnesium deficiency may cause dyslipidemia and insulin hypersecretion [by Ko and Tsai et al. [5, 6]

There is evidence for the administration of melatonin for the prevention of GD. Melatonin is considered to lower bile cholesterol by reducing the rate of its absorption by the intestinal epithelium and by increasing the rate of its conversion to bile acids by Koppisetti et al. [7] Of great importance in the prevention of recurrent gallstones are the following factors: (1) to avoid inactivity by Volzke and Kharitonova et al. [8, 9] Patients with GD are recommended to exercise (graduated walking of at least 1 km daily; daily exercises associated with the tension of prelum abdominal and the elevation of intraabdominal pressure); (2) to keep a dietary pattern (frequent, fractional) and low-cholesterol diet.

II. Therapy of Gallstone Disease: What It Was, What It Is, What It Will Be [10]

Cholesterol gallstone disease is a common clinical condition influenced by genetic factors, increasing age, female gender, and metabolic factors. Although laparoscopic cholecystectomy is currently considered the gold standard in treating patients with symptomatic gallstones, new perspectives regarding medical therapy of cholelithiasis are currently under discussion, also taking into account the pathogenesis of gallstones, the natural history of the disease and the analysis of the overall costs of therapy. A careful selection of patients may lead to successful nonsurgical therapy in symptomatic subjects with a functioning gallbladder harboring small radiolucent stones. The classical oral litholysis by ursodeoxycholic acid has been recently paralleled by new experimental observations, suggesting that cholesterol-lowering agents which inhibit cholesterol synthesis (statins) or intestinal cholesterol absorption (ezetimibe), or drugs acting on specific nuclear receptors involved in cholesterol and bile acid homeostasis, might be proposed as additional approaches for treating cholesterol gallstones. In this review Portincassa et al. discuss old, recent and future perspectives on medical treatment of cholesterol cholelithiasis.

The prevalence of gallstones increases with age, and is associated with a number of major risk factors (Table 5.2.1) by Portincassa, Katsika and Kratzer et al. [11-13] In westernized countries, well known risk factors are: obesity, type 2 diabetes, dyslipidaemia, and hyperinsulinaemia, which are often components of the metabolic syndrome by Grundy, Eckel and Tsai et al. [14-18]

Table 5.2.1. Non-genetic risk factors for gallbladder stones

Age
Female gender
High-calorie, low-fiber diet
High-carbohydrate diet, dietary glycemic load
Obesity
Physical inactivity
Rapid weight loss/surgery for obesity
Total gastrectomy with lymph node dissection
Spinal cord injury
Infections: enterohepatic *Helicobacter* species, malaria
Biliary strictures
Drugs: estrogens, calcineurin inhibitors, fibrates, octreotide, ceftriaxone
Total parenteral nutrition
Duodenal diverticulum
Extended ileal resection (black pigment stones)
Vitamin B12/folic acid deficient diet (black pigment stones)
Pancreatic insufficiency
CholanCgitis (brown pigment bile duct stones)

Adapted from Portincasa et al. [1] and Grünhage et al. [160] with permission.

Although the majority of stones in the gallbladder remain "silent" and do not require medical or surgical treatment, gallstone disease is still one of the most common digestive diseases requiring hospital admission and financial resources, since its prevalence ranges from 10% to 15% in adults and medical expenses for gallstone treatment exceeded $6 billion in the year 2000 in the United States by Wang, Everhart and Sandler et al. [11, 19-21] To know exactly the composition of gallstones is an essential step to select patients responsive to oral litholysis with bile acids.

In principle, the only gallstones amenable to litholysis are cholesterol-enriched, calcium-free stones. Cholesterol gallstones represent about 75% of the gallstones in westernized countries by Diehl and Attili et al. [22-24] and can be dissolved when no calcium has deposited in the stones. [11, 25] Historically, the Renaissance physician, botanist, alchemist and astrologer Paracelsus (Philippus Aureolus Theophrastus Bombastus von Hohenheim) was the first one to hypothesize that gallbladder concrements were originating from the precipitation of solid material made of tartaric acid by Theophrastus Bombastus and Poertrincassa et al. [26, 27] To date, we know that specific pathogenetic factors contributing to the formation of cholesterol gallstones must include: hepatic hypersecretion of cholesterol into bile leading to a supersaturated bile, accelerated nucleation/ crystallization of cholesterol, defective gallbladder motility (a form of leiomyopathy) leading to gallbladder stasis, increased absorption of intestinal cholesterol, and influence of *LITH* genes by Wang, Portincassa and Lammert et al. [11, 28-33] Genetic predisposition. The remning gallstones are pigment stones that contain less than 30% cholesterol, i.e., black pigment stones which are about 20% of all gallstones found in the gallbladder and/or bile duct (containing mainly insoluble bilirubin pigment polymer mixed with calcium phosphate and carbonate, and cholesterol) and brown pigment stones which are about 5% of all gallstones, found in bile ducts (containing calcium bilirubinate, calcium palmitate, stearate and cholesterol) by Sherlock and Dooley. [34] patients presenting with a typical colicky pain ("symptomatic") do need treatment because of the high rates of complications (e.g., acute cholecystitis, acute biliary pancreatitis or cholangitis), and early recurrence of symptoms. The high costs of both surgical and medical therapeutic interventions and the natural history of the disease indicate restricting the treatment to a subgroup of symptomatic patients with specific symptoms by Portincassa et al. [11, 32, 35] The first cholecystectomy was performed in 1882 by Carl Langenbuch in Berlin by Langenbuch and Ammon et al, [36, 37] which was the first milestone in the treatment of gallstones. Initial experiments on the dissolution of gallstones were already happening at the end of the 19th century by Dabney and Schiff et al. [38, 39] and in the first half of the 20th century. [40] However, it was Danzinger et al. [41] in 1972 who reported that the primary bile acid chenodeoxycholic acid (CDCA) could dissolve cholesterol gallstones in humans when given orally for 6 mo. These days, oral litholysis by ursodeoxycholic acid (UDCA) plays a limited role in cholesterol gallstone treatment. However, some novel and interesting therapeutic options have been suggested by data from pathogenetic and pharmacological studies by Portincassa et al, [11] in particular in subjects permanently or temporarily at risk for gallstone disease (Table 5.2.1). Experimental data on the capacity of the Niemann-Pick C1-like 1 (NPC1L1) protein inhibitor ezetimibe to reduce intestinal absorption of cholesterol by Hou et al.,[42] the effects of statins to inhibit cholesterol synthesis by Istvan and Deisenhofer, [43] or drugs acting on specific nuclear receptors (NRs) involved in cholesterol and bile acid homeostasis [44] may offer an integrate, potent and innovative strategy for the medical treatment of cholesterol gallstones by Wang et al. [4] Major updated therapeutic aspects in patients with gallstones will be reviewed.

Managing Gallstone Disease

The therapeutic option of gallstone disease is based on few crucial steps, i.e., presence/absence of typical symptoms (i.e., colicky pain), presence of complications, and gallbladder function, as well as composition and size of gallstones (Figure 5.2.1). Bearing in mind data on epidemiology and overall costs of both medical and surgical therapies, it is not routinely recommended to treat asymptomatic gallstone patients by Hofman, Tait and Johnston et al. [45-47] Therefore, an expectant management (medical attention) is currently considered the most appropriate choice in patients with gallstones of any type without specific symptoms (i.e., biliary colic). Indeed, approximately 60%-80% of patients with gallstones are completely asymptomatic by Gibney, Jorgensen and Festi et al. [48-50] and stones are frequently found during routine abdominal ultrasonography by Gibney, Jorgensen and Festi et al. [48-50].

In general, the risk of developing typical biliary pain is low (2.0%-2.6% per year by Thistle, Friedman and Gracie et al. [51-54] although microlithiasis or biliary sludge in the gallbladder lumen puts patients at risk for colicky pain or acute pancreatitis [55, 56] Nevertheless, the overall risk rate for complications (yearly incidence 0.3%) and gallbladder cancer (0.02%) are very low by Paumgartner and Brugge et al. [57, 58] If biliary pain and/or complications are present, cholecystectomy represents the gold standard (see below), as oral litholysis with hydrophilic bile acids have a limited role, and are reserved to symptomatic patients with small radiolucent gallstones in a well-functioning gallbladder with a patent cystic duct by Portincassa et al. [11, 32]

Before cholecystectomy, however, careful medical attention and analgesia are often required. Major features of the uncomplicated biliary colic are depicted in Table 5.2.2, concerning pathogenesis, onset, intensity, localization, duration, radiation, associated features, relief of pain, and therapeutic aspects. The chemical formula of drugs currently used to induce analgesia in patients with colicky pain is depicted in Figure 5.2.2.

Cholecystectomy

Cholecystectomy can be performed by laparoscopy, by a small-incision (< 8 cm in length), or by open operation, and several meta-analyses indicate surgical procedures as the gold standard for the treatment of symptomatic gallstones by Keus et al. [59-61] Laparoscopic cholecystectomy, or alternatively, small incision cholecystectomy by Keus et al., [61] are both safe with a similar mortality rate ranging from 0.1% to 0.7% by Keus and Lammert et al. [60-62] Both these procedures are cost-effective compared with open cholecystectomy. [60] Hospital stay and convalescence are shorter, as is the total cost lower for laparoscopic

cholecystectomy compared with open cholecystectomy by Lammert et al. [62] The overall incidence of bile duct injuries requiring corrective surgery varies between 0.1% and 0.3% by Giger, Tuveri and Duca et al. (63-65) and both laparoscopic and open cholecystectomies yield similar complication rates by Keus and Lammert et al. [60, 62] Principally due to the low rate of complications, it is currently under discussion if cholecystectomy may be suggested also for patients with asymptomatic gallstones, but it is generally conceived that surgical procedures are not recommended routinely in symptom-free patients (Figure 5.2.1). Few indications for prophylactic cholecystectomy in asymptomatic patients with gallstones are reported in Table 5.2.3. For example, cholecystectomy should be considered in children with asymptomatic gallstones by Pokorny et al. [66] in particular with sickle cell disease by Gumiero and Bogue et al. [67, 68] spherocytosis and elliptocytosis) who are exposed to the risk of pain and complications. In this group the natural history of gallstones is not well known by Chan et al., [69] although a recent study suggests that clinically silent gallstones in children and infants are associated with low rates of complications and can be therefore managed conservatively by Bogue et al., [68] as in adults.

Table 5.2.2. Major features of the uncomplicated biliary colic

Pathogenesis	Visceral pain caused by the impaction of the stone in the cystic duct or the ampulla of Vater, followed by distension of the gallbladder and/or biliary tract with activation of visceral sensory neurons[161]
Onset	Not exclusively postprandial, typically intermittent
Intensity	Mean visual analogue scale of 9 cm on a 0-10 cm scale
Localization	Most frequently right upper quadrant of the abdomen and/or the epigastrium (representative dermatomes T8/9)
Duration	Generally longer than 15-30 min. Can last several hours and be associated non-specific symptoms of indigestion
Radiation	Angle of the right scapula and/or shoulder (about 60% of cases), retrosternal area (less than 10% of cases)
Associated features	Urgency to walk[162] (two-third of patients), nausea or vomit[42,161,162]
Relief	If the stone returns into the gallbladder lumen, passes through the ampulla of Vater into the duodenum or migrates back to the common bile duct[26]
First-line therapy	If the stone returns into the gallbladder lumen, passes through the ampulla of Vater into the duodenum or migrates back to the common bile duct [26] Fast-acting narcotic analgesics (meperidine[163]) or non-steroidal anti-inflammatory drugs (NSAIDs) (im or iv ketorolac or ibuprofen po) which could also reduce the risk of evolution towards acute cholecystitis[164-167]
Second-line therapy	Antispasmodic (anticholinergic) agents like hyoscine (scopolamine). Less effective than NSAIDs[164]
Recommendations	Fasting, to avoid release of endogenous cholecystokinin and further gallbladder contraction

Adapted with permission.

Old and New Non-Surgical Options

There is no established medical therapy for dissolution of pigment stones or calcified stones of any type. For oral litholysis with bile acids (see below). Medical therapies alternative to oral bile acids have been proposed in the past, including direct stone dissolution with methyl tert-butyl ether (MTBE), a potent organic cholesterol solvent by Bonatsos et al., [77] extracorporeal shock-wave lithotripsy (ESWL) by Thistle et al., [78] or in combination Sauerbruch et al.,[79] followed by oral litholysis with bile acids. The interest in such options, however, has vanished due to their invasiveness, potential toxicity (MTBE) or traumatic

(ESWL) side effects and, for both, the high post-dissolution recurrence rate by Portincassa, Veegunst and Sackman et al. [11, 80, 81] Novel treatments to be discussed include statins, ezetimibe, and agonists/ antagonists of NRs.

Table 5.2.3. Indications of: "prophylactic" cholestectomy (i.e., for asymptomatic patients with high risk of becoming symptomatic)

Children (because they are exposed to the long-term physical presence of stones[58])
Morbid obese patients undergoing bariatric surgery (high risk to become symptomatic during rapid weight loss[62])
Increased risk for gallbladder cancer[63]
Patients with large gallstones (greater than 3 cm)[64,65]
A "porcelain" gallbladder[66] or gallbladder polyps rapidly growing or larger than 1 cm
Native Americans with gallstones (risk of gallbladder cancer 3 to 5 percent)[67]
Gallstone patients with sickle cell anemia (formation of calcium bilirubinate gallstones due to chronic hemolysis.
Patients may become symptomatic with recurrent episodes of abdominal pain[68])
Coexistence of small gallstones and gallbladder dysmotility (increased risk of pancreatitis[47])

Adapted with permission.

Other groups in which prophylactic cholecystectomy must be considered are the morbidly obese undergoing bariatric surgery, patients at high risk for gallbladder cancer, patients with sickle cell anemia, and coexistence of small gallstones and gallbladder dysmotility by Randi, Sleigsenger, Ashur, Amaral and GREPCO et al. [55, 70-76] A totally different approach is necessary in the case of complicated biliary colic, as also shown in Table 5.2.4.

Table 5.2.4. Major features of complicated biliary colic

Additional findings compared to uncomplicated biliary pain
Leukocytosis, nausea, jaundice, vomiting, fever
Underlying potential complications
Acute pancreatitis, acute cholecystitis, biliary obstruction and cholangitis, gallbladder perforation, abscess formation, mucocele of the gallbladder
Decision quick admission to the hospital
Therapies Antibiotics or invasive procedures with or without surgical procedures (Figure 1)
Early laparoscopic cholecystectomy recommended

Adapted with permission.

Oral Dissolution Therapy

The first successful dissolution of cholesterol gallstones was achieved in 1972 by oral administration of the natural primary tri-hydroxy bile acid CDCA [41] (Figure 5.2.3). The use of CDCA was abandoned because side effects were noticed, including a dose-dependent increase in serum liver enzymes, an increase in serum low-density lipoprotein (LDL) cholesterol, and diarrhea. A further step was to use the more hydrophilic trihydroxy bile acid UDCA by Pauletzki et al. [82] UDCA is more hydrophilic and less toxic than CDCA, and is currently employed for oral litholysis of small cholesterol gallstones in patients with a functioning gallbladder (Figure 5.2.3). This bile acid, in a dose of 10-14 mg/kg per day, increases its proportion in the bile acid pool (it originally accounts for less than 8%-10% of the biliary bile acid pool in healthy subjects), inducing a decreased hepatic secretion of biliary cholesterol and the formation of unsaturated gallbladder bile (cholesterol saturation index of less than 1) by Makino and van Erpecum et al., [83-85] the key factor which promotes the dissolution of cholesterol crystals and gallstones.

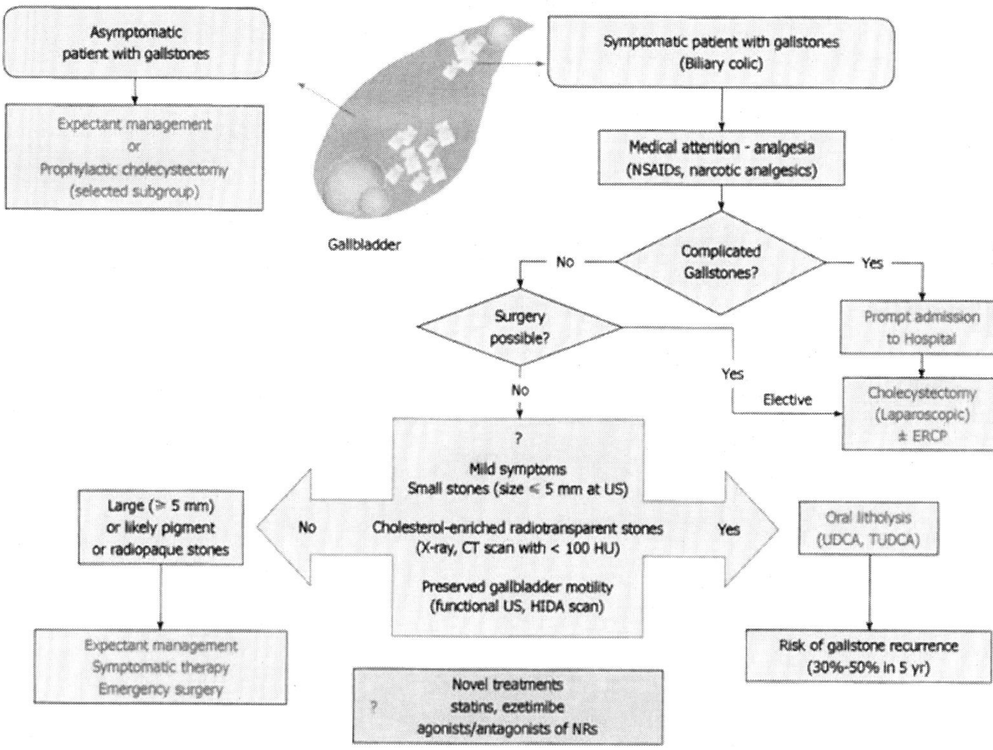

Figure 5.2.1. Flow-chart depicting the standard therapies of gallstone disease (adapted from Portincasa et al [1,15,23,148]). As a starting point, at the top the gallbladder containing "supersaturated" biliary cholesterol is depicted. Typical solid plate-like monohydrate cholesterol crystals form first and aggregate after, to grow as cholesterol stones. Left: flow-chart reserved to asymptomatic patients with gallstones (i.e., when stones/crystal aggregates are not impacted within the cystic duct). Best choice is expectant management, while few indications for prophylactic cholecystectomy exist and are reported in Table 5.2.2; Right: the complex flow-chart reserved to symptomatic gallstone patients is shown. This is the case when stones/crystal aggregates are impacted within the cystic duct. A key step is to identify the "symptomatic" patients with or without complications. In this respect, documenting the presence of biliary colic is of key importance. Meta-analyses indicate that surgery (cholecystectomy) is the gold standard for treating symptomatic gallstones [51-53]. For treatment of uncomplicated and complicated biliary colic, see also Tables 5.2.3 and Tables 5.2.4. CT: Computed tomography; ERCP: Endoscopic retrograde cholangiopancreatography; HIDA: 99mTc-N-(2,6-dimethylacetanilide)-iminodiacetic acid; HU: Hounsfield Unit; NSAIDs: Non-steroidal anti-inflammatory drugs; NRs: Nuclear receptors; TUDCA: Tauroursodeoxycholic acid; UDCA: Ursodeoxycholic acid; US: Abdominal ultrasonography. The HU is an arbitrary unit of X-ray attenuation used for CT scans. Each voxel is assigned a value on a scale in which air has a value of -1000; water, 0; and compact bone, +1000. *Courtesy of World J Gastrointest Pharmacol Ther, Baishideng Publishing Group.*

The fine mechanisms involved in UDCA-induced dissolution of cholesterol stones are rather complex. The so-called ternary phase diagram is used to explain the molecular effects of UDCA on bile composition and cholesterol solubility by Portincassa et al. [86] A group of the equilibrium phase diagram of cholesterol-lecithin-taurine-conjugated bile acid systems (37°C, 0.15 M NaCl, pH 7.0, total lipid concentration 7.5 g/dL) are drawn to display varied positions and configuration of crystallization regions due to decreasing bile acid hydrophobicity, with the lipid components being expressed in moles percent. At the bottom, the ne-phase micellar zone exists (i.e., high bile acid-lecithin moles percent), while above this zone two-phase zones exist on both sides from a central three phase zone. The study of solid and liquid crystallization sequences present in bile shows that different regions exist within each zone, i.e., A, B in the left two-phase, C, D in the central three-phase regions, and E in the right -phase zone.

The number of phases given represents the equilibrium state and develop as cholesterol monohydrate crystals and saturated micelles for crystallization regions A and B; cholesterol monohydrate crystals, saturated micelles and liquid crystals for regions C and D; and liquid crystals of variable compositions and saturated micelles for region E. [86].

As the bile acid hydrophobicity decreases, the maximum micellar cholesterol solubility is reduced and crystallization pathways A-E move to the left. This change results in an enlarged region E that extends to the left and overlaps pathophysiological compositions as examplified in the tauroursodeoxycholate (TUDC)-lecithin-cholesterol system. This event induces a greatly reduced chance for the formation of solid plate-like cholesterol monohydrate crystals in bile.

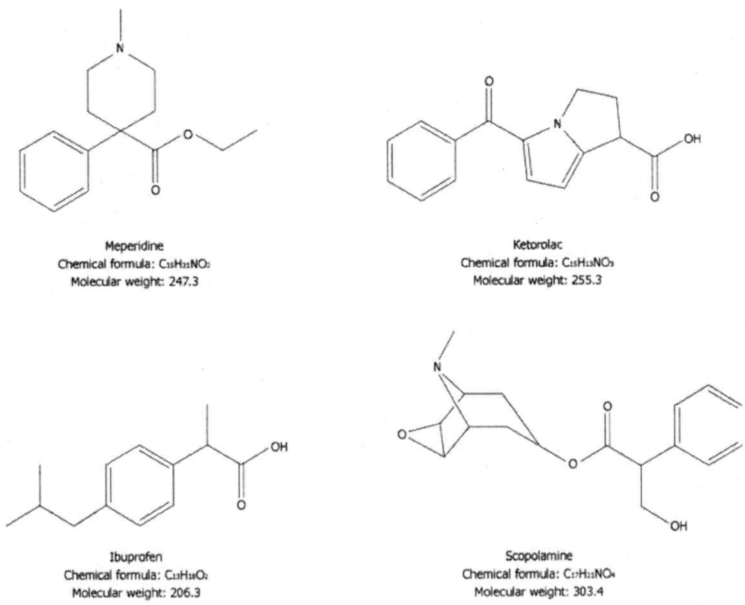

Figure 5.2.2. Chemical formula of drugs currently used to induce analgesia in patients with colicky pain. The three categories are: narcotic analgesics, nonsteroidal anti-inflammatory drugs, and antispasmodics. *Courtesy of World J Gastrointest Pharmacol Ther, Baishideng Publishing Group.*

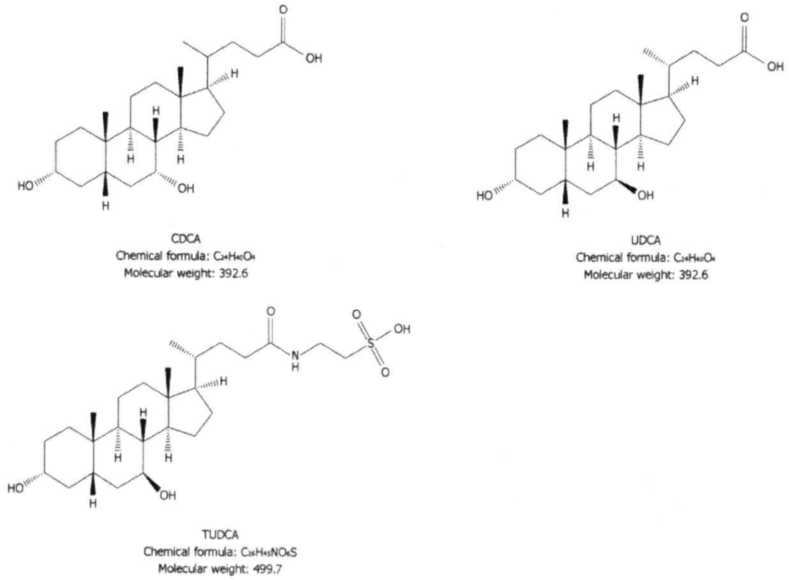

Figure 5.2.3. Chemical formula of bile acids used for oral litholysis of small, radiotransparent, cholesterol-enriched gallstones in a functioning gallbladder with a patent cystic duct of patients with symptomatic gallstones. CDCA: Chenodeoxycholic acid; UDCA: Ursodeoxycholic acid; TUDCA: Tauroursodeoxycholic acid. *Courtesy of World J Gastrointest Pharmacol Ther, Baishideng Publishing Group Co.*

A bedtime administration of UDCA or TUDCA, is recommended since it maintains hepatic bile acid secretion rate overnight, thus reducing secretion of supersaturated bile and increasing the dissolution rate by Wang and Kupfer et al. [87, 88] The hydrophilic bile acid UDCA is also able to act as a litholytic agent through the reduction of intestinal cholesterol absorption by Lanzini, Hardison and Uchida et al. [89-91] and as a possible "prokinetic" agent capable of ameliorating postprandial gallbladder emptying as suggested by observations *in vitro* on isolated gallbladder smooth muscle strips from both animals and gallstone patients by Wang and Heijning et al. [92, 93] the improvement of gallbladder smooth muscle contractility probably also results from the prevention of the impairment of smooth muscle contractility induced by the more hydrophobic and toxic deoxycholate by Guarino and Xiao et al. [94, 95].

Nevertheless, although the majority of gallstones (about two-thirds) in westernized countries are mainly composed of cholesterol, only a minority of patients (less than 10% of total) with cholesterol-enriched gallstones is amenable to oral dissolution therapy with UDCA or with its taurine- conjugates TUDCA Portincassa et al. [11, 35] Indeed, dissolution therapy with oral bile acids can be only suggested to symptomatic gallstone patients who are unfit for surgery and have small (equal to or less than 5 mm in size), uncalcified (radiolucent), and cholesterol-enriched (i.e., more than 80%) stones in a functioning gallbladder with a patent cystic duct by Stolk et al. [96] A number of diagnostic techniques provide essential information for appropriate selection of patients. Gallbladder ultrasonography allows the accurate visualization of gallstone number, size, burden, biliary sludge by Paumgartner and Leopold et al. [47, 97, 98] and explores the morphology and contractile property of the gallbladder, the features of the gallbladder wall with respect to the (acute-chronic) inflammatory status, and the patency of the cystic duct by Portincassa, Venneman, Pauletzki and Festi et al. [99-105] An abdominal plain radiography or a computed tomography (CT) scan by Portincassa and Pereira et al. [106, 107] are needed to exclude the presence of calcified stones by `. [34] By CT scan, in particular, values of < 00 Hounsfield Units predict radiolucent cholesterol rich, dissolvable stones [108] (see also Figure 1 for explanation). An accurate selection of gallstone patients with the characteristics described above offers a higher (99-105) chance of successful oral litholysis alone or after ESWL inducing stone fragmentation by Portincassa, Pauletzki, Hussaini and Venneman et al, [101-104, 109] with an expected dissolution rate of about 1 mm decrement in stone diameter per month by Sackman et al. [110] The complete disappearance of stones with a diameter of less than 5 mm has been described after 6 months of UDCA administration in about 90% of cases by Senior et al. [111] The chance of dissolution is significantly lower (less than 40%-50% after 1 year of the treatment) in patients with larger or multiple stones by Jasraei et al. [57, 112] Main limits of the dissolution therapy by oral bile acids are the possibility of gallstone recurrence (about 10% per year up to 5 years by Paumgartner and Lanzini et al. [113, 114]) and the risk of appearance of a surface calcification on cholesterol gallstones during bile acid therapy in about 10% of cases by Rabenstein et al. [115] A recurrence rate of 30%-50% at 5 years is seen after bile acid therapy or lithotripsy by Bateson, Sackman and Villanova et al,(102, 116-118) particularly in patients with multiple gallstones by Sackman et al. [117] After gallstone disappearance, the persistence of the same pathogenetic factors inducing gallstone formation is principally responsible for their recurrence by Portincassa et al. [11] It has to be underlined, however, that recurrent gallstones respond well to a re-treatment by Petroni et al. [107, 119] Although limited to a relatively small subgroup of patients, the dissolution therapy with UDCA or TUDCA still remains at present an interesting tool in patients who form gallstones as a consequence of transient and nongenetic risk factors (i.e., pregnancy, convalescence from abdominal surgery, obese patients during rapid weight loss by Portincassa, Petroni, O'Leary and Gilat et al, [11, 120-122] Table 5.2.1) and, thus, have a minimum risk of recurrence. Early non-randomized or placebo-controlled studies by Sugerman, Tint and Meredith et al. [123-125] suggested that UDCA might also reduce the risk of biliary colic. A large randomized, double-blind, placebo-controlled trial on the effects of UDCA in highly symptomatic gallstone patients scheduled for cholecystectomy, nevertheless, found that UDCA was ineffective on biliary colic. In fact, the likelihood of remaining colic-free is comparable in patients with strong or weak baseline gallbladder contraction as determined by ultrasonography after a standard mixed meal by Tomida et al. [126].

Cholesterol Lowering Agents

Bile supersaturation with cholesterol is a key factor for cholesterol gallstone formation, and it is principally related to a sustained hepatic hypersecretion of cholesterol depending on the source; from hepatic cholesterol biosynthesis, intestinal cholesterol absorption and HDL-derived cholesterol. [28] As a consequence, all drugs targeting these steps are potentially able to influence both cholesterol gallstone formation and dissolution. Statins and ezetimibe have interesting effects.

Statins are competitive inhibitors of 3-hydroxy-3- methyl-glutaryl-CoA (HMG-CoA) reductase, a rate-limiting enzyme for cholesterol biosynthesis, and they are able to reduce biliary cholesterol independently of their ability to suppress hepatic cholesterol synthesis by Venneman and Loria et al. [127-130] Several statins are being used (Figure 5.2.4) and their pharmacological properties modulate cholesterol homeostasis both in bile and in the liver, potentially leading to a reduction of cholesterol gallstone formation by Hanson, Saunders and Smit et al, [131-133] as clearly demonstrated by animal studies by Tazuma and Abedin et al. [134, 135] In humans, by contrast, the potential beneficial effects of statins on cholesterol gallstones are not so clear. The risk of cholecystectomy decreased slightly in a cohort of US women self-reporting long-term use of statins by Davis et al. [136] Similar results were suggested by a case-control analysis using the UK-based General Practice Research Database and evaluating incident patients between 1994 and 2004. In this study the long-term use of statins (1 to 1.5 years) was associated with a decreased risk of gallstones followed by cholecystectomy, compared with patients without statin use Tsai et al. [137] Furthermore, a recent population-based control study using medical databases from northern Denmark showed a decreased odds ratio for gallstone disease in current statin users (1-2 years of statin use), as compared with nonusers by Bodmer et al. [138] Nevertheless, experimental studies show controversial results, since a decreased biliary cholesterol concentration, a reduced gallstone formation, or gallstone dissolution has been found by some by Erichsen, Chapman, Porsch-Ozcurumez and Smith et al. [139-142] but not all studies by Wilson, Smit, Sharman, Miettinen and Caroli-Bosc et al. [143-147] Recent advances underscore the role of intestinal factors as a key factor for cholesterol absorption, biliary secretion and cholesterol gallstones by Portincassa and Gonzalez-Perez et al. [11, 148] In fact, it has been found experimentally that if dietary cholesterol is absent, all biliary cholesterol derives mainly from a limited *de novo* synthesis (less than 15%).

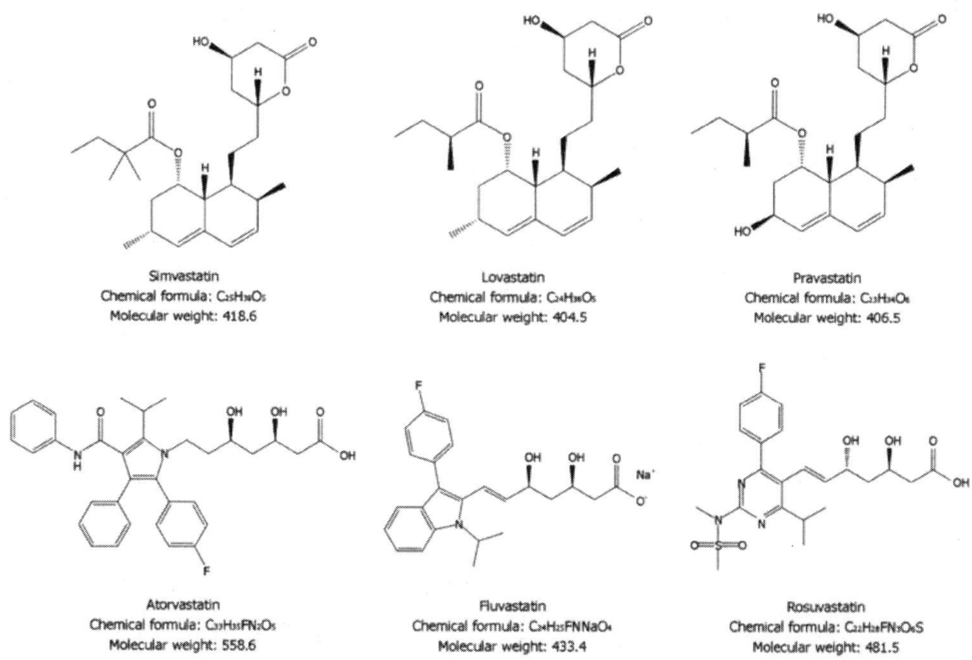

Figure 5.2.4. Chemical formula of different statins used to inhibit hepatic cholesterol synthesis.
Courtesy of World J Gastrointest Pharmacol Ther, Baishideng Publishing Group Co.

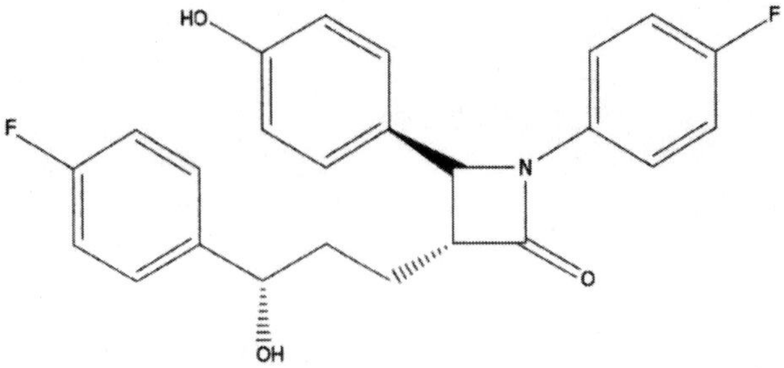

Ezetimibe
Chemical formula: $C_{24}H_{21}F_2NO_3$
Molecular weight: 409.4

Figure 5.2.5. Chemical formula of ezetimibe, the specific inhibitor of the Niemann-Pick C1-like 1 protein. *Courtesy of World J Gastrointest Pharmacol Ther, Baishideng Publishing Group.*

Thus, the small intestine must be seen as a unique organ providing dietary and reabsorbed biliary cholesterol to the body by Gonzalez-Perez et al. [148]. This step plays a crucial role in cholesterol gallstone pathogenesis, since animal studies demonstrate that there is a significant positive correlation between the efficiency of intestinal cholesterol absorption and the prevalence of cholesterol gallstone formation. [31] Ezetimibe, in this respect, is an interesting drug since it has novel hypocholesterolemic effect. By Wang [149] (Figure 5.2.5). Ezetimibe has a strong inhibitory effect on intestinal cholesterol absorption; cholesterol is indeed the most effective substrate of the NPC1L1 protein, the protein that governs intestinal absorption of cholesterol by recycling between the endocytic recycling compartment and plasma membrane by Davis et al. [150] NPC1L1 is highly expressed in the small intestine and localized along the brush border in both humans and mice by Wang and Davis et al., [151, 152] but also present in the human liver by Davis and Altman et al. [152, 153] In mice, ezetimibe largely reduces cholesterol, and to some extent phospholipid content, but not the bile acid content in gallbladder bile. However, all crystallization pathways and phase boundaries on the bile phase diagram are essentially similar, regardless of whether animals are treated with or without ezetimibe. (4) By inhibiting both the cholesterol absorption in the intestine and the hepatic uptake of chylomicron remnants, ezetimibe might lower biliary cholesterol secretion and saturation by Davis et al. [154 Furthermore, it has been also demonstrated that increasing doses of ezetimibe lead the relative lipid composition of gallbladder bile to a progressive shift down and to the left of the phase diagram, which goes into the one-phase (protective) micellar zone, with an abundance of unsaturated micelles but never solid cholesterol crystals or liquid crystals. As a consequence, in gallbladder bile the micellar cholesterol solubility is increased, with more cholesterol molecules transferred from the cholesterol monohydrate surface into unsaturated micelles. In this environment, gallstones are reduced in size and can be completely dissolved. [3, 4]. Ezetimibe might therefore act as a new tool in treating/preventing cholesterol gallstones [2] but also induce amelioration of gallbladder motility, as a consequence of bile desaturation [4]. Ezetimibe is also effective in humans, since it has been demonstrated in a Mexican population that this drug in a dosage of 20 mg po/d for 1 month, is able to significantly reduce cholesterol saturation and cholesterol saturation index and to retard cholesterol crystallization in gallstone patients. In the near future, well designed experimental studies might confirm the efficacy of statins and ezetimibe, alone and/or in association with hydrophilic bile acids, in symptomatic patients without genetic risk of gallstone formation but in the presence of several predisposing conditions (Table 5.2.1). Obesity, in particular, is associated with an increased cholesterol biosynthesis in the liver, mostly due to higher levels of HMG-CoA reductase activity. Thus, in obese patients, the administration of statin might be potentially useful to prevent gallstone formation by Di Ciaula et al. [155] It may be also useful in patients with rapid weight loss, a condition characterized by an increased hepatic secretion of biliary cholesterol, an increase in mucin production by the gallbladder epithelium, and a significant impairment of gallbladder motility [149].

Agonists and Antagonists of NRS

Multiple physiological, developmental, and toxicological processes in the body are regulated by sets of genes, which are coordinated and activated by ligand-activated transcription factors, the NRs. [156] Lipid sensing NRs drive lipid homeostasis in the hepatobiliary and gastrointestinal systems. A key function is exerted by the oxysterol receptor liver X receptor (LXR) and by the bile acid receptor farnesoid X receptor (FXR); both are involved in the molecular regulation of hepatic and biliary lipid metabolism, and modulate bile flow and cholesterol gallstone formation. LXR acts as the intracellular "sensor" of cholesterol by Mangelsdort et al, [157] while FXR is the intracellular sensor of bile acids by Janowski and Parks et al. [158, 159] To maintain lipid homeostasis, cells synthesize oxysterols under conditions of cholesterol overload, and oxysterols, in turn, bind and activate LXR, which acts to reduce the systemic cholesterol burden by Makishima et al. [160] In the enterohepatic system, FXR highly determines expression levels of genes involved in the maintenance of cholesterol, bile acid and triglyceride homeostasis by Repa et al. [161] FXR also up-regulates hepatic expression of bile acid and lipid transporters on the canalicular membrane of hepatocytes and increases activity of regulatory enzymes responsible for bile acid detoxification. These biochemical properties characterize FXR as a potential suitable target for drugs to be employed in the treatment of both cholestasis and cholelithiasis by Kalalay et al. [162] Animal studies confirmed a direct role of LXR and FXR in the processes leading to cholesterol precipitation in bile. FXR-null mice are prone to cholesterol gallstone formation, while the activation of FXR *via* specific synthetic ligands such as GW4064 restores a normal homeostasis between cholesterol, bile acids and phospholipids in bile. [163] This mechanism depends on FXR-induced activity of the energy dependent ATP-Binding Cassette (ABC) transporters ABCB11 for bile acids and ABCB4 for phospholipid by Modica et al. [164] and it is linked to a better cholesterol solubilization in bile, thus preventing the formation of cholesterol crystals and gallstones. The activation of FXR promotes an increase in cholesterol secretion by a direct up-regulation of the main hepatocyte canalicular transporters (ABCG5 and ABCG8) leading to increased biliary cholesterol saturation and precipitation of cholesterol crystals, gallstone formation and growth by Uppal et al. [165]. Such innovative and intriguing results from animal studies have not been confirmed in humans, so far. Future studies are required to assess the usefulness and safety of synthetic, liver-specific FXR agonists and LXR antagonists in humans, not only targeting gallstone disease but also type II diabetes, dyslipidaemia and several cancers [35].

Conclusion

The gold standard for treating symptomatic gallstones remains laparoscopic cholecystectomy. Oral litholysis (basically restricted to few oral hydrophilic bile acids) has a limited role in a scant subgroup of selected patients with symptomatic cholesterol gallstones, but is complicated by the high rate of gallstone recurrence after dissolution treatment and a negative cost-benefit balance. As a consequence of novel and recent animal and human studies, the research agenda in the field of non-surgical therapy of cholesterol cholelithiasis is filled with several possibilities.

Drugs affecting cholesterol synthesis and intestinal absorption (i.e., statins, ezetimibe) and agonists/antagonists of the NRs FXR/LXR involved in biliary lipid secretion may offer, in the near future, promising agents to treat cholesterol gallstones or to prevent their formation in populations at risk.

III. Effect of Ezetimibe on the Prevention and Dissolution of Cholesterol Gallstones [4]

Cholesterol cholelithiasis is one of the most prevalent and most costly digestive diseases in developed countries and its incidence has markedly increased in Asian countries due to the adoption of Western-type dietary habits. Because animal experiments showed that high efficiency of intestinal cholesterol absorption contributes to gallstone formation, Wang et al. explored whether the potent cholesterol absorption inhibitor ezetimibe could prevent gallstones and promote gallstone dissolution in mice and reduce biliary cholesterol content in humans.

Male gallstone-susceptible C57L mice were fed a lithogenic diet and concomitantly administered with ezetimibe at 0, 0.8, 4 or 8 mg/kg/day for 8 or 12 weeks. Gallbladder biles and gallstones were examined by microscopy. Gallbladder emptying in response to CCK-8 was measured gravimetrically. Biliary lipid outputs were analyzed by physical-chemical methods. Cholesterol absorption efficiency was determined by fecal dual-isotope ratio and mass balance methods. Lipid changes in gallbladder biles of gallstone patients vs. overweight subjects without gallstones were examined before (day 0) and at 30 days after ezetimibe treatment (20 mg/day).

Ezetimibe prevented gallstones by effectively reducing intestinal cholesterol absorption and biliary cholesterol secretion, and protected gallbladder motility function by desaturating bile in mice. Treatment with ezetimibe promoted the dissolution of gallstones by forming an abundance of unsaturated micelles. Furthermore, ezetimibe significantly reduced biliary cholesterol saturation and retarded cholesterol crystallization in biles of patients with gallstones.

Ezetimibe is a novel approach to reduce biliary cholesterol content and a promising strategy for preventing or treating cholesterol gallstones by inhibiting intestinal cholesterol absorption.

Cholesterol gallstone formation represents a failure of biliary cholesterol homeostasis in which the physical-chemical balance of cholesterol solubility in bile is disturbed by Portincassa and Wang et al. [11, 19]. Lithogenic bile is mainly caused by persistent hepatic hypersecretion of biliary cholesterol, which has both hepatic and small intestinal components. Obviously, in a person receiving no dietary cholesterol, all biliary cholesterol could be derived mainly from *de novo* synthesis. However, the contribution of *de novo* cholesterol synthesis to biliary cholesterol secretion is small, possibly less than 15% by Liu and Turley et al. [166, 167]. The small intestine is a unique organ providing dietary and reabsorbed biliary cholesterol to the body. [31] Epidemiological investigations have demonstrated that cholesterol cholelithiasis is prevalent in cultures consuming a "Western" diet consisting of high total calories, cholesterol, saturated fatty acids, refined carbohydrates, proteins, and salt, as well as low fibers, and its incidence in North and South American as well as European populations is significantly higher than that in Asian and African populations by Wang et al. [22, 168] Several clinical studies have found an association between the increased incidence of cholesterol gallstones in China and a "westernization" of the traditional Chinese diet by Mendez-Sanchez, Zhu and Huang et al. [169-171] In Japan, cholesterol cholelithiasis once was rare, but over the past 40 years with the adoption of Western-type dietary habits, the incidence has increased markedly by Nagase et al. [172, 173] Because biliary cholesterol hypersecretion is an important prerequisite for cholesterol gallstone formation by Portincassa et al, [11, 19] it is reasonable to assume that by inhibiting cholesterol absorption and/or hepatic uptake of chylomicron remnants, biliary cholesterol secretion and saturation could be significantly reduced. More recently, we observed that there is a significant and positive correlation between the efficiency of intestinal cholesterol absorption and the prevalence of cholesterol gallstone formation in 15 strains of inbred mice, suggesting that high efficiency of intestinal cholesterol absorption and high dietary cholesterol are two independent risk factors for cholesterol gallstone formation. In this study, we investigated whether the potent cholesterol absorption inhibitor ezetimibe could prevent the formation of cholesterol gallstones, and facilitate the dissolution of gallstones in gallstone-susceptible C57L mice carrying *Lith1* and *Lith2* genes. Also, we studied whether ezetimibe may act as a potent biliary cholesterol-desaturating agent in patients with gallstones.

In the materials and methods section, male C57L/J mice, 6–8 weeks old, were purchased from The Jackson Laboratory (Bar Harbor, ME). All mice were provided free access to water and normal rodent chow containing trace (<0.02%) cholesterol (Harlan Teklad F6 Rodent Diet 8664, Madison, WI). For gallstone prevention studies, mice were divided into five groups (n=20 per group) fed 8 or 12 weeks with a lithogenic diet (1% or 2% cholesterol plus 0.5% cholic acid and 15% butter fat) supplemented with ezetimibe (Merck/Schering-Plough Pharmaceuticals, North Wales, PA) in doses of 0, 0.8, 4, or 8 mg/kg/day. We previously observed that at 12 weeks on 2% cholesterol plus 0.5% cholic acid and 15% butter fat, 100% of C57L mice formed cholesterol gallstones. For gallstone dissolution experiments, additional groups (n=20 per group) of mice that have formed cholesterol gallstones due to the 12-week feeding of 2% cholesterol plus 0.5% cholic acid and 15% butter fat, were fed the chow diet supplemented with ezetimibe in doses of 0, 0.8, 4, or 8 mg/kg/day for 8 weeks. All procedures were in accordance with current National Institutes of Health guidelines and were approved by the Institutional Animal Care and Use Committee of Harvard University (Boston, MA).

Human Study Design

To observe whether ezetimibe reduces bile cholesterol content and saturation in humans, Wang et al. studied patients with gallstones (n=7; 40.3±14.5 years old; 1 male and 6 females) and overweighed subjects without gallstones (n=5; 38.2±13.6 years old; 2 males and 3 females). All participants were examined by ultrasonography, which confirmed the existence of gallstones in the gallbladder. All subjects took 20 mg/day of ezetimibe daily for 30 days. During the study period, daily dietary cholesterol intake was approximately 500 mg. Gallbladder bile samples were collected endoscopically before (day 0) and at day 30 after medication. In brief, after an overnight fast and during a routine upper endoscopy, the tip of the endoscope was advanced to the second portion of the duodenum and the ampulla of Vater was visualized. Bile samples were harvested by stimulating gallbladder emptying using an intraduodenal infusion of 30 ml of an 80 g/L amino acid solution.14 A 20- to 30-ml sample of duodenal bile was obtained from each subject. Bile samples were frozen and stored at −20°C for further lipid analyses. Cholesterol saturation indexes (CSI) were determined after biliary cholesterol, phospholipid and bile salt concentrations, as well as bile salt species were measured by Carey and Wang et al. [31, 174] Detection times of plate-like cholesterol monohydrate crystals were investigated in these bile samples according to published methods.16 These studies were approved by the Human Subjects Committees at The Medica Sur Clinic and Foundation (Mexico City, Mexico), as conforming to the ethical guidelines of the 1975 Declaration of Helsinki. Written informed consent was obtained from all participants before entry.

Microscopic Studies of Gallbladder Biles and Gallstones

At 8 or 12 weeks on the lithogenic diet supplemented with various doses of ezetimibe, a cholecystectomy was performed in overnight fasted mice (n=20 per group). Fresh gallbladder bile were examined for mucin gel, liquid crystals, plate-like cholesterol monohydrate crystals, sandy stones, and real gallstones, all of which were defined according to previously established criteria by Nakayama et al. [175]

Determination of Biliary Lipid Outputs and Bile Salt Pool Sizes

The first hour collection of hepatic biles in additional groups of mice (n=5 per group) were used for biliary lipid secretion studies as described previously by Wang et al. [176].

Lipid Analyses

Biliary cholesterol, phospholipid, total and individual bile salts, bile cholesterol, cholesterol content in chow and gallstones, and fecal neutral steroids were determined as described previously by Nakayama, Wang et al. [86, 175-178] The CSI values in gallbladder and hepatic biles were calculated from the critical tables by Nakayama et al. [174].

Measurement of Intestinal Cholesterol Absorption by Fecal Dual-Isotope Ratio Method

Nonfasted and nonanesthetized mice (n=10 per group) were given by gavage an intragastric bolus of 150 μl of medium-chain triglyceride containing 1 μCi of [14C] cholesterol and 2 μCi of [3H] sitostanol. The ratios of the two radiolabels in the fecal extra

Cholesterol Balance Analysis

Because high dietary cholesterol exerts the effect of the radioisotope dilution on specific activity of cholesterol in the upper small intestine, we used cholesterol balance analysis by

Wang et al. [177] to determine cholesterol absorption efficiency in mice challenged to the lithogenic diet. Mice (n=5 per group) were fed the lithogenic diet supplemented with various doses of ezetimibe for 7 days. After cholecystectomy was performed and the common bile duct was cannulated, hepatic bile was collected for the first hour of biliary secretion. Percent cholesterol absorption was calculated as described previously by Wang et al. [177]

Quantitative Real-time PCR Assay

Total RNA was extracted from fresh jejunum tissues of mice (n=4 per group) using RNAse Midi (Qiagen, Valencia, CA). Primer Real-time PCR assays of *Npc1l1*, *Abcg5* and *Abcg8* for all samples were performed in triplicate by Duan et al. [178]. To obtain a normalized target value, the target amount was divided by the endogenous reference amount of rodent *Gapdh* as the invariant control.

Gallbladder Contraction Study

To explore whether ezetimibe has a protective effect on gallbladder motility function, we measured gallbladder contraction in response to exogenously administered sulfated CCK octapeptide (CCK-8) in mice (n=5 per group) fed the lithogenic diet supplemented with varying doses of ezetimibe for 8 weeks according to published methods. [179] Gallbladder contractile function was determined by comparing the areas under the curves of bile flow rates and bile salt outputs, respectively, in the collected samples with mixed gallbladder and hepatic biles.

Statistical Method

All data are expressed as means ± SD. Statistically significant differences among groups of mice were assessed by Student's *t*-test, Mann-Whitney U-tests, or Chi-square tests. If the F-value was significant, comparisons among groups of mice were further analyzed by a multiple comparison test. Analyses were performed with a *Super ANOVA* software (Abacus Concepts, Berkeley, CA). Statistical significance was defined as a two-tailed probability of less than 0.05.

In the results section, concerning effect of ezetimibe on biliary cholesterol secretion in mice and humans, at 8 weeks on the lithogenic diet, administration of ezetimibe to mice resulted in a clear dose dependent decrease in biliary cholesterol outputs during the first hour of biliary secretion of interrupted enterohepatic circulation. Similarly, biliary phospholipid outputs were significantly reduced in a dose-dependent fashion. Nevertheless, hepatic outputs of biliary bile salts varied slightly and were not significantly different among four groups of mice (Figure 5.4.1C). They also observed a dose-dependent decrease in cholesterol/phospholipid ratios and cholesterol/bile salts ratios, indicating that bile cholesterol saturation was significantly reduced by ezetimibe. At day 30 after ezetimibe treatment, plasma concentrations of total cholesterol in overweight subjects without gallstones and LDL cholesterol in gallstone patients were significantly reduced. Other parameters of plasma lipids were decreased slightly and did not reach significant statistical differences. Furthermore, mole percent cholesterol and cholesterol saturation index were significantly reduced in patients with gallstones, and to some extent, in overweighed subjects without gallstones. As a result, crystal detection times were significantly retarded in patients with gallstones and overweight subjects without gallstones. Mole percent phospholipid and bile salts in gallbladder biles were not influenced in humans treated with ezetimibe at 20 mg/day.

Prevention of Cholesterol Gallstones by Ezetimibe

Administration of ezetimibe induced a significant dose-dependent inhibition of intestinal cholesterol absorption in chow-fed mice as measured by the fecal dual-isotope ratio method. Compared with the chow diet, cholesterol absorption efficiency was significantly increased in mice fed the lithogenic diet, because of the dietary cholic acid as discussed elsewhere by Carey. [91, 180] Nevertheless, there was a significant dose-dependent inhibitory effect on intestinal cholesterol absorption by ezetimibe in mice challenged to the lithogenic diet, as measured by the mass balance method. As expected, the lithogenic diet significantly increased mole percent cholesterol in gallbladder biles. [175] In contrast, mole percent cholesterol in biles was gradually decreased with increasing doses of ezetimibe. Thus, the CSI values of pooled gallbladder biles were obviously reduced from 1.56 to 0.37 by ezetimibe (Table 3). As a result, there was a dose-dependent decrease in gallstone prevalence rates from 80% to 10% in mice treated with ezetimibe from 0 to 4 mg/kg/day. Of special note is that no gallstones were found in mice treated with the highest dose of ezetimibe at 8 mg/kg/day. This protective effect of ezetimibe was also observed in mice fed the lithogenic diet with even higher (2%) amounts of cholesterol for a longer (12 weeks) period.

Physical-Chemical Analysis of Gallbladder and Hepatic Biles

Analyses of individual bile salt species by HPLC revealed that all bile salts in gallbladder and hepatic biles of mice were taurine conjugated with a similar distribution of bile salt compositions. In mice challenged to the lithogenic diet, taurocholate (58.7–70.1%) was the major bile salt of biliary pool, followed by taurodeoxycholate (6.9–17.6%) and taurochenodeoxycholate (7.8–14.0%). There was a low concentration in tauro-β-muricholate (2.9–6.4%), tauro-ω-muricholate (1.7–4.1%) and tauroursodeoxycholate (2.4–4.0%). Hydrophobicity indexes of bile salts in biles were essentially similar (−0.01 to +0.10) among four groups of mice. These results indicate that ezetimibe does not influence bile salt species in bile. The relative lipid compositions of pooled gallbladder biles from mice fed the lithogenic diet supplemented with ezetimibe at 0 or 0.8 mg/kg/day were located in the central three-phase area denoted Region C (Figure5.4.4). These biles were composed of solid cholesterol monohydrate crystals, liquid crystals and saturated micelles. Further, with an increase in doses of ezetimibe, the relative lipid compositions of pooled gallbladder biles progressively shifted downward and to the left of the phase diagrams. These alterations were caused by a significant reduction in cholesterol content. Consequently, administration of ezetimibe at 8 mg/kg/day resulted in the biliary lipid compositions plotted within the one-phase micellar zone. By phase analysis, these biles were composed of one phase, namely micellar bile, exactly as was observed experimentally in model biles. It indicates that the highest dose of ezetimibe can successfully prevent the formation of cholesterol gallstones in mice challenged to high dietary cholesterol.

Dissolution of Cholesterol Gallstones by Ezetimibe

At 12 weeks on the lithogenic diet containing 2% cholesterol, 100% of male C57L mice formed cholesterol gallstones, with stone size being 0.72±0.33 mm. After the diet was changed to the normal rodent chow diet, gallstones were still present in 85% of mice, with stone diameters in 0.63±0.28 mm. This indicates that spontaneous dissolution of gallstones did not occur after the lithogenic diet was replaced with the chow diet for 8 weeks. When the chow diet was added with ezetimibe at 0.8 mg/kg/day, some mucin gel, solid and liquid crystals, sandy stones, and tiny real gallstones (0.27±0.14 mm in diameter) were observed in 5% of mice. Although preexisting cholesterol gallstones were completely dissolved by ezetimibe at 4 mg/kg/day, an abundance of liquid crystals and cholesterol monohydrate crystals were still detected in biles. In contrast, in mice treated with ezetimibe at 8 mg/kg/day, gallbladder biles were transparent and their examination by polarizing light microscopy revealed no solid cholesterol crystals or gallstones. It indicated that treatment with the highest dose of ezetimibe for 8 weeks resulted in complete gallstone dissolution rates of 100%. Compared with the chow diet, the CSI values, cholesterol/phospholipid ratios, and mole percent cholesterol of pooled gallbladder biles were decreased markedly by ezetimibe in a dose-dependent manner. In addition, no differences in bile salt species and the hydrophobicity indexes were found in biles of these mice. Figure 5.4.2C plots the relative lipid compositions of pooled gallbladder biles before (day 0) and at week 8 after ezetimibe treatment on a taurocholate-rich bile phase diagram. The lipid compositions of pooled gallbladder biles with preexisting cholesterol gallstones in chow-fed mice still fell in the central three-phase zone. In contrast, the relative lipid compositions of biles from mice fed the highest dose of ezetimibe were located on the one-phase micellar zone in which bile is composed of unsaturated micelles.

Amelioration of Gallbladder Contraction by Ezetimibe

Under lithogenic diet feeding conditions, gallbladder sizes were significantly increased compared with the chow diet. In the lithogenic state, gallbladder sizes were still enlarged in mice treated even with a low (0.8 mg/kg/day) dose of ezetimibe. Nevertheless, these lithogenic effects on gallbladder dynamics were fully blocked by ezetimibe in doses of higher than or equal to 4 mg/kg/day. Because CCK-8 stimulated gallbladder emptying and concentrated gallbladder bile was released, biliary bile salt output and bile flow rate were increased sharply and significantly only in mice treated with the highest (8 mg/kg/day) dose of ezetimibe. In contrast, these parameters were decreased when the doses of ezetimibe were reduced from 4 to 0 mg/kg/day. These alterations suggested that during lithogenesis, gallbladder motility function was impaired completely in mice fed the lithogenic diet and partially in mice treated with lower doses ($\leq$4 mg/kg/day) of ezetimibe. In contrast, the administration of CCK-8 induces complete gallbladder emptying in mice treated with ezetimibe at 8 mg/kg/day.

Effect of Ezetimibe on Gene Expression of Intestinal Sterol Transporters

Relative to the mRNA levels of intestinal lipid transporters in mice fed the lithogenic diet and receiving no ezetimibe, and their relative expression levels are set at 1. Treatment of ezetimibe at 8 mg/kg/day resulted in significant decreases in expression levels of the intestinal *Abcg5*, *Abcg8* and *Acat2* genes in mice on the lithogenic diet. It is highly likely that these changes are a secondary phenomenon due to reduced amounts of the absorbed cholesterol entering the enterocyte in ezetimibe-treated mice. Moreover, ezetimibe treatment significantly reduced expression levels of *Npc1l1* in the small intestine.

In the **discussion** section, cholesterol cholelithiasis is a multifactorial disease influenced by a complex interaction of genetic and environmental factors by Portincassa et al. (11, 19) In mouse studies, targeted deletion of the acyl- CoA:cholesterol acyltransferase gene 2 (*Acat2*) results in the lack of cholesterol ester synthesis in the small intestine. This causes a marked reduction in intestinal cholesterol absorption and complete resistance to diet-induced cholesterol gallstones by Wang et al. [154, 181] Further, absence of expression of intestinal APO-B48, but not APO-B100, reduces biliary cholesterol secretion and cholelithogenesis, possibly by decreasing intestinal absorption and hepatic bioavailability. [182] Reduced gallstone prevalence in lithogenic diet-fed apolipoprotein E knockout mice may be explained by decreased availability of chylomicron-derived cholesterol in the liver for biliary secretion by Carey. [180] These studies by Wang et al. [154, 181, 182] support the notion that high dietary cholesterol through the chylomicron pathway could provide an important source of excess cholesterol molecules for secretion into bile, thereby inducing cholesterol-supersaturated bile and enhancing cholelithogenesis. Since ezetimibe significantly suppresses cholesterol absorption from the small intestine via the NPC1L1 pathway by Buhman et al, [183] possibly a transporter-facilitated mechanism, this should diminish the cholesterol content of the liver, which in turn decreases bioavailability of cholesterol for biliary secretion. Indeed, we observed that ezetimibe induces a significant dose dependent reduction in intestinal cholesterol absorption efficiency, coupled with a significant dose-dependent decrease in biliary cholesterol outputs and gallstone prevalence rates. In particular, even under high dietary cholesterol loads, cholesterol gallstones can be prevented in C57L mice treated with the highest dose of ezetimibe at 8 mg/kg/day. They observed that although ezetimibe primarily reduces cholesterol content and to some extent phospholipid content but not in bile salt content in gallbladder bile, all crystallization pathways and phase boundaries on the bile phase diagram are essentially similar, regardless of whether mice are treated with or without ezetimibe. Of special note is that the relative lipid compositions of gallbladder biles from mice treated with varying doses of ezetimibe become appreciably less saturated with cholesterol and also contain relatively lower mole percent phospholipid. As a result, in company with increased doses of ezetimibe, the relative lipid compositions of pooled gallbladder biles are progressively shifted down and to the left of the phase diagram, as well as entering the one-phase micellar zone when the dose of ezetimibe is the highest at 8 mg/kg/day. The micellar zone contains an abundance of unsaturated micelles but never solid cholesterol crystals or liquid crystals. [86] Under these circumstances, the micellar cholesterol solubility is dramatically increased in gallbladder bile. Thus, the cholesterol molecules could be transferred from the cholesterol monohydrate surface into unsaturated micelles so that gallstones become smaller and eventually dissolved. This provides an excellent physical-chemical explanation for the absence of solid cholesterol crystal formation in mice treated with the highest dose of ezetimibe (8 mg/kg/day) at week 8 of gallstone dissolution treatment. In humans, the gallbladder is another key player in gallstone pathogenesis because enlarged fasting gallbladder volume, together with impaired postprandial and interdigestive gallbladder emptying, are frequent and distinctive features in gallstone patients by Amigo et al. [100, 184] This type of "gallbladder stasis" provides time for nucleation of cholesterol crystals and their aggregation into macroscopic stones by Portincassa et al. [11, 19, 29] It has become increasingly evident that the gallbladder epithelium could actively modify the lipid compositions of bile by secretion and absorption of lipids and water. [184, 185] Cholesterol-supersaturated bile facilitates gallbladder absorption of cholesterol and enhances the accumulation of excess cholesterol in the gallbladder wall. Because gallbladder absorptive cells apparently cannot assemble lipoproteins for lipid transport into plasma, the absorbed cholesterol is converted to cholesteryl ester and stored in the mucosa and lamina propria. Henceforth, excess cholesterol in smooth muscle cells could stiffen sarcolemmal membranes and decouple the G-protein-mediated signal transduction that usually ensues when CCK binds to its receptor, thereby further paralyzing gallbladder contractile function and consequently impairing gallbladder emptying function. In contrast, these lithogenic effects on gallbladder motility function can be totally blocked by ezetimibe in the highest dose at 8 mg/kg/day, mostly attributable to decreased biliary cholesterol content in bile by Portincassa et al. [186] The hydrophilic bile acid, ursodeoxycholic acid (UDCA) has been recommended as first-line pharmacological therapy in a subgroup of symptomatic patients with small, radiolucent cholesterol gallstones, [11, 187] and its long-term administration has been shown to promote the dissolution of cholesterol gallstones and to prevent the recurrence of gallstones after extracorporeal shock wave lithotripsy.35 Despite major improvements in the treatment of cholesterol gallstones, optimal use of UDCA is not always achieved in clinical practice, because of failure to titrate the dose adequately. On the basis of animal studies, the natural trihydroxy hydrophilic bile acid of rodents, β-muricholic acid has recently been proposed for the prevention and the treatment of cholesterol gallstones. It should be emphasized that the cholelitholytic mechanism of ezetimibe is different from that of hydrophilic bile acids such as β-muricholic acid and UDCA. These hydrophilic bile acids favor the formation of vesicles in bile so that the growth of liquid crystals on the cholesterol monohydrate surface and their subsequent dispersion might occur during gallstone dissolution. Resultantly, liquid crystalline dissolution allows the transport of a great amount of cholesterol from stones. Our results indicate, therefore, that ezetimibe and hydrophilic bile acids promote the dissolution of cholesterol gallstones by two distinct mechanisms via the formation of an unsaturated micelle and a liquid crystalline mesophase, respectively. Of note is that the *NPC1L1* gene is expressed in livers of humans, but not in mice. More recently, Temel et al. [188] found that mice transgenic for a human *NPC1L1* gene display an increase in biliary cholesterol concentrations. This suggests that inhibition of NPC1L1 in the liver by ezetimibe may rescue biliary cholesterol secretion and increase CSI values in bile. However, in this study we observed that at day 30 after the medication, ezetimibe at 20 mg/ day can significantly reduce cholesterol concentrations and CSI values of gallbladder biles in patients with gallstones, mostly attributable to its inhibitory effect on intestinal cholesterol absorption by Buhman et al. [152, 183] As a result, cholesterol crystallization is retarded so that detection time of cholesterol monohydrate crystals is significantly delayed. Recent research on molecular transporters responsible for biliary lipid secretion suggests that the secretion efficiency of biliary cholesterol is most likely determined by the net effect between efflux and influx of cholesterol molecules across the canalicular membrane of the hepatocyte, which could be regulated by the ABCG5/G8-dependent and independent pathways as well as the NPC1L1 pathway [37]. One possible reason for the results is that because biliary cholesterol secretion is a unique path for excretion of cholesterol from the body in humans and animals, hepatic ABCG5/G8 may play a stronger role in the regulation of biliary cholesterol secretion than NPC1L1. Another possible explanation is that in the gut-liver axis, the intestinal NPC1L1 plays a significant role in providing dietary and reabsorbed biliary cholesterol to the body and the inhibition of its functions by ezetimibe significantly reduces cholesterol absorption. So, the bio-availability of cholesterol from intestinal sources for biliary secretion is decreased markedly. In contrast, the blockage of the hepatic NPC1L1 by ezetimibe has a weak effect on biliary cholesterol secretion and CSI values, as we found in this study. Nevertheless, we are performing clinical studies to observe whether gallstones may completely dissolve after treating patients with ezetimibe for a longer period. To evaluate treatment time, response rate and overall cost-benefit analysis, a more detailed, long-term human study is requested as well. Furthermore, on the basis of our mouse study, it is highly likely that cholesterol gallstones could be dissolved faster by combination therapy of ezetimibe and UDCA in patients. Again, further studies are required to confirm this hypothesis. Overall, our results show that ezetimibe prevents cholesterol gallstones through inhibiting intestinal cholesterol absorption so that biliary cholesterol secretion is reduced, and gallbladder motility function is preserved by desaturating bile in gallstone-susceptible C57L mice challenged to the lithogenic diet. Also, ezetimibe promotes the dissolution of cholesterol gallstones through a greater capacity to form an abundance of unsaturated micelles. Therefore, they conclude that ezetimibe is a novel and potential cholelitholytic agent for preventing or treating cholesterol gallstone disease. Our findings suggest a novel strategy for the prevention of cholesterol gallstones by inhibiting intestinal cholesterol absorption in humans.

IV. Ezetimibe: Its Novel Effects on the Prevention and the Treatment of Cholesterol Gallstones and Nonalcoholic Fatty Liver Disease [189]

The cholesterol absorption inhibitor ezetimibe can significantly reduce plasma cholesterol concentrations by inhibiting the Niemann-Pick C1-like 1 protein (NPC1L1), an intestinal sterol influx transporter that can actively facilitate the uptake of cholesterol for intestinal absorption. Unexpectedly, ezetimibe treatment also induces a complete resistance to cholesterol gallstone formation and nonalcoholic fatty liver disease (NAFLD) in addition to preventing hypercholesterolemia in mice on a Western diet. Because chylomicrons are the vehicles with which the enterocytes transport cholesterol and fatty acids into the body, ezetimibe could prevent these two most prevalent hepatobiliary diseases possibly through the regulation of chylomicron-derived cholesterol and fatty acid metabolism in the liver. It is highly likely that there is an intestinal and hepatic cross-talk through the chylomicron pathway. Therefore, understanding the molecular mechanisms whereby cholesterol and fatty acids are absorbed from the intestine could offer an efficacious novel approach to the prevention and the treatment of cholesterol gallstones and NAFLD.

The small intestine is a unique organ providing dietary and reabsorbed biliary cholesterol to the body by Wang and Temel et al. [148, 178, 190] High plasma total and low-density lipoprotein (LDL) cholesterol concentrations are an important risk factor for cardiovascular diseases. The restriction of dietary calories, cholesterol, and saturated fat has been used as the primary initial therapeutic modality for the treatment of patients with dyslipidemia by de Bari et al. (191) Nevertheless, the reduction of dietary cholesterol is frequently not associated with a significant decrease in circulating LDL cholesterol levels, despite significant restrictions in dietary intake. Therefore, pharmacological intervention aimed to reduce intestinal cholesterol absorption is potentially an effective way of lowering plasma total and LDL cholesterol concentrations by Temel et al. [190] The use of cholesterol absorption inhibitors for treating hypercholesterolemia has a long history, and several classes of compounds such as hydrophilic bile acid ursodeoxycholic acid (UDCA) by Temel et al., [190] the bile acid sequestrants, specific lipase inhibitors, the intestinal acyl-CoA: cholesterol acyltransferase (ACAT) inhibitors by Lammert and Manhas et al., [192, 193] and cholesterol ester transfer protein inhibitors(194) have been developed, and some of them are currently being evaluated in clinical trials. Recently, the discovery and [193] development of ezetimibe, a novel, selective, and potent inhibitor that effectively blocks intestinal absorption of dietary and biliary cholesterol, opened a new door to the treatment of hypercholesterolemia by Grundy, Davidson, Knopp and Dujovne et al. [190, 195-198] Ezetimibe, which can be administered either as monotherapy or in combination with statins, has been shown to be a safe and efficacious treatment for hypercholesterolemia, potentially enabling more patients to reach recommended LDL cholesterol standards set by the National Cholesterol Education Program Adult Treatment Panel III guidelines. [199] Unexpectedly, it was found that ezetimibe treatment can induce a complete resistance to cholesterol gallstone [190] Journal of Lipids formation [181] and nonalcoholic fatty liver disease (NAFLD) in addition to its effect on hypercholesterolemia in mice on a Western diet by Dujovne et al. [200] Furthermore, ezetimibe can prevent gallstones by effectively reducing intestinal cholesterol absorption and biliary cholesterol secretion and protecting gallbladder motility function by desaturating bile in mice. Treatment with ezetimibe also promotes the dissolution of gallstones by forming an abundance of unsaturated micelles in bile. Furthermore, ezetimibe significantly reduces biliary cholesterol saturation and retards cholesterol crystallization in biles of patients with gallstones. [4] It is also found that ezetimibe could prevent fatty liver by reducing hepatic lipogenesis in mice on a high-fat diet and attenuating diet induced insulin resistance, a state known to drive hepatic lipogenesis through elevated circulating insulin levels by Ballantyne et al. [201] Therefore, it is highly likely that ezetimibe could be a novel approach to reduce biliary cholesterol content and hepatic triglyceride accumulation, and thus a promising strategy for preventing or treating cholesterol gallstones and NAFLD, by inhibiting intestinal cholesterol absorption. [4] In this paper, they will review recent progress in understanding the biochemical and physical-chemical mechanisms, whereby ezetimibe could prevent or treat cholesterol gallstones and NAFLD, the two most prevalent hepatobiliary diseases that constitute a considerable health care burden in the USA.

1. Chemistry and Pharmacology of Ezetimibe

Ezetimibe (SCH 58235), 1-(4-fluorophenyl)-(3*R*)-[3-(4-fluorophenyl)-(3*S*)-hydroxypropyl]-(4*S*)-(4-hydroxyphenyl)-2- azetidinone, and an analog, SCH 48461, (3*R*)-(3-Phenylpropyl)- 1, (4*S*)-bis(4-methoxyphenyl)-2-azetidinone, are highly selective intestinal cholesterol absorption inhibitors. They can effectively and potently prevent the absorption of cholesterol by inhibiting the uptake and transport of dietary and biliary cholesterol across the apical membrane of enterocytes. [202] It has been found that the 2-azetidinones are able to inhibit cholesterol absorption at very low doses and induce significant reductions in plasma cholesterol concentrations in humans and in a series of different animal models by Temel, Rosenblum, Burnett and Clador et al. [190, 203-205] After oral administration, ezetimibe undergoes rapid monoglucuronidation in enterocytes and the liver during its first pass. Because ezetimibe and its glucuronide are enterohepatically recirculated, it is most likely that they could repeatedly produce an inhibitory action on the Niemann-Pick C1-like 1 protein (NPC1L1) on the apical membrane of enterocytes, exhibiting multiple peaks of serum drug concentrations with an elimination half-life of approximately 22 hours by Kosoglou et al. [206] This may explain why ezetimibe has a longer duration of action and why its therapeutic effects persist for several days after its cessation. These observations support the notion that once-daily dosing should be sufficient for an adequate therapeutic effect. It has also been demonstrated that 12 hours after oral administration of the glucuronide (SCH-60663), more than 95% of the compound still can be found in the intestine. Because the glucuronide is more potent in inhibiting cholesterol absorption than ezetimibe, it confirms that ezetimibe acts directly in the intestine as glucuronide. [193] Studies with [125I]-labeled ezetimibe glucuronide and [14C]-labeled cholesterol have found that the glucuronide could block the cholesterol uptake into the enterocytes [190] because it is often detected in the brush border membrane, a site predominantly associated with cholesterol uptake and transepithelial transport. Furthermore, ezetimibe and its analogs are relatively small molecules that may not be able to change the physical-chemical nature of the intraluminal environment, nor affect the enterohepatic flux of bile acids by Temel et al. [190] A careful analysis of 399 patients receiving either placebo- or ezetimibe-doses of 0.25, 1, 5, or 10 mg once daily found a median percentage reduction of plasma LDL cholesterol levels of 0%, 12.7%, 14.7%, 15.8%, and 19.4%, respectively by Kosoglou et al. [206] Ten milligrams of ezetimibe daily reduces intestinal cholesterol absorption by 54% compared with placebo. This effect is accompanied by a decrease in plasma LDL cholesterol levels of 20%, a compensatory increase of 89% in hepatic cholesterol biosynthesis (versus placebo) and is also associated with a decrease in the absorption of plant sterols that are highly structurally related to cholesterol by Sudhop and Davidson et al. [207, 208] During ezetimibe treatment, there is a marked compensatory increase in cholesterol biosynthesis in the liver, but not in the extrahepatic organs, and an accelerated loss of cholesterol in the feces with little or no change in the rate of conversion of cholesterol to bile acids. Therefore, the combined administration of the cholesterol absorption inhibitor (ezetimibe) and the 3-hydroxy-3-methylglutaryl oenzyme A (HMG-CoA) reductase inhibitors (e.g., atorvastatin or simvastatin) produces an enhanced reduction in plasma total and LDL cholesterol levels, as well as provides a complementary treatment strategy for high-risk patients, including patients with homozygous familial hypercholesterolemia by Kosoglou et al. [206] These results showed that ezetimibe in combination with HMG-CoA reductase inhibitors would be particularly effective at reducing plasma cholesterol levels in humans. In the early studies, it was reported that ezetimibe may not affect intestinal absorption of triglycerides, fatty acids, bile acids, or fat-soluble vitamins, including vitamins A, D, E, and α- and β-carotenes by Jandacek et al. [209]. More recently, intestinal fatty acid absorption was carefully reexamined by a sensitive and physiologically accurate method, the sucrose polybehenate technique in mice by Jandacek and Labonte et al. [210, 211] Instead of monitoring the appearance in plasma of digestion products from an acutely delivered bolus of oil, fecal excretion of dietary fat is measured by this technique and normalized to the excretion of a nonabsorbable fat, sucrose polybehenate, incorporated into the diet by Lbonte et al. [211] It is observed that on the chow diet, dietary fatty acid absorption is significantly reduced from approximately 95% in control mice to about 87% in ezetimibetreatedmice. Moreover, ezetimibe treatment can significantly reduce intestinal absorption of saturated fatty acids in a graded manner that correlates with chain length. Thus, intestinal absorption of palmitate (16 : 0) and stearate (18 : 0) is reduced from approximately 90% and 70% in control mice to 80% and 50% in ezetimibe-treatedmice, respectively. Intestinal absorption efficiency of medium-chain saturated fatty acids is more moderately affected, possibly because medium-chain fatty acid absorption is less dependent on the chylomicron pathway. Myristate (14 : 0) absorption is reduced by 7–10% and laurate (12 : 0) absorption by 4% in ezetimibe-treated mice as compared with control mice by Labonte et al. [211] These experiments strongly indicate that ezetimibe can reduce intestinal absorption efficiency of not only cholesterol but also long-chain fatty acids in mice. Additionally, it has been found that besides plasma total and LDL cholesterol concentrations, ezetimibe reduces liver cholesteryl ester levels in a dose-dependent fashion in cholesterol-fed hamsters, rats, and monkeys by inhibiting intestinal cholesterol absorption. Nevertheless, ezetimibe does not significantly affect plasma HDL cholesterol or triglyceride levels. It was found from an indirect measurement of chylomicrons from plasma, but not lymph, that cynomolgus monkeys fed a single high cholesterol meal and treated with an ezetimibe analogue displayed a significant reduction in the chylomicron cholesterol content, but not in the triglyceride content by van Heek et al. [212]. These results suggest that it may be important to carefully investigate the absorption and lymphatic transfer of cholesterol and fatty acids in lymph-fistula animal models. Because chylomicrons and chylomicron remnants may be atherogenic by Havel, [213] further investigation of this phenomenon might shed more light on the mechanism of the antiatherogenic effect of ezetimibe. It will also be important to investigate whether ezetimibe could influence the lipid and lipoprotein composition of chylomicrons and their physical structure, as well as their assembly and secretion by the enterocytes into the lymph in animals and humans. Of note is that while statins may increase the clearance of chylomicron remnants, they do not reduce the cholesterol content of chylomicrons. Therefore, the combination of a statin and ezetimibe could be highly effective in reducing the atherogenic potential of chylomicrons by Catapano. [214].

2. Mechanisms of Ezetimibe Action on Intestinal Absorption of Cholesterol and Fatty Acids

Although ezetimibe reduces intestinal cholesterol absorption, it does not influence intestinal gene expression levels of *Abcg5*, *Abcg8*, *Sr-b1*, and *Abca1* in mice. [190, 215]

Employing a genomic-bioinformatics approach, Altmann et al. [152] identified transcripts containing expression patterns and structural characteristics anticipated in cholesterol transporters (e.g., sterol-sensing and transmembrane domains, extracellular signal peptides) and established a strong candidate for the ezetimibe-sensitive cholesterol transporter, the awkwardly named Niemann-Pick C1-like protein 1 (NPC1L1). NPC1L1 has 50% amino acid homology to NPC1, [152] which is defective in the cholesterol storage disease Niemann-Pick type C and functions in intracellular cholesterol trafficking by Catapano et al. [216] However, in contrast to *NPC1* that is expressed in any tissue by Repa and Carstea et al, [217, 218] *NPC1L1* is expressed predominantly in the gastrointestinal tract with peak expression in the proximal jejunum. Subfractionation of brush border membrane suggests that NPC1L1 is associated with the apical membrane fraction of enterocytes. Further, NPC1L1 deficient ice show a ~65% reduction in intestinal cholesterol absorption (16%) compared with wild-type mice (45%). e cholesterol absorption efficiency in NPC1L1 deficient ice is unaffected by ezetimibe or cholic acid, supporting the presence of redundant alternative pathways. [152] These studies strongly suggest that NPC1L1 could be an ezetimibe-sensitive target protein and is responsible for cholesterol uptake by the enterocyte for intestinal absorption (Figure 5.4.1). [152] any of the details of how ezetimibe prevents cholesterol absorption have been elucidated, and recently a molecular echanism for cholesterol uptake mediated by the NPC1L1 as been proposed. The NPC1L1 protein recycles between the plasma membrane facing the extracellular space and he endocytic recycling compartment. [155] If the cholesterol oncentration in the intestinal lumen is high, it is corporated into the plasma membrane and is sensed by NPC1L1 that is localized on the surface of apical membrane of the enterocytes by Carstea et al. [218] Both NPC1L1 and cholesterol are then internalized together through clathrin/AP2-mediated endocytosis. [150] The clathrin-coated globular vesicles are transported along microfilaments to the endocytic recycling impartment where large quantities of cholesterol and NPC1L1 are subsequently stored. [150, 219] If the intracellular cholesterol level is low, endocytic recycling compartment-localized NPC1L1 free of cholesterol moves back to the plasma membrane along microfilaments to transfer new cholesterol as it is absorbed by the enterocytes. The key role of the NPC1L1 inhibitor ezetimibe s to prevent NPC1L1 from entering the AP2-mediated clathrin-coated vesicles. At this stage, the endocytosis of NPC1L1 is inhibited and cholesterol absorption is decreased. [150] although it has been observed that ezetimibe can reduce intestinal fatty acid absorption in mice, the molecular mechanism of this action is still unclear. As reviewed above, the deletion of the *Npc1l1* gene also reduces intestinal bsorption of fatty acids, especially long-chain fatty acids. Potential mechanism may be that inhibition of intestinal cholesterol absorption by ezetimibe could somehow influence intestinal expression of genes involved in fatty acid uptake and transport. It is well known that hydrolysis and absorption of dietary fat (mainly triglycerides) are extremely efficient processes (>90%). Nevertheless, it remains a matter of debate whether intestinal fatty acid absorption occurs solely by passive diffusion or also by protein-facilitated transport. Some studies have suggested that fatty acid transporter/cluster determinant 36 (FAT/CD36) may play role in intestinal fatty acid absorption by Drover and Nassir et al. [220, 221] Therefore, it has been hypothesized that ezetimibe may have potential inhibitory effects on "protein-facilitated" absorption of fatty acids by enterocytes. [211] As found by Western blot analysis, protein concentrations of fatty acid transport protein 4 FATP4) in the small intestine are significantly reduced by approximately 50% in ezetimibe-treated mice compared with control mice (Figure 5.4.1), which is associated with reduced intestinal absorption of long-chain saturated fatty acids. [26, 40] It is unclear whether this inhibitory effect in intestinal FATP4 is induced by ezetimibe through a direct or indirect action pathway. Another explanation is hat ezetimibe treatment significantly reduces cholesterol absorption so that the physical structure of chylomicrons may be modified and their assembly, and/or secretion into the lymphatics may be impaired. Because chylomicrons are a crucial vehicle for the transfer of cholesterol and fatty acids as triglyceride from the intestinal lumen to the lymph, impairing their formation by reducing cholesterol availability may induce a secondary action on fatty acid absorption. Because of this possible mechanism of action, it will be important to examine the physical structure of chylomicrons and their assembly and secretion into lymph to prove this hypothesis.

3. Physical-Chemistry of Bile, Physical Forms of Cholesterol Carrier, and Pathophysiology of Cholesterol Gallstones

Cholesterol, phospholipids, and bile salts are three major lipid components of bile in animals and humans. [28] Because cholesterol is virtually insoluble in an aqueous medium such as bile, specialized transport mechanisms are required to maintain it in solution and the mechanism for its solubilization in bile is complex. Similarly, phospholipids re insoluble in water and require carrier vehicles in bile. Bile salts have the property of amphiphilicity with both hydrophilic and hydrophobic areas of the molecules and are soluble in aqueous solutions to varying degrees, depending on the number and characteristics of hydroxy groups and side chains, as well as the composition of the particular aqueous solution. Bile salt monomers can aggregate spontaneously to form simple micelles when their concentration exceeds the critical micellar concentration. [19]

As defined, a micelle is a colloidal aggregation of molecules of an amphipathic compound (e.g., bile salt) in which the hydrophobic portion of each molecule faces onward and the hydrophilic groups point outward. [41] The formation of simple micelles of bile salts alone depends primarily on the concentration of bile salts. Therefore, micelles are formed at, but not below, a critical micellar concentration of bile salts in bile, which is approximately 2 mmol/L. [28] The formation of micelles is also influenced by the concentrations of biliary solids and counter ions, by the type of bile salt (i.e., by its degree of hydroxylation and whether it is conjugated with taurine or glycine or not), and by the temperature and pH of the bile. These simple micelles (~3 nm in diameter) are small, thermodynamically stable aggregates that are principally composed of bile alts by Wang et al. [222] The cholesterol can be solubilized within the hydrophobic center of the micelle. Also, simple micelles of bile salts are capable of solubilizing and incorporating phospholipids. This enables the micelles—then referred to as mixed micelles—to solubilize at least three times the amount of cholesterol solubilized by simple micelles. The solubility of cholesterol in mixed micelles is enhanced when the concentration of total lipids (bile salts, phospholipids, and cholesterol) in bile is high. Moreover, maximal solubility occurs when the molar ratio of phospholipids to bile salts is between 0.2 and 0.3.[28] Mixed micelles (~4–8 nm in diameter) large, thermodynamically stable aggregates that are composed of bile salts, cholesterol, and phospholipids. Their size varies depending on the relative proportion of bile salts and phospholipids. The shape of a mixed micelle is that of a lipid bilayer with the hydrophilic groups of the bile salts and phospholipids aligned on the "outside" of the bilayer, interfacing with the aqueous bile, and the hydrophobic groups on the "inside".

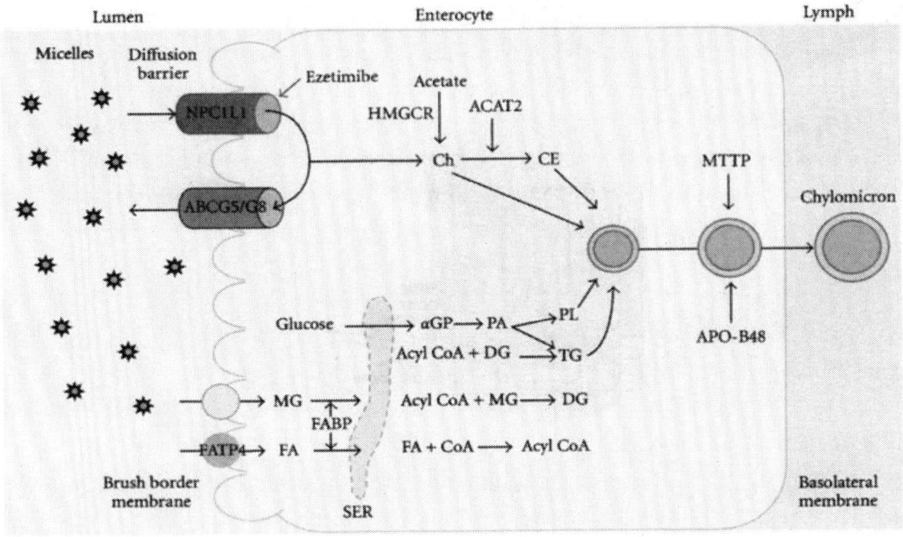

Figure 5.4.1. Within the intestinal lumen, the micellar solubilization of sterols facilitates movement through the diffusion barrier overlying the surface of the absorptive cells. In the presence of bile acids, large amounts of the sterol molecules are delivered to the aqueous-membrane interface so that their uptake rate is greatly increased. The Niemann-Pick C1-like 1 protein (NPC1L1), a newly identified sterol influx transporter, is located at the apical membrane of the enterocyte and may actively facilitate the uptake of cholesterol and plant sterols by promoting the passage of these molecules across the brush border membrane of the enterocyte. In contrast, ABCG5/G8 promote active efflux of cholesterol and plant sterols from the enterocyte into the intestinal lumen for excretion. The combined regulatory effects of NPC1L1 and ABCG5/G8 play a critical role in modulating the amount of cholesterol that reaches the lymph from the intestinal lumen. Ezetimibe may reduce cholesterol uptake by the enterocytes through the NPC1L1 pathway, possibly a transporter-facilitated mechanism. Absorbed cholesterol as well as some that is newly synthesized from acetate by 3-hydroxy-3-methylglutaryl-CoA reductase (HMGCR) within the enterocyte is esterified by acyl-CoA:cholesterol acyltransferase isoform 2 (ACAT2) to form cholesteryl esters. It is likely that fatty acids (FA) and monoacylglycerol (MG) could be taken up into enterocytes by facilitated transport. With the assistance of fatty acid binding protein 4 (FABP4), fatty acids and monoacylglycerol are transported into the smooth endoplasmic reticulum (SER) where they are used for the synthesis of diacylglycerol (DG) and then triacylglycerol (TG). Glucose is transported into the SER for the synthesis of phospholipids (PL) through the phosphatidic acid (PA) pathway (abbreviation: α-GP, α-glycerophosphate). All of these lipids participate in the formation of chylomicrons, a process which also requires the synthesis of apolipoprotein (APO)-B48 and the activity of microsomal triglyceride transfer protein (MTTP). As observed in lymph, the core of the secreted chylomicrons contains triglycerides and cholesteryl esters and the surface of the particles is a monolayer containing phospholipids, mainly phosphatidylcholine, unesterified cholesterol and apolipoproteins including APO-B48, APO-AI, and APO-AIV. Therefore, intestinal cholesterol absorption is a multistep process that is regulated by multiple genes. *Courtesy of Journal of Lipids, Hindawi Publishing Corporation.*

Cholesterol molecules and, therefore, be solubilized on the inside of the bilayer way from the aqueous areas on the outside. The amount of cholesterol that can be solubilized in micelles depends on the relative proportions of bile salts and phospholipids, with additional phospholipids aiding in cholesterol solubilization. [28] Studies using techniques such as quasielastic light-scattering spectroscopy (QLS) and electron microscopy to investigate the physical-chemistry of model and native bile samples have defined more complex mechanisms of cholesterol solubilization in bile by Mazer and Somjen et al. [28, 223, 224] Beside simple and mixed micelles, biliary vesicles, nonmicellar carriers of cholesterol, do exist in bile for the solubilization of cholesterol. Vesicles are unilamellar spherical structures and contain phospholipids, cholesterol, and little, if any, bile salts. thus, vesicles (~40 to 100nm in diameter) are substantially larger than either simple or mixed micelles, but much maller than liquid crystals (~500nm in diameter) that are composed of multilamellar spherical structures. Vesicles are present in large quantities in hepatic bile and are presumably secreted by the hepatocyte. [28] Vesicles in bile have one of two distinct origins. Those formed at the canalicular membrane of hepatocytes are unilamellar and rich in phosphatidylcholines compared with cholesterol (i.e., contain one cholesterol molecule per three phosphatidylcholine molecules). Because of increasing bile salt concentrations in the biliary tree, these vesicles rapidly undergo structural rearrangements and are therefore detectable only in bile specimens analyzed immediately after collection. A second type of vesicle forms spontaneously in bile when the capacity of mixed and simple micelles to solubilize cholesterol is exceeded. These unilamellar or multilamellar vesicles are cholesterol-rich, with cholesterol content reaching as high as two cholesterol molecules per phosphatidylcholine molecule. When concentrations of bile salts are relatively low, vesicles are relatively stable, especially in dilute hepatic bile. Moreover, vesicles may transform or convert completely to mixed micelles when bile salt concentrations in concentrated gallbladder bile are increased. When the bile salt concentration is not high enough, only some vesicles convert to micelles. Because relatively more phospholipids than cholesterol can be transferred from vesicles to mixed micelles, the residual vesicles, now remodeled, may be rich in cholesterol relative to the phospholipids. If the remaining vesicles havea relatively low cholesterol/phospholipid ratio (<1), they are relatively stable. However if the cholesterol/phospholipid ratio in vesicles is >1, vesicles become increasingly unstable by van Erpecum et al. (225) These cholesterol-rich vesicles may transfer some cholesterol to less cholesterol-rich vesicles or to micelles, or may fuse or aggregate to form larger (~500nm in diameter) multilamellar vesicles that may now be termed liposomes or liquid crystals. (28) Liquid crystals are visible by polarizing light microscopy as lipid droplets with birefringence in the shape of a Maltese cross. Liquid crystals are inherently unstable and may form solid cholesterol monohydrate crystals, which is termed cholesterol nucleation. As a result, the nucleation of cholesterol monohydrate crystal induces a decrease in the amount of cholesterol contained in vesicles but not of cholesterol in micelles, supporting the concept that vesicles could serve as the primary source of cholesterol during cholesterol nucleation and crystallization. [28] It is well known that cholesterol cholelithiasis is a multifactorial disease influenced by a complex interaction of genetic and environmental factors by Portincassa et al. [4, 11, 19] Based on recent studies on humans and mouse models, a novel concept has been proposed that interactions of five defects could play an important role in determining the formation of cholesterol gallstones (Figure 5.4.2), which are considered in terms of *LITH* genes (genetic defect), thermodynamics solubility defect, kinetics (nucleation defect), stasis (residence time defect), and lipid sources (metabolic defect). [226]

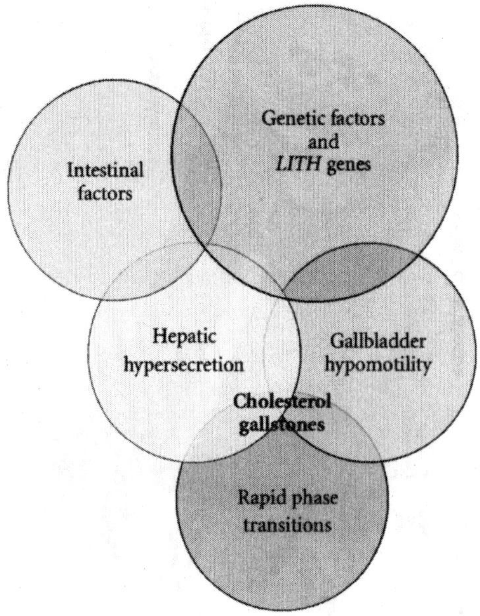

Figure 5.4.2. Venn diagram of five primary defects: genetic factors and *LITH* genes, hepatic hypersecretion, gallbladder hypomotility, rapid phase transitions, and intestinal factors. The hypothesis proposed is that hepatic cholesterol hypersecretion into bile is the primary defect and is the outcome in part of a complex genetic predisposition. The downstream effects include gallbladder hypomotility and rapid phase transitions. A major result of gallbladder hypomotility is alteration in the kinetics of the enterohepatic circulation of bile salts, resulting in increased cholesterol absorption and reduced bile salt absorption that lead to abnormal enterohepatic circulation of bile salts and diminished biliary bile salt pool size. Not only does gallbladder hypomotility facilitate cholesterol nucleation/crystallization, but also it allows the gallbladder to retain cholesterol monohydrate crystals. Although a large number of candidate *Lith* genes have been identified in mouse models, the identification of human *LITH* genes and their contributions to gallstones require further investigation.

Furthermore, cholesterol gallstone formation represents a failure of biliary cholesterol homeostasis in which the physical-chemical balance of cholesterol solubility in bile is disturbed. The liver is the source of cholesterol supersaturated bile in the gallbladder with cholesterol gallstones. Thus, gallstones can be viewed in one sense as a liver disease because some metabolic defects or a combination of defects within the liver result in hypersecretion of biliary cholesterol. As noted, supersaturated bile is a prerequisite for cholesterol gallstone formation, and hypersecretion of biliary cholesterol is the primary metabolic abnormality responsible or initiating cholelithiasis. However, the gallbladder and intestine also conspire as part of a "vicious cycle" that creates physical-chemical instabilities in bile and culminates in the formation of cholesterol gallstones. Therefore, the formation of cholesterol gallstones is the final consequence of excess secretion of cholesterol from the liver into bile. [19, 167] It has been hypothesized that reducing cholesterol availability in the liver for biliary secretion can prevent the formation of cholesterol gallstones and promote the solution of cholesterol crystals and gallstones. This information on the physical-chemistry of bile and the physical forms of cholesterol carriers can help us in understanding why ezetimibe could have a potential therapeutic effect on cholesterol gallstones.

4. Effects of Ezetimibe on the Prevention and the Treatment of Cholesterol Gallstones

Although some, but not all, studies found that high dietary choleerol is associated with increased hepatic secretion of biliary cholesterol, epidemiological investigations have clearly demonstrated that cholesterol cholelithiasis is prevalent in cultures consuming a "Western" diet consisting of high total calories, cholesterol, saturated fatty acids, refined carbohydrates, proteins, and salt, as well as low fiber content.

Many studies have found that the gallstone incidence in North and South American as well as European populations is significantly higher than that in Asian and African populations. [4, 22, 168] Furthermore, several clinical studies ave found an association between the increased incidence of cholesterol gallstones in China and a "westernization" of the traditional Chinese diet. In Japan, cholesterol cholelithiasis once was rare, but over the past 40 years with the adoption of Western-type dietary habits, the incidence has increased markedly. [4,172, 173] Moreover, it has been observed that there is a significant and positive correlation between the efficiency of intestinal cholesterol absorption and the prevalence of cholesterol gallstone formation in mice, suggesting that high efficiency of intestinal cholesterol absorption and high dietary cholesterol are two independent risk factors in the formation of cholesterol gallstones. [91] In addition, in mouse studies, targeted deletion of the acyl- CoA:cholesterol acyltransferase gene 2 (*Acat2*) resulted in the lack of cholesterol ester synthesis in the small intestine. This causes a marked reduction in intestinal cholesterol absorption and a complete resistance to diet-induced cholesterol gallstones. [4, 181] Furthermore, the absence of expression of intestinal APO-B48, but not APO-B100, reduces biliary cholesterol secretion and cholelithogenesis, possibly by decreasing intestinal absorption and hepatic inavailability. [179, 154, 182] Reduced gallstone prevalence in lithogenic diet-fed apolipoprotein E knockout mice may be explained by decreased availability of chylomicron-derived cholesterol in the liver for biliary secretion. [180, 179] These studies support the notion that high dietary cholesterol through the chylomicron pathway could provide an important source of excess cholesterol molecules for secretion into bile, thereby inducing cholesterol-supersaturated bile and enhancing cholelithogenesis. [179] Indeed, because biliary cholesterol hypersecretion is an important prerequisite for cholesterol gallstone formation by Portincassa et al., [179, 11, 19] inhibition of cholesterol absorption in the intestine, or hepatic uptake of chylomicron remnants has become an attractive alternative to decrease biliary cholesterol secretion and saturation. [179] Since ezetimibe significantly suppresses intestinal cholesterol absorption via the NPC1L1 pathway, [183, 179] possibly a transporter-facilitated mechanism,(218)(179) this should reduce the cholesterol content of the liver, which in turn decreases bioavailability of cholesterol for biliary secretion. [179] It has been found that ezetimibe induces a significant dose-dependent reduction in intestinal cholesterol absorption efficiency, coupled with a significant dose-dependent decrease in biliary cholesterol outputs and gallstone prevalence rates. (Figure 5.4.3) In particular, even under high dietary cholesterol loads, cholesterol gallstones can be prevented by ezetimibe in C57L mice carrying the *Lith1* and *Lith2* genes that predispose to cholesterol stone formation. [179]. Although ezetimibe substantially reduces cholesterol concentrations and to some extent phospholipid concentrations, but not bile acid concentrations in gallbladder bile, all crystallization athways and phase boundaries on the bile phase diagram are not influenced by ezetimibe. Further, in company with increased doses of ezetimibe, the relative lipid compositions of pooled gallbladder bile samples are progressively shifted down and to the left of the phase diagram, entering the one-phase micellar zone where there is an abundance of unsaturated micelles, but never solid cholesterol crystals or liquid crystals. Because the micellar cholesterol solubility is dramatically increased in gallbladder bile, the cholesterol molecules can be transferred from the cholesterol monohydrate surface into unsaturated micelles. as a result, gallstones become smaller and eventually dissolved (Figure 5.4.4). [179]

This excellent physical-chemical mechanism could explain, in part, how ezetimibe treatment prevents cholesterol gallstone formation in mice. Enlarged fasting gallbladder volume, together with impaired postprandial and inter digestive gallbladder emptying, is a frequent and distinctive feature in gallstone patients, [179, 29, 100] indicating that the gallbladder is another key player in cholelithogenesis. This type of "gallbladder stasis" provides time for nucleation of cholesterol crystals and their aggregation into macroscopic stones. [179, 11, 19, 29] Under conditions of cholesterol-supersaturated bile, the gallbladder absorbs a large amount of cholesterol, thereby resulting in the accumulation of excess cholesterol in the gallbladder wall. Because gallbladder absorptive cells apparently cannot assemble lipoproteins for lipid transport into plasma, the absorbed cholesterol is converted to cholesteryl ester and stored in the mucosa and lamina propria. As a result, excess cholesterol in smooth muscle cells could stiffen sarcolemmal membranes and decouple the G-protein-mediated signal transduction that usually occurs when CCK binds to its receptor, thereby further paralyzing gallbladder contractile function and consequently impairing gallbladder emptying function. These lithogenic effects on gallbladder motility function can be completely inhibited by ezetimibe. [179, 186] This effect of ezetimibe on protecting gallbladder motility can mostly be attributed to the desaturation of bile. Ursodeoxycholic acid (UDCA) is currently used as a first-line pharmacological therapy to treat only a subgroup of symptomatic patients with small, radiolucent cholesterol stones by Portincassa et al. [179, 11, 187] Extensive clinical studies have shown that long-term administration of UDCA promotes the dissolution of cholesterol gallstones and prevents the recurrence of gallstones after extracorporeal shock wave lithotripsy. [179, 80] However, because of a failure to titrate the dose adequately, optimal use of UDCA is not always achieved n clinical practice [179].

It should be pointed out that the hydrophilic bile acid UDCA can greatly favor the formation of vesicles in bile, which can enhance the growth of liquid crystals on the cholesterol monohydrate surface and their ubsequent dispersion might occur during gallstone dissolution. Consequently, liquid crystalline dissolution allows the transport of a great amount of cholesterol from stones. [179] Because the cholelitholytic mechanism of ezetimibe is totally different from that of hydrophilic bile acids such as UDCA, it has been proposed that a combined therapy of ezetimibe and UDCA could be a faster means to promote the dissolution of cholesterol gallstones, because of the two distinct mechanisms via the formation of unsaturated micelles by ezetimibe and a liquid crystalline mesophase by DCA,(179) respectively. Clinical study has been performed to examine whether ezetimibe would reduce biliary cholesterol concentrations in gallstone patients compared to overweight subjects without gall stones. [179] It was observed that 30 days after starting the medication, ezetimibe at 20mg/day significantly reduced cholesterol concentrations and cholesterol saturation indexes (CSIs) of gallbladder biles in gallstone patients (Table 5.4.1), similar to the results as observed in mouse studies. [179] Consequently, cholesterol crystallization was retarded and detection time of cholesterol monohydrate crystals was significantly delayed as analyzed by polarized light microscopy. Although similar results between mice and gallstone patients have been observed regarding the effect of ezetimibe on the reduction in bile cholesterol concentrations and cholesterol crystallization, a long-term human study is needed to observe whether ezetimibe can reduce gallstone prevalence and completely dissolve gallstones. [179]

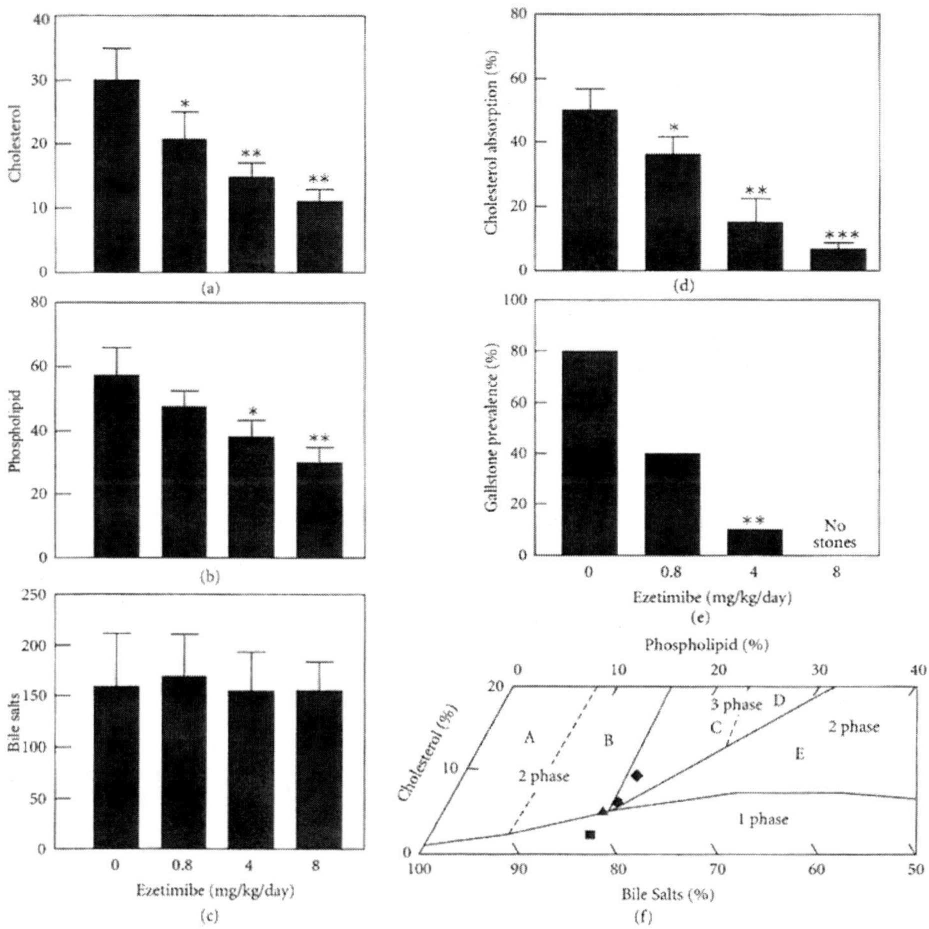

Figure 5.4.3. Effect of ezetimibe on the prevention of cholesterol gallstones. Ezetimibe significantly reduced, in a dose-dependent fashion, hepatic output of (a) biliary cholesterol and (b) phospholipid, but not (c) bile salts. $*P < 0.05$, $**P < 0.01$, and $^{***}P < 0.001$, compared with mice fed the lithogenic diet and receiving no ezetimibe. (d) There is a clear dose-dependent reduction in intestinal cholesterol absorption efficiency from 50 ± 6% to 4 ± 2% in chow-fed with mice, as measured by the fecal dual-isotope ratio method. (e)When doses of ezetimibe are increased from 0 to 4 mg/kg/day, gallstone prevalence rates are reduced from 80% to 10% in mice fed with the lithogenic diet for 8 weeks. no gallstones are found in mice treated with ezetimibe at 8 mg/kg/day. (f) The relative lipid composition of pooled gallbladder bile from mice fed with the lithogenic diet and receiving no ezetimibe are located in the central three-phase zone, where bile is composed of solid cholesterol monohydrate crystals, liquid crystals, and saturated micelles at equilibrium. In contrast, administration of the highest dose (8 mg/kg/day) of ezetimibe resulted in the relative biliary lipid composition of pooled gallbladder bile plotted in the one-phase micellar zone, even upon the lithogenic diet feeding for 8 weeks. By phase analysis, these bile samples are composed of unsaturated micelles at equilibrium. A symbol _represents relative lipid composition of pooled gallbladder bile at 8 weeks on the lithogenic diet supplemented with ezetimibe at 0; 0.8; 8mg/kg/day. *Courtesy of Journal of Lipids, Hindawi Publishing Corporation.*

Table 5.4.1. Plasma and biliary lipids before (day 0) and at day 30 after ezetimibe treatment in humans (20 mg/day)[a]

Parameter	Overweight subjects without gallstones		Gallstone patients	
	Before	After	Before	After
BMI (kg/m^2)	31.5 ± 3.8	31.4 ± 3.4	27.0 ± 2.8	27.1 ± 2.3
Plasma lipid concentrations				
Total Ch (mg/dl)	220 ± 41	168 ± 29[b]	223 ± 32	193 ± 26
LDL Ch (mg/dL)	144 ± 53	99 ± 36	145 ± 26	115 ± 23[b]
HDL Ch (mg/dL)	44 ± 13	37 ± 13	45 ± 11	45 ± 11
TG (mg/dL)	164 ± 88	160 ± 104	166 ± 64	165 ± 76
Biliary lipid compositions of gallbladder biles				
Ch (mole%)	7.4 ± 0.7	6.8 ± 1.9	9.3 ± 1.9	7.2 ± 1.2[b]
PL (mole%)	20.2 ± 2.4	21.8 ± 2.5	19.3 ± 2.8	20.0 ± 3.5
BS (mole%)	72.4 ± 2.9	71.4 ± 3.9	71.4 ± 4.3	72.8 ± 4.2
Ch/PL ratio	0.37 ± 0.03	0.31 ± 0.08[c]	0.48 ± 0.05	0.37 ± 0.06
Ch/BS ratio	0.10 ± 0.01	0.10 ± 0.03	0.13 ± 0.03	0.10 ± 0.02
[TL] (g/dL)	5.3 ± 0.4	5.0 ± 0.9	5.5 ± 0.7	5.3 ± 0.8
CSI	1.2 ± 0.1	1.0 ± 0.2	1.6 ± 0.2	1.3 ± 0.2[b]
CDT (days)	6.4 ± 1.1	10.4 ± 1.1[c]	4.0 ± 1.2	7.0 ± 1.3[c]

[a]Values were determined from overweight subjects without gallstones (n = 5) and gallstone patients (n = 7).

[b]$P < 0.05$ and [c]$P < 0.01$, compared with before ezetimibe treatment (paired t test).

BMI: body mass index; TG: triglycerides; Ch: cholesterol; PL: phospholipids; BS: bile salts; [TL]: total lipid concentrations; CSI: cholesterol saturation index; CDT: crystal detection time.

Reproduced with slightly modifications and with permission from [15].

It should be emphasized that there is a difference in issue distribution of NPC1L1 between mice and humans. In mice, NPC1L1 is expressed only in the intestine, while in humans, it can be detected in both the intestine and iver. [218] Because of this, it has been hypothesized that ezetimibe may have different effects on biliary cholesterol output in humans than in mice. It has been found that the secretion efficiency of biliary cholesterol is most likely determined by the net effect between efflux and influx of cholesterol molecules across the canalicular membrane of the hepatocyte, which could be regulated by the ABCG5/G8- dependent and independent pathways as well as the NPC1L1 pathway. [154, 179] Indeed, ezetimibe treatment can reduce bile cholesterol content and CSIs and prolong detection times of cholesterol monohydrate crystals in humans.

One possible reason for these results in humans is that because biliary cholesterol secretion is a unique path for excretion of cholesterol from the body in humans and animals, hepatic ABCG5/G8 may play a stronger role in the regulation of biliary cholesterol secretion than NPC1L1. Another possible explanation is that in the gut-liver axis, the intestinal NPC1L1 may play a significant role in providing dietary and reabsorbed biliary cholesterol to the body, and the inhibition of its functions by ezetimibe significantly reduces cholesterol absorption. So, the bioavailability of cholesterol from intestinal sources for biliary secretion is decreased markedly.

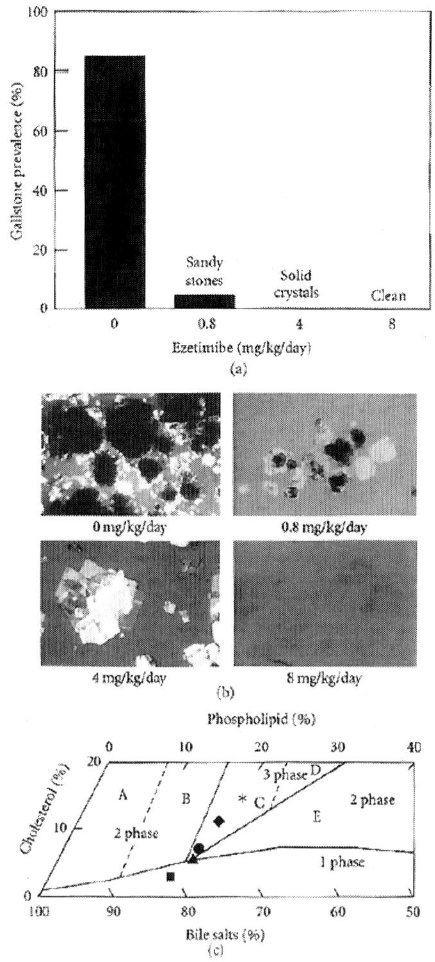

Figure 5.4.4. Effect of ezetimibe on the dissolution of cholesterol gallstones. (a) For gallstone dissolution experiments, mice with preexisting allstones were fed a chow diet alone for 8 weeks, which does not result in a spontaneous dissolution of gallstones. In contrast, treatment with ezetimibe at 0.8 to 8mg/kg/day induces rapid dissolution of gallstones. Gallstones were completely dissolved by the highest (8 mg/kg/day) dose of ezetimibe. (b) Representative photomicrographs of mucin gel, liquid crystals, cholesterol monohydrate crystals, and gallstones as observed in gallbladder biles at week 8 after ezetimibe treatment. All magnifications are ×800, except for ezetimibe treatment at 0 and .8mg/kg/day, which are ×400, by polarizing light microscopy. (c) The relative lipid composition of pooled gallbladder bile from mice fed 8 weeks with the chow diet supplemented with varying doses of ezetimibe is plotted on a condensed phase diagram. Because of a 12- week feeding period of the lithogenic diet, the relative lipid composition of pooled gallbladder bile from mice that have formed cholesterol gallstones is located in the central three-phase zone. Although the lithogenic diet is replaced with the chow diet for 8 weeks, the relative biliary lipid composition of bile is still in region C, where at equilibrium the bile is composed of solid cholesterol crystals, liquid crystals, and saturated micelles. By feeding varying doses of ezetimibe, the relative lipid composition of pooled gallbladder bile gradually shifts down and, finally, enters the one-phase micellar zone. These alterations explain that gallstones are dissolved through an unsaturated micelle mechanism. symbol * represents relative lipid composition of pooled gallbladder bile from mice that have preexisting gallstones and before ezetimibe treatment; _ relative lipid composition of pooled gallbladder bile at the end of the gallstone dissolution study at week 8 of feeding the chow iet only (control); • 0.8; 4; 8mg/kg/day of ezetimibe. *Courtesy of Journal of Lipids, Hindawi Publishing Corporation.*

In contrast, inhibition of the hepatic NPC1L1 by ezetimibe has a weak effect on biliary cholesterol secretion and CSI values. [179] More interestingly, similar to humans, he Golden Syrian hamster displays the abundance of NPC1L1 in the small intestine that far exceeds that in other regions of the gastrointestinal tract such as liver and gall bladder. [227]. The tissue distribution pattern of NPC1L1 s nearly similar between hamsters and humans. It was found that the ezetimibe-induced reduction in intestinal cholesterol absorption is coupled with a decrease in the absolute and relative cholesterol levels in bile in hamsters fed a high-cholesterol diet. [227] These results are consistent with a recent finding that ezetimibe treatment significantly reduces biliary cholesterol saturation in patients with gallstones. Overall, ezetimibe treatment can prevent cholesterol gallstones mainly through inhibiting intestinal cholesterol absorption so that hepatic secretion of biliary cholesterol is reduced, and gallbladder motility function is preserved by desaturating bile (Figure 5.4.5). Also, ezetimibe promotes the dissolution of cholesterol gallstones through a greater capacity to form an abundance of unsaturated micelles. Therefore, ezetimibe is a novel and potential cholelitholytic gent for both preventing and treating cholesterol gallstones [179].

5. Pathophysiology of Nonalcoholic Fatty Liver Disease (NAFLD)

Nonalcoholic fatty liver disease (NAFLD) is a chronic liver disease, which includes a spectrum of hepatic pathology ranging from simple triglyceride accumulation in hepatocytes hepatic steatosis) to hepatic steatosis with inflammation steatohepatitis), fibrosis, and cirrhosis in the absence of alcohol abuse and other causes. (228-230) NAFLD is characterized pathologically by macrovesicular steatosis, mild diffuse lobular mixed acute and chronic inflammation, perivenular and zone 3 perisinusoidal collagen deposition, hepatocyte ballooning, poorly formed Mallory-Denk bodies, glycogen nuclei in periportal hepatocytes, lobular lipogranulomas, and PAS-diastase-resistant Kupffer cells. [231, 232].

AFLD was once proposed to be the result of two distinct but related "hits" to the hepatocyte. (233, 234) The first "hit" is the development of lipid accumulation and hepatic steatosis because of an imbalance of hepatic lipid metabolism, which leads to either excessive lipid influx, decreased lipid clearance, or both. (231) At this point, steatosis s potentially reversible and does not necessarily induce permanent hepatic injury. Although it is less common and occurs in approximately 5% of individuals with steatosis, he second "hit" is more virulent, being an inflammatory recess that is induced probably by oxidative stress, lipid peroxidation, and cytokine action by van Erpecum et al. [235]. The resulting lobular inflammation causes ballooning degeneration and perisinusoidal fibrosis, which promote apoptosis, and hepatocellular death.

These alterations eventually induce scarring and progression to nonalcoholic steatohepatitis (NASH) by Wang et al. [236] However, many studies have been unable to prove that either oxidant stress or lipid peroxidation is necessary for the development of steatohepatitis in humans. Recently, the lipotoxicity model of NASH pathogenesis has emerged based on evidence showing that triglyceride often accumulates in the liver as a parallel rather than pathogenic process during lipotoxic hepatocellular injury (Figure 5.4.6) by Valasek et al. [237]

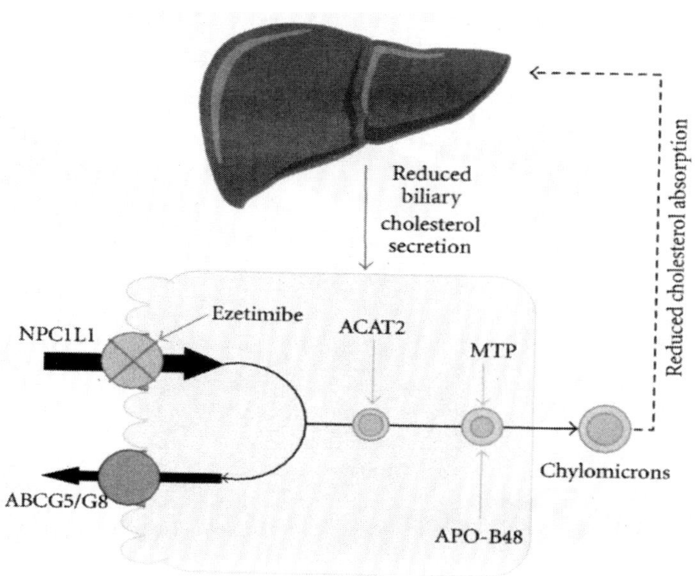

Figure 5.4.5. Pathway underlying the absorption of cholesterol from the intestinal lumen and its delivery to the liver. High dietary cholesterol delivery through the chylomicron pathway could provide an important source of excess cholesterol molecules for hepatic secretion into bile, thereby inducing cholesterol-supersaturated bile and enhancing cholesterol gallstone formation. Ezetimibe significantly suppresses cholesterol absorption from the small intestine via the Niemann-Pick C1-like 1 (NPC1L1) pathway, possibly by a transporter-facilitated mechanism. This effect of ezetimibe could significantly diminish the cholesterol content of the liver, which in turn remarkably decreases bioavailability of cholesterol for hepatic secretion into bile. ABCG5/G8: ATP-binding cassette (transporters) G5 and G8; ACAT2: acyl- CoA:cholesterol acyltransferase isoform 2; APO-B48: apolipoprotein B48; MTTP: microsomal triglyceride transfer protein. *Courtesy of Journal of Lipids, Hindawi Publishing Corporation.*

Therefore, it has been hypothesized that metabolites f unesterified fatty acids play a critical role in inducing ipotoxic injury in the liver. The generation of lipotoxic metabolites of fatty acids typically occurs in parallel with the accumulation of triglyceride droplets (steatosis), resulting in a phenotype recognized as NASH, where steatosis and features of cellular injury are present together by Valasek et al. [237] Metabolic abnormalities predisposing to lipotoxic injury include an increased supply or impaired disposal of unesterified fatty acids.

More importantly, insulin resistance could play a central role in these processes by allowing unsuppressed lipolysis in adipocytes resulting in an excessive flow of fatty acids from adipose tissues and also impairing peripheral glucose disposal [236]. *De novo* lipogenesis in the liver using excessive dietary carbohydrate as a substrate for fatty acid synthesis is also a significant contributor to the burden of saturated fatty acids in the liver. Fatty acid disposal in the liver occurs through oxidative pathways and through the formation of triglyceride which is either stored temporarily s lipid droplets or secreted as VLDL by Wang et al. [236] Additional actors, including oxidative stress, mitochondrial dysfunction, nut-derived lipopolysaccharide and adipocytokines, may promote further hepatocellular damage by Adams and Augulo et al. [238, 239] These processes can lead to inflammation, necrosis, apoptosis and lipogenesis, which may ultimately lead to cirrhosis, liver failure, hepatocellular carcinoma and death by Zheng et al. [240].

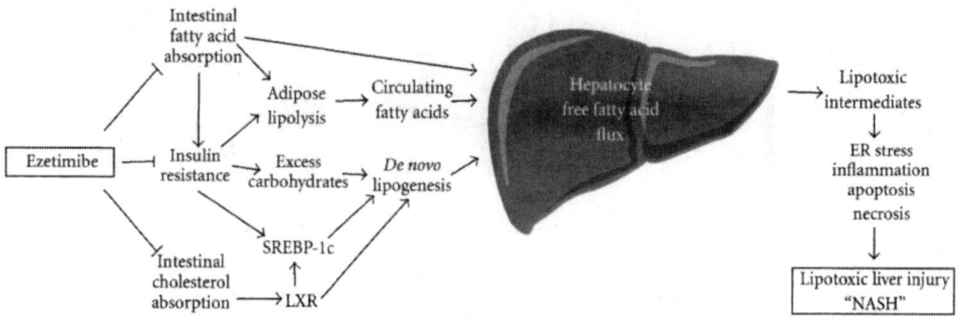

Figure 5.4.6. Potential therapeutic effects of ezetimibe on nonalcoholic fatty liver disease and steatohepatitis (NAFLD and NASH). On the basis of the lipotoxicity model of NAFLD and NASH [51], it has been proposed that metabolites of unesterified fatty acids may induce lipotoxic hepatocellular injury manifested as ER stress, inflammation, apoptosis, necrosis, and dysmorphic features such as ballooning and Mallory-Denk body formation. The generation of lipotoxic metabolites of fatty acids often takes place in parallel with the accumulation of triglyceride droplets (steatosis) in the liver. A high-fat diet often causes insulin resistance, a state that is associated with hyperinsulinemia and hyperglycemia. Because insulin resistance promotes an excessive flow of fatty acids from adipose tissue and also impairs peripheral glucose disposal, these alterations increase the need for fatty acid disposal in the liver through oxidative pathways and through the formation of triglyceride which is then either stored temporarily as lipid droplets or secreted as VLDL. Furthermore, elevated blood insulin and glucose activate transcription factors SREBP-1c to increase hepatic lipogenic gene expression. In addition, intestinal cholesterol absorption promotes hepatic lipogenesis via cholesterol-dependent activation of LXR. Ezetimibe treatment could block (i) intestinal fatty acid absorption, which could reduce a delivery of fatty acids from the gut to the adipose tissue through the chylomicron pathway; (ii) diet-induced insulin resistance in part by reducing intestinal fatty acid absorption; (iii) cholesterol-driven lipogenesis by inhibiting intestinal cholesterol absorption, which together may substantially reduce the burden of fatty acids on the liver. ER: endoplasmic reticulum; LXR: liver X receptor; SREBP-1c: sterol regulatory element-binding protein-1c. *Courtesy of Journal of Lipids, Hindawi Publishing Corporation.*

6. Potential Therapeutic Effects of Ezetimibe on NAFLD

Although the role of dietary fat in the pathogenesis of AFLD continues to be investigated, evidence from animal studies supports the concept that fat overconsumption plays an important role in the etiology of hepatic steatosis. [201] t has been found that feeding a high-fat diet can induce significant accumulation of lipids in the liver of animals such as mice and rats by Oosterveer et al. [241] In humans, a large amount of dietary fat could result in the accumulation of triglyceride n the liver, but stable isotope studies found that up to only 5% of lipids accumulated in the liver are derived directly from dietary fat by Utzschneider and Donnely [242, 243]. In contrast, a low-carbohydrate diet, which is otherwise rich in protein and fat, has been used as treatment for NAFLD by Tendler et al. [244] Furthermore, long-term overconsumption of fat could increase risk for obesity and insulin resistance, which enhances susceptible to NAFLD by Gronbaek et al. [245] Indeed, mice and rats develop hepatic steatosis in response to a high-fat diet and their livers are enlarged and appear grossly pale. Histopathological studies from these livers reveal that hepatocytes are filled with multilocular droplets of varying sizes (Figure 5.4.7). [3].

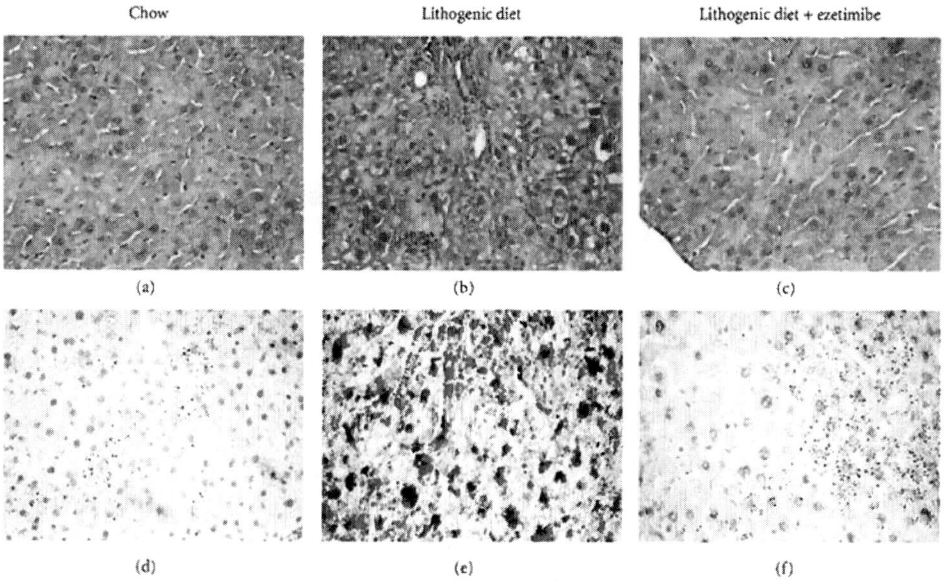

Figure 5.4.7. Histological characterization of the hepatic response to ezetimibe in mice fed a chow versus a lithogenic diet for 4 weeks. The liver samples from mice fed with different diets and treated with or without ezetimibe were isolated and subjected to histological analysis. Panels (a)–(c) show representative liver histology with hematoxylin-eosin staining and panels (d)–(f) show Oil Red O staining. (a) and (d) Mice fed with the chow diet. (b) and (e) Mice fed with the lithogenic diet without ezetimibe. (c) and (f) Mice fed with the lithogenic diet with ezetimibe. The lithogenic diet induced a significant accumulation of triglyceride and cholesteryl ester in the liver as well as hepatocyte damage and inflammation. Interestingly, ezetimibe treatment markedly reduced the accumulation of lipids and prevented hepatic inflammation. *Courtesy of Journal of Lipids, Hindawi Publishing Corporation.*

Strikingly, these diet-induced pathological abnormalities are completely absent in livers not only from ezetimibe-treated mice, butalso from NPC1L1 deficient mice. [201]. In addition, no signs f inflammatory cell infiltration are found in these livers. Hepatic concentrations of both triglyceride and cholesteryl ester are significantly reduced in ezetimibe-treated mice compared with chow-fed control mice. (201) although a high-fat diet may promote fat accumulation n the liver by simply providing more substrate for triglyceride synthesis, an important mechanism whereby a highfat diet may drive hepatic steatosis is by causing selective insulin resistance by Shulman et al. [201, 246] The increased circulating insulin ails to suppress hepatic gluconeogenesis but can promote hepatic lipogenesis. In contrast, ezetimibe treatment could prevent diet-induced hepatic steatosis, weight gain, and insulin resistance. [201]. These alterations are associated with reduced circulating insulin levels, hepatic *de novo* fatty acid synthesis, and hepatic levels of mRNAs for lipogenic genes including glucokinase, an enzyme critical in conversion of glucose to fat. Because elevated blood insulin increases hepatic lipogenic gene expression via transcription factors such as SREBP-1cChen and Uyeda et al. [201, 247, 248] and glucokinase is an important mediator in this lipogenic pathway by Dentin et al., [201, 249] ezetimibe treatment may protect against diet-induced hepatic steatosis by reducing hepatic lipogenesis, mostly through preventing diet-induced insulin resistance and the associated hyperinsulinemia. because excessive amounts of cholesterol are lipogenic through activation of LXR by its metabolites, [157, 201,

250] reduced intestinal cholesterol absorption by ezetimibe could significantly decrease cholesterol content in the liver. This way prevent diet-induced hepatic steatosis in part by reducing cholesterol-dependent LXR activation in the liver. [201] Nevertheless, ezetimibe treatment indeed plays a significant role in preventing diet-induced fatty liver in animals such as mice and rats; however, its therapeutic effect on AFLD needs to be further investigated and proven in humans.

7. Future Research Directions and Clinical Applications

Ezetimibe is a highly potential and selective cholesterol absorption inhibitor that prevents absorption of cholesterol from dietary and biliary sources by suppressing uptake and transport of cholesterol through the enterocytes. Although here is clear evidence showing that ezetimibe can inhibit cholesterol absorption through the NPC1L1 pathway, careful and systematic studies are needed to confirm whether ezetimibe could reduce intestinal absorption of fatty acids in animal models by direct measurement of their absorption and lymphatic transport and studies need to be undertaken in humans by a balance method of intestinal fatty acid absorption.

Because of significantly reduced absorption of intestinal cholesterol and fatty acids, the physical structure of chylomicrons and their metabolism in adipose tissues and liver could be influenced by ezetimibe treatment. To valuate treatment duration, clinical response rates and the overall cost-benefit analysis on cholesterol gallstones and AFLD, long-term human studies are needed. Similar to atherosclerosis, the risk for cholesterol gallstone formation and NAFLD increases with dyslipidemia, hyperinsulinemia, obesity, diabetes, sedentary lifestyle, and aging. It is highly likely that the long-term administration of ezetimibe may benefit this group of subjects who could have a high redisposition to cholesterol gallstones and NAFLD.

V. Reactive Oxygen Species and the Hypomotility of the Gallbladder As Targets [7]

Free radical-mediated damage of the gallbladder epithelium predisposes to the development of both gall bladder inflammation and gallstone formation, which often coexist. Melatonin, a pineal and gut secretory product, due to its antioxidant activity along with its effect on the aging gall bladder myocytes, inhibits gallstone formation. Melatonin reduces the biliary levels of cholesterol by inhibiting cholesterol absorption across the intestinal epithelium and by increasing the conversion of cholesterol to bile acids. The incidence of gallstones is increasing and is expected to rise dramatically with the increase in the longevity and the risk factors such as obesity. The change in the prevalence of cholelithiasis is associated with a proportionate rise in the incidence of cholangiocarcinoma. In an attempt to improve the quality of life of the rapidly increasing aging population, this article reviews up-to-date information on the pathophysiology of the gall bladder function and discusses the development of new therapies with potential good patient compliance and lower cost than the current treatments.

Cholelithiasis was first described in 1507 by a Florentine pathologist, Antonio Benivenius. [251] Gallstone disease remains one of the most common medical problems requiring surgical intervention. Every year, approximately 700,000 cholecystectomies are performed 1993 NIH Consensus. [252] with cholelithiasis affecting approximately 10–15% of the adult population in the US. It is well documented that the presence of gallstones increases with age. The most effective treatment against gallstones is cholecystectomy while medical treatment is limited to those individuals not amenable to surgery. Current medical treatment is aimed at dissolving cholesterol stones, which are composed of salts of acids naturally occurring in bile. However, nonsurgical therapy is effective only against cholesterol stones and is followed by stone recurrence in 50% of the treated cases. Recent studies show a lack of the beneficial effects of medical therapy with ursodeoxycholic acid when used in symptomatic patients awaiting elective cholecystectomy. There is a clear and pressing need for the development of additional agents which act through alternate mechanisms, which would enhance the rate of response and which would be broadly applicable to individuals susceptible to and those with cholelithiasis. Reactive oxygen species (ROS) are involved in several enteric pathologies, including cholelithiasis by Cross et al. [253] This article reviews the stages in the pathology of gallstone formation and potential mechanisms of inhibition by melatonin, a potent antioxidant, at the respective steps of gallstone formation. Gallstone Types and Their Formation Gallstones are composed principally of cholesterol monohydrate crystals (cholesterol stones) or of the acid salt of calcium bilirubinate (pigment stones). Cholesterol stones and the black variety of pigment gallstones form in sterile gallbladder bile whereas brown pigment gallstones form in infected bile. The key pathological events in the formation of gallstones are the increase in the cholesterol:bile acid ratio, gall bladder hypomotility, and an increase in the nucleating factors. Biliary supersaturation with cholesterol is the principal pathophysiological defect in the formation of gallstones. Bile salts maintain cholesterol in the form of micelles, which are soluble. The presence of cholesterol in excess of the bile salts is a result of metabolic and dietary causes or a reduction in the hepatic release of the bile acids resulting in a rise in cholesterol vesicles, which are insoluble. This leads to the formation of cholesterol crystals that coalesce, forming large cholesterol stones by Ahmed et al. [254] In cholesterol gallstone disease, the human gallbladder epithelium loses its capacity to selectively and efficiently absorb cholesterol and phospholipids from bile. This epithelial dysfunction eliminates the positive effect that the normal gallbladder exerts on cholesterol solubility in bile by Corradini et al. [255] The abnormalities of gallbladder epithelial function involved in cholesterol gallstone pathogenesis are (a) impaired biliary lipid absorption and (b) increased secretion of mucin gel.

Hypercholesterolemia As a Risk Factor for Gallstone Formation

Hypercholesterolemia is one of the risk factors for the formation of gallstone (Table 1). Several studies have shown the effect of a high-cholesterol diet in the formation of both cholesterol and pigment stones by Caroli-Bosc et al. [256] However, biliary supersaturation with cholesterol occurs frequently in healthy individuals by Holzbach et al. [257] suggesting that microcrystals can be flushed into the duodenum during normal postprandial gallbladder contraction. In patients with gallstones, pronucleating factors such as biliary glycoproteins and mucin by Jirsa et al [258] as well as impaired gallbladder motility [105] allow these microcrystals to be retained and eventually to grow into macroscopic gallstones. The lithogenicity of bile decreases following the administration of statins due to a reduction in the total low-density lipoprotein (LDL) cholesterol without affecting the bile acid synthesis as measured by the total bile acid excretion in feces by Hooger Brugge-vd Linden et al. [259] The effect of a high-cholesterol diet in the formation of pigment stones was documented by an in vivo experiment conducted by LaMorte et al.. [260] Guinea pigs fed with a high cholesterol diet formed calcium bilirubinate crystals. These animals also had a higher fasting gall bladder volume with an increase in the gall bladder dry mass without any documented biliary obstruction. Melatonin affects cholesterol homeostasis by reducing the intestinal absorption of cholesterol by Hussain et al. [261] Effects of melatonin on cholesterol metabolism were examined in rats with hypercholesterolemia secondary to high-fat diet and due to hypothyroidism. [262] Melatonin, when administered in doses of 12.5 mg/kg i.p., reduced total serum cholesterol concentration and total LDL cholesterol. It also induced an increased catabolism of cholesterol to bile acids as shown by a rise in fecal bile acid excretion. In rats with hypercholesterolemia secondary to hypothyroidism induced by 2-thiouracil, melatonin increased the high-density lipoprotein (HDL) to very low-density lipoprotein (VLDL) + LDL cholesterol ratio. Melatonin also augmented the hypocholesterolemic effect of statins by Hussain et al. [263] The beneficial effect of this indole includes a reduction in the serum total cholesterol, triglycerides, LDL, VLDL, and an increase in the HDL levels by Hussain, Al-Mahabashi and Isnail et al. [263-265] Long-term treatment with melatonin also modifies the fatty acid composition of plasma and liver lipids and reduces arterial fatty infiltration induced by cholesterol by Gomez-Pipilla et al. [266].

Decreased Gall Bladder Motility with Aging

The unexplained relation between increased incidence of gall bladder disease and aging was explored by Gomez- Pinilla et al. [266] In an in vitro study with isolated guinea pig gall bladder smooth muscle, they found that aging influences gall bladder smooth muscle, mainly by affecting membrane L-type and capacitative calcium entry (CCE) Ca^{2+} channels, which may contribute to the reduction in contractility in response to KCl, CCE, and cholecystokinin (CCK). CCK induces Ca^{2+} entry into L-type and CCE Ca^{2+} channels after releasing Ca^{2+} from intracellular stores. [267, 268] Aging also reduces neurogenic contractions, which are associated with the impairment of the nitrergic innervations and with an elevated responsiveness of capsaicin-sensitive relaxant nerves. There is general agreement that aging compromises gallbladder function as a result of changes in the inhibitory neuromodulation of smooth-muscle contractility and by reducing its myogenic response to contractile agonists. The reduced gall bladder motility is associated with an elevated incidence of cholesterol gall stones by van Erpecum, Portincassa, Xu and Chen et al. [92, 269-272] The studies by Gomez Pinilla and coworkers [266] showed that treatment of guinea pigs for 4 weeks with melatonin(2.5 mg/kg/day) induccd a total recovery of the contractile response to Ca^{2+} influx activation and electrical field stimulation; moreover, there was also a reversion of the age induced changes in efferent and sensory innervation as a result of melatonin administration. Treatment with melatonin increased the release of CCK in a dose-dependent manner by Jaworek et al. [273] The indolamine also reverses the age-mediate loss in the sensitivity of the gall bladder smooth muscle cells to CCK by increasing the F-actin content by Gomez-Pinilla et al. [266]. Uncommonly high physiological levels of melatonin are found in the gall bladder bile by Tan and Messner et al. [274, 275] In support of its action in the function of the gall bladder, the expression and the localization of MT1 melatonin receptors in the gallbladder epithelium has been defined using reverse transcription polymerase chain reaction (RT-PCR) by Aust et al. [276] Also, MT1 mRNA is present in gall bladder epithelial cells, during cholelithiasis, and in gall bladder cancer cells. The presence of a melatonin receptor in the gall bladder along with the known actions of melatonin as a free-radical scavenger and anti-inflammatory agent suggests the possibility that melatonin may have receptor-dependent and receptor-independent actions in this organ. Considering the exceptionally high concentration of melatonin in bile, the receptor-independent free-radical scavenging effect may far outweigh the receptor-mediated actions of melatonin in this organ by van Gall et al. [277] Gall bladder motility is impaired in many high-risk situations that precipitate gallstone formation; these situations include pregnancy, obesity, rapid weight loss in obese patients, diabetes mellitus, and total parenteral nutrition van Erpecum et al. [278] Other risk factors for gallstone formation are summarized.

Inflammation and Increase in Pronucleating Factors

Inflammatory changes in gall bladder mucosa are often associated with cholelithiasis. One of the mechanisms of hypercholesterolemia-induced cholelithiasis is the induction of inflammatory changes in gall bladder epithelium. [279] Inflammatory processes lead to the generation of reactive oxygen species (ROS) which influence cell function by Kourie et al. [280] The occurrence of inflammation in advance of the formation of gallstone/cholesterol monohydrate crystals has been reported in several publications by Lee and Scott et al. [281-283] The changes are characterized by acute inflammatory reactions (granulocyte infiltration, edema), mucus hypersecretion (increased number of apical granules), accumulation of mucus gel, glandular hyperplasia, and cell proliferation by Lee et al. [281] Increased gall bladder mucin is associated with the formation of gallstones of both the pigment and cholesterol variety by Scott, Lee, Burstein and Bouchier et al. [282, 284-286] In in vitro experiments, this increase in mucin production by gall bladder epithelial cells is cyclooxygenase (COX)-2-mediated by Kim et al. [287] Lipopolysaccharide (LPS) stimulation causes the expression of the COX-2 isoenzyme, the inducible form of COX, which initiates the synthesis of prostaglandin E2 (PGE2), leading to elevated mucin production Kim et al. [287] The mucin gel is the only biliary protein with a confirmed pathogenetic role in cholesterol gallstone disease. Gallbladder mucin has the ability to bind lipids and bile pigment. MUC2, MUC3, MUC4, MUC5B, and MUC5AC are the mucin genes expressed by normal gall bladder epithelial cells by van Klink and Lee et al. [288, 289] MUC5B is the prominent mucin MUC5AC and MUC5B, the most common gall bladder epithelial mucin, are secreted into bile. MUC5AC gene expression increases with inflammation of gall bladder epithelium and in the presence of pigment gallstones by Vilkin et al. (290) The expression of both MUC4 and MU5AC mRNA is increased in cholangiocarcinomas and in the dysplastic cells of stone-containing intrahepatic bile Ducts by Lee et al. [289] The mucin gel is thought to enhance gallstone formation by binding to biliary lipids and promoting cholesterol crystal precipitation and aggregation by Nunes et al. [291] The interaction between gall bladder mucin and calcium binding protein favors the formation of calcium phosphate pigment stones by Afdhal et al. [292] The hydrophobic binding sites in the polypeptide core of mucin may provide an optimal environment for nucleation of cholesterol monohydrate from supersaturated bile. The stimulus for gallbladder mucin hypersecretion appears to be a component of lithogenic bile. Prostaglandins regulate mucin release from gallbladder epithelium in vitro and probably in vivo. In the cholesterol-fed prairie dog, blockade of mucin release with aspirin inhibits gallstone formation by LaMont et al [293] since mucin release is mediated via the COX-2 pathway. In a randomized control study involving 55 patients with gallstones similar results were seen by Rhodes et al. [294] The subjects taking aspirin at a dose of 300 mg/day showed a significant reduction in the production of mucin by the gall bladder epithelium. Prostaglandins also decrease the motility of gall bladder and the cystic duct by affecting biliary smooth muscle by Chapman et al. [295]. This reduces gall bladder emptying, which predisposes to cholelithiasis. The role of mucin in cholecystitis is supported by changes in the mucin core proteins in the gall bladder epithelium with inflammation. The reactivity of MUC2 gene, which is absent in normal gall bladder, is significantly elevated in acute cholecystitis specimens by Ho et al. [296] Celecoxib, a selective COX-2 inhibitor, results in a reduction in gallstone formation by [279] This study assessed the degree of mucosal inflammation and the level of COX- 2 expression in the gall bladder mucosa of three groups of rabbits after feeding one of the groups with a high-cholesterol diet, a second with a high-cholesterol diet followed by Celecoxib administration while a control group was fed a normal diet. This study documented increased mucosal inflammation and COX-2 expression in rabbits fed with the high-cholesterol diet and a significant reduction in the animals given the high-cholesterol diet in combination with Celecoxib. The inflammatory stimulus caused enteric nitric oxide (NO) production (via iNOS), which in turn initiates PGE-2 generation (via COX-2); finally, PGE-2 acts as a powerful stimulus for an active secretomotor reflex in which vasoactive intestinal peptide (VIP) is used as a final mediator. VIP induces the elevated secretion of inflammatory fluid by Jansson et al. [297] The inhibitory effect exerted by melatonin in gallstone formation is due to its dual function as a COX-2 inhibitor and a free-radical scavenger by Shiesh et al. [266, 298] The anti-inflammatory activity of melatonin and its metabolites, N1-acetyl-N2- formyl-5-methoxykynuramine (AFMK) and N1-acetyl-5-methoxykynuramine (AMK), are secondary to the inhibition of COX-2 at the transcription level by Mayo and Wu et al. [299, 300] COX-2 (also called prostaglandin endoperoxide synthase- 2) is the essential enzyme in acute and chronic tissue inflammation; it has been implicated in several diseases, including cancer. COX-2 catalyzes the two sequential steps in the biosynthesis of PGs, which are important components in the regulation of vascular function under physiological conditions. Melatonin at 1 mM inhibits LPS or LPS/interferon (IFN)-c-induced COX-2 promoter activity by *50% by Wu et al. [300] The 50-flanking region of the genes for COX-2 and iNOS have several regulatory elements responsive to LPS and cytokines, among which the jB and CCAAT/enhancer binding protein (C/EBP) elements are essential for the activation of the promoter region of these genes by Xie, Lowenstein, Wadleigh and Herschman et al. [301-304] LPS upregulates binding of NF-jB and C/EBPb to thcsc two sitcs, respectively. There are five isoforms of NF-jB, three belonging to the Rel family (RelA, RelB, and C-Rel) and two to the NF-jB family (NF-jB1 or p50 and NF-jB2 or p52) by Dixit et al. [305] Melatonin selectively inhibits the binding of p52 to the NF-jB enhancer element, thereby suppressing LPS-induced iNOS and COX-2 expression by Wu et al. [300] p52 binding to the jB enhancer element is regulated by acetylation of p52 by p300 histone acetyl transferase (HAT). p300 overexpression also augments the LPS/IFNc-induced p52 binding both to COX-2 and iNOS promoter sites. Melatonin reduces p52 acetylation by inhibiting p300 (HAT) activity. [300] These studies suggest that melatonin inhibits COX-2 gene expression at the transcription level by reducing the acetylation and also the binding of p52 to its promoter region. Role of Free Radicals in Cholesterol and Pigment Stones Inflammation is followed by increased blood flow, which promotes lithogenic bile in cholesterol monohydrate crystals by Conter et al. [306] The mucosal inflammation, in part, involves its infiltration with phagocytes by Nash et al.,[307] which are associated with the generation of ROS. Further, free radicals indirectly favor cholesterol monohydrate crystal formation by stimulating mucus hypersecretion by Hale et al. (308) Lichtenberg et al. [309] argued that the increased concentrations of ROS makes bile increasingly more lithogenic. Nucleation time is the time (in days) to the first appearance of typical, rhomboid cholesterol monohydrate crystals in bile. [310] Eder et al. [311] conducted in vitro studies to measure the effect of ROS on the propensity of model bile to form cholesterol crystals and to define the mechanisms by which ROS may induce cholesterol crystal formation. The mechanism of toxicity by oxygen-derived free radicals is via peroxidation of phospholipids; these are major components of the cell membrane which cause cell death due to loss of cell wall integrity by Weiss et al. [312] Phospholipids are also major components of the bile required for cholesterol solubilization. Peroxidation of biliary phospholipids is, therefore, the likely mechanism of ROS-induced pronucleating activity. The in vitro study by Eder et al. [311] supports the hypothesis that an elevation in the peroxidation of phospholipids in the bile is caused by free radicals, as measured by malonaldehyde (MDA) levels, with elevated phospholipid peroxidation favoring shortening of nucleation time. The hydroxyl radical (•OH) is an extremely powerful oxidant that reacts with virtually all biological substrates. A notable characteristic of •OH is its ability to abstract hydrogen atoms from polyunsaturated fatty acids, which initiates lipid peroxidation. The Fenton reaction, which leads to the generation of •OH is, therefore, considered to be a prominent mechanism for the initiation of lipid peroxidation in biological systems. This is supported by evidence that the addition of the iron chelator, deferral, which binds free iron and prevents lipid peroxidation, was shown to inhibit •OH generation from H2O2. [311] Treatment with the iron chelator also proved extremely efficient in inhibiting both lipid peroxidation and cholesterol crystal formation in bile. Lipid peroxidation generates proinflammatory agents such as free fatty acids, lipid peroxides or aldehydes, including MDA and 4-hydroxynonenal (4-HNE). This is consistent with results which show that inflammation was enhanced by chemotactic agents and granulocyte stimulating activity [313] •OH stimulates the release of glucoproteins from gall bladder epithelium by Hale et al. [308] resulting in the promotion of cholesterol crystal formation. An in vivo study by Shiesh et al. [298] is based on the in vitro findings supporting the role of free radicals in lipid peroxidation and the induction of cholesterol stone formation. Koppisetti et al.'s study was aimed at finding the relation between oxidative stress and pigment gallstone formation and the role of melatonin as a free-radical scavenger in inhibiting both. Gallstone formation was induced by ligation of the common bile duct for 14 days in guinea pigs with (1 mg/kg daily) and without melatonin treatment. Oxidative stress was measured by the changes of MDA levels and total antioxidant activity in the biliary sludge in animals on days 7, 9, 12, and 14 after duct ligation. The sludge showed the presence of calcium bilirubinate, whose peak height per milligram gradually increased with time after ligation. The bile of ligated guinea pigs showed a reduction in the total antioxidant activity with an increase in pH, bile salts, and MDA when compared to sham-operated controls. In the melatonin- treated guinea pigs there was not only a significant reduction in the incidence of pigment gallstone formation but the level of the oxidative parameters were reduced to those in the control animals. These results confirmed previous observations and documented the inhibitory effect of melatonin on pigment stone formation. The protective action of melatonin was believed to be related to its antioxidant and anti-inflammatory actions. The effect of oxidative stress on gall bladder mucosa in the pathogenesis of gallstones was also studied by comparing the levels of lipid peroxides, lipid hydroperoxides (LPH), and conjugated dienes from the mucosal scrapings obtained from 30 patients with gallstones who underwent cholecystectomy. Antioxidant enzymes including catalase, superoxide dismutase, glutathione peroxidase, glutathione transferase, and glutathione reductase were assessed. The activity levels of functional enzymes alkaline phosphatase, adenosine triphosphatase, and protease were also estimated. The data document a significant increase in the levels of conjugated dienes, LPH, and oxidized lipid in gall bladder mucosa, with lower levels of glutathione and glutathione- related enzymes, catalase and superoxide dismutase, and a reduction in the activities of functional enzymes when compared with these values in the mucosa of gallstone-free gall bladders by Geetha et al. [314] Melatonin is a multifaceted free-radical scavenger. It detoxifies a variety of reactive oxygen and nitrogen species. The highly toxic •OH is scavenged by melatonin, resulting in the formation of cyclic 3-hydroxymelatonin and N-acetyl-N-formyl-5-methoxykynuramine by Haedeland et al. [315] One molecule of melatonin and its metabolites may have the capacity to scavenge up to ten free radicals and associated reactants. The antioxidant effects of melatonin are certainly in part related to its secondary and tertiary metabolites by Reiter et al. [316] The potential utility of melatonin in the treatment of enteric pathology due to its free-radical scavenging effect is well supported by previously published studies by Osturk, Bilici, Qi, Sener-Muratoglou, Sener, Bubenic and Contuk et al. [317-323]. Other Antioxidants Used The benefits of antioxidants in the treatment of gallstones has been observed in several investigations. The results of a pilot study by Worthington et al. [324] showed that an insufficiency of dietary antioxidants contributes to the formation of cholesterol gallstones. [324] Also, the administration of the antioxidants vitamins E and C reduces the concentration of unconjugated bilirubin along with calcium, resulting in the reduction of pigment gallstones by Lin and Vagner et al. [325, 326]. A study involving 157 patients with cholelithiasis and chronic liver disease documented a loss in catalase activity in liver and serum. In the presence of liver pathology, such as hepatic cirrhosis or chronic hepatitis, treatment with nonenzymatic antioxidants including ascorbic acid or alpha-tocopherol is suggested in order to compensate for the decrease in the naturally occurring protective antioxidant actions of the liver by Vagner et al. [326] The potency of melatonin as an antioxidant is at least ten times greater than that of vitamins C or E by Tan et al. [327]. A traditional Mexican medicine, Larrea tridentate (chaparral) is used in the treatment of gallstones; its efficacy was proven by the in vivo experiment with hamsters. The dry ethanolic extract of the leaves at a level of 0.5% of diet fed to the hamsters completely inhibited the formation of cholesterol gallstones by Arteaga et al. [328] Chaparral contains nordihydroguaiaretic acid, which makes it effective not only in treating cholesterol gallstones but also in repairing the free radical- induced damage caused by drugs such as amphetamine and cocaine. It also inhibits the enzyme lipoxygenase in the inflammatory pathway by Abou-Gazar et al. [329] Nevertheless, routine use of chaparral is controversial due to its hepatotoxicity by Arteaga et al. [328] Current Treatments for Cholelithiasis About 50–80% of gallstones are asymptomatic at some point. [254] Once symptomatic, the incidence of recurrence of the symptoms is 38–50% per year. [51] The most common treatment for symptomatic gallstones is cholecystectomy, although there are contraindications for this procedure. Nevertheless, the increased waiting period for elective cholecystectomy is associated with elevated risk for biliary colic and other complications by Lawrentzschek, Olson, Rutledfe and Salman et al. [330-333] Medical therapy is restricted to those with contraindications to surgery. The drugs ursodiol and chenodiol work best for small cholesterol stones. Months to years of treatment are necessary for the stones to dissolve. Both drugs cause mild diarrhea, and chenodiol is associated with a temporary rise in the levels of blood cholesterol and the liver enzyme transaminase [4]. Extracorporeal shockwave lithotripsy plus oral bile acids for symptomatic gallstones was introduced two decades ago. [78] However, subsequent studies proved the recurrence of gallstones in 30–50% of cases 5 years after bile salt therapy or lithotripsy. [80, 117]. The medical treatment alternatives to gall bladder surgery leave the organ intact; thus, stone recurrence is a major drawback. Incomplete emptying of the gall bladder is one of the important factors for the recurrence of gallstones. [334] Ursodeoxycholic acid (UDCA) is also used to alleviate biliary pain in patients waiting for elective cholecystectomy.

UDCA has been reported to reduce the risk of biliary colic by Bachrach et al [123-125, 335] by decreasing gall bladder motility. However, recent studies by Vennmann et al. [126] involving symptomatic patients with gallstones showed no beneficial effect of UDCA. Also, a 5% increase in the rate of complications was found among the symptomatic patients. These medical treatment options have remained more or less the same over time with cholecystectomy being the cornerstone of therapy by Thistle, Schoenfield, Anderson and Lee et al. [41, 336-340] Complications Acute cholecystitis is a major complication of cholesterol gallstones and is due to supersaturation of bile with cholesterol by Strasberg and Womack et al. [272, 341, 342] With the increased incorporation of cholesterol into the plasma membrane of the gall bladder muscle cells, the response to CCK and acetylcholine is impaired, resulting in reduced contraction of the gall bladder; this leads to an elevation in the concentration of the biliary contents and cholestasis. [94] The hydrophobic bile salts diffuse across the mucosa into the smooth-muscle layer and generate ROS, which damage the transmembrane receptors. [94] Increased cholesterol levels in the plasma membrane also impairs the cytoprotective effect exerted by PGE2 which the muscle cells use to protect themselves against injury from concentrated bile and free radicals by Xiao et al. [343] Cholestasis, one of the complications of cholelithiasis, is due to blockade to the outflow of bile due to gallstones. Not only does this lead to increased concentration of bile acids but also gastric and hepatic injury and systemic hypotension by Lane et al. [344] The increased concentrations of bile acids induce lipid peroxides due to the stimulation of phagocytic activity of polymorphonuclear leukocytes and inflammatory cells which are present after biliary tract obstruction by Canturk and Montilla et al. [345, 346] Protec [45-347] Administration of melatonin to rats at a dose of 500 *l*g/kg body weight daily beginning the first day after bile duct ligation resulted in a significant decrease in lipid peroxidation and free-radical-induced gastric ulceration by Polat et al. [347] The degree of hepatic injury following experimentally induced cholestasis by bile duct ligation was studied using a number of markers of hepatic injury. The parameters considered were the hepatic levels of thiobarbituric acid reactive substances as an index of lipid peroxidation, reduced glutathione (GSH) levels, and the activity of hepatic myeloperoxidase (MPO), an index of tissue neutrophil infiltration. These were found to be elevated in rats with bile duct ligation when compared with sham-operated controls. Melatonin administration in therapeutic doses showed a significant reduction in all of the measured parameters by Ohta et al. [348, 349] A comparative study between melatonin and alpha-tocopherol in alpha-naphthyl isothiocyanate- induced hepatotoxicity resulted in a more potent effect of melatonin in terms of antioxidant and anti-inflammatory activities by Ohta et al. (350) Other complications occur when gallstone disease is untreated. Chronic gallstone disease may lead to fibrosis, mucosal trauma, and loss of function of the gall bladder, which predisposes it to cancer by Vitetta et al. [351] The strong association between gallstones and the gall bladder cancer was observed among Chileans, where the risk of this disease is the highest worldwide by Nervi et al. [352] This was apparent by the increase in the incidence of gall bladder cancer in Chile during the 1970s and 1980s when the rate of cholecystectomy was reduced by Srerra et al. [353] The risk of gallbladder cancer is approximately 4–5 times higher in patients with gallstones than without gallstones, especially in susceptible populations such as the natives of South and North America and the Maori population of New Zealand by Lowenfels et al. [354] A retrospective analysis by Lam and coworkers [355] concluded an increase in gallbladder cancer presenting with acute cholecystitis to be higher when compared with the same finding in patients undergoing elective cholecystectomy for cholelithiasis. Not only can an untreated case of cholelithiasis present clinically with the recurrence of the same symptoms, leading to chronic cholecystitis, but it can also lead to a variety of other complications, the most common being acute cholecystitis, acute pancreatitis, ascending cholangitis, and gangrenous gallbladder by Abou-teif, [356] Less frequently Mirizzi syndrome, cholecystocholedochal fistula, choledocholithiasis, biliary-enteric fistulas, hydrops, limy bile or porcelain gallbladder occur by Tucker et al. [357] It can also lead to gallbladder empyema or a localized perforation of gallbladder with diffuse peritonitis. The perforation of intestinal wall by large stones leads to an occlusion of the gastrointestinal tract and results in a gallstone ileus by Losanof et al. [358] Concluding Remarks Gallstone disease is a common gastroenterological disease seen in the aging population. With an estimated 20% of the elderly population developing gallstones in the next 50 years by Prevention CFDC, [359] there is an urgent need to reduce the associated morbidity. With increasing age, biliary secretion and intestinal absorption of cholesterol increases. These are associated with a reduction in hepatic synthesis and biliary secretion of bile salts and reduction in gallbladder contractility, all of which increase susceptibility to cholesterol cholelithiasis by Wang et al. [272, 360] Although it is well established that pineal melatonin production decreases with age by Karasek et al., [361, 362] there is no specific information available regarding the changes in biliary or gastrointestinal melatonin. If gastrointestinal melatonin and specifically biliary concentrations are also reduced with age, the pathological conditions associated with aging of the hepatobiliary system in general and the gallbladder in particular would likely increase due to melatonin deficiency. The restoration of gallbladder contractility in response to melatonin treatment in aged guinea pigs is consistent with this hypothesis. [266] Though the exact sequence in the formation of gallstones is as yet unknown, considering the known actions of melatonin, there is a need for a thorough investigation of the role of this indole in the reduction of gallstone formation. Also, it would be important to examine changes in the biliary concentrations of melatonin with age. The prevalence of gall bladder disease is high in minority populations, e.g., in Native Americans and Hispanics due to the presence of the more predisposing factors. [363].

A study by Puppala et al. [364] revealed major susceptibility loci for gall bladder disease on chromosome 1p and other genetic locations, with evidence of linkage to symptomatic gallstone disease. The global rise in the incidence of gallstones is associated with a rise in the incidence of cholangiocarcinoma [351]. The prevention of gallstone formation can, hence, decrease the prevalence of unresectable gall bladder disease. The growing global epidemic of obesity and metabolic syndrome will increase the prevalence of gallstone disease worldwide. Melatonin and its metabolites are potent antioxidants by Man, Madonado Tan and Manda et al. [365-368] and anti-inflammatory agents by Cuzzufreas, Rodrigeuz and Nosal'ova et al. [369-371] Melatonin is available in pure form as an over-the-counter supplement. It has minimal acute or chronic side-effects and is inexpensive. Melatonin has been widely used by patients to successfully treat a variety of conditions including ulcerative colitis by Madonado., [365] sepsis in premature newborns by Gitto et al., [372] chronic respiratory infection by Gitto et al, [373, 374] functional dyspepsia by Klupinska et al., [375] free-radical responses associated with tooth removal by Cutando et al., [376] and many other clinical conditions. Its benefits in the prevention of gallstones is evidenced by studies in mouse and guinea pig models and human subjects. If prophylactically useful in the prevention of gallstone formation, as the data published to date indicate, it could have a significant beneficial effect for the aging population.

References

[1] Reshetnyak, V.I. 2012. Concept of the pathogenesis and treatment of cholelithiasis. *World J Hepatol* 4:18-34.

[2] Ahmed, M.H. 2010. Ezetimbe as potential treatment for cholesterol gallstones: the need for clinical trials. *World J Gastroenterol* 16:1555-1557.

[3] Zuniga, S., Molina, H., Azocar, L., Amigo, L., Nervi, F., Pimentel, F., Jarufe, N., Arrese, M., Lammert, F., and Miquel, J.F. 2008. Ezetimibe prevents cholesterol gallstone formation in mice. *Liver Int* 28:935-947.

[4] Wang, H.H., Portincasa, P., Mendez-Sanchez, N., Uribe, M., and Wang, D.Q. 2008. Effect of ezetimibe on the prevention and dissolution of cholesterol gallstones. *Gastroenterology* 134:2101-2110.

[5] Ko, C.W. 2008. Magnesium: does a mineral prevent gallstones? *Am J Gastroenterol* 103:383-385.

[6] Tsai, C.J., Leitzmann, M.F., Willett, W.C., and Giovannucci, E.L. 2008. Long-term effect of magnesium consumption on the risk of symptomatic gallstone disease among men. *Am J Gastroenterol* 103:375-382.

[7] Koppisetti, S., Jenigiri, B., Terron, M.P., Tengattini, S., Tamura, H., Flores, L.J., Tan, D.X., and Reiter, R.J. 2008. Reactive oxygen species and the hypomotility of the gall bladder as targets for the treatment of gallstones with melatonin: a review. *Dig Dis Sci* 53:2592-2603.

[8] Volzke, H., Baumeister, S.E., Alte, D., Hoffmann, W., Schwahn, C., Simon, P., John, U., and Lerch, M.M. 2005. Independent risk factors for gallstone formation in a region with high cholelithiasis prevalence. *Digestion* 71:97-105.

[9] Kharitonova, L. 2003. Cholelithiasis in children: issues of choice of therapeutic tactics. *Russkiy Meditsinskiy Zhurnal* 11:4.

[10] Portincasa, P., Ciaula, A.D., Bonfrate, L., and Wang, D.Q. 2012. Therapy of gallstone disease: What it was, what it is, what it will be. *World J Gastrointest Pharmacol Ther* 3:7-20.

[11] Portincasa, P., Moschetta, A., and Palasciano, G. 2006. Cholesterol gallstone disease. *Lancet* 368:230-239.

[12] Katsika, D., Grjibovski, A., Einarsson, C., Lammert, F., Lichtenstein, P., and Marschall, H.U. 2005. Genetic and environmental influences on symptomatic gallstone disease: a Swedish study of 43,141 twin pairs. *Hepatology* 41:1138-1143.

[13] Kratzer, W., Mason, R.A., and Kachele, V. 1999. Prevalence of gallstones in sonographic surveys worldwide. *J Clin Ultrasound* 27:1-7.

[14] Grundy, S.M., and Barnett, J.P. 1990. Metabolic and health complications of obesity. *Dis Mon* 36:641-731.

[15] Grundy, S.M., Cleeman, J.I., Daniels, S.R., Donato, K.A., Eckel, R.H., Franklin, B.A., Gordon, D.J., Krauss, R.M., Savage, P.J., Smith, S.C., Jr., et al. 2005. Diagnosis and management of the metabolic syndrome: an American Heart Association/National Heart, Lung, and Blood Institute Scientific Statement. *Circulation* 112:2735-2752.

[16] Grundy, S.M. 2005. Metabolic syndrome scientific statement by the American Heart Association and the National Heart, Lung, and Blood Institute. *Arterioscler Thromb Vasc Biol* 25:2243-2244.

[17] Eckel, R.H., Grundy, S.M., and Zimmet, P.Z. 2005. The metabolic syndrome. *Lancet* 365:1415-1428.

[18] Tsai, C.J., Leitzmann, M.F., Willett, W.C., and Giovannucci, E.L. 2004. Prospective study of abdominal adiposity and gallstone disease in US men. *Am J Clin Nutr* 80:38-44.

[19] Wang, D.Q., and Afdhal, N.H. 2004. Genetic analysis of cholesterol gallstone formation: searching for Lith (gallstone) genes. *Curr Gastroenterol Rep* 6:140-150.

[20] Everhart, J.E., Khare, M., Hill, M., and Maurer, K.R. 1999. Prevalence and ethnic differences in gallbladder disease in the United States. *Gastroenterology* 117:632-639.

[21] Sandler, R.S., Everhart, J.E., Donowitz, M., Adams, E., Cronin, K., Goodman, C., Gemmen, E., Shah, S., Avdic, A., and Rubin, R. 2002. The burden of selected digestive diseases in the United States. *Gastroenterology* 122:1500-1511.

[22] Diehl, A.K. 1991. Epidemiology and natural history of gallstone disease. *Gastroenterol Clin North Am* 20:1-19.

[23] Attili, A.F., Carulli, N., Roda, E., Barbara, B., Capocaccia, L., Menotti, A., Okoliksanyi, L., Ricci, G., Capocaccia, R., Festi, D., et al. 1995. Epidemiology of gallstone disease in Italy: prevalence data of the Multicenter Italian Study on Cholelithiasis (M.I.COL.). *Am J Epidemiol* 141:158-165.

[24] Attili, A.F., Capocaccia, R., Carulli, N., Festi, D., Roda, E., Barbara, L., Capocaccia, L., Menotti, A., Okolicsanyi, L., Ricci, G., et al. 1997. Factors associated with gallstone disease in the MICOL experience. Multicenter Italian Study on Epidemiology of Cholelithiasis. *Hepatology* 26:809-818.

[25] Portincasa, P., Di Ciaula, A., Wang, H.H., Moschetta, A., and Wang, D.Q. 2009. Medicinal treatments of cholesterol gallstones: old, current and new perspectives. *Curr Med Chem* 16:1531-1542.

[26] Theophrastus Bombastus, v.H. 1589. *Das Buch von den tartarischen Krankheiten nach dem alten Namen vom Stein/sand und Gries.* Basel:: Conrad Waldkirk. 5 pp.

[27] Portincasa, P. 1995. Gallbladder and bile in health and gallstone disease: The role of motility, gallstones and bile lipid composition. Utrecht: Utrecht University. Wang, H., Portincasa, P., and Wang, D. 2008. Molecular pathophysiology and physical chemistry of cholesterol gallstones. *Front Biosci* 13:23.

[28] Portincasa, P., Di Ciaula, A., Wang, H.H., Palasciano, G., van Erpecum, K.J., Moschetta, A., and Wang, D.Q. 2008. Coordinate regulation of gallbladder motor function in the gut-liver axis. *Hepatology* 47:2112-2126.

[29] Lammert, F., and Sauerbruch, T. 2005. Mechanisms of disease: the genetic epidemiology of gallbladder stones. *Nat Clin Pract Gastroenterol Hepatol* 2:423-433.

[30] Wang, D.Q., Zhang, L., and Wang, H.H. 2005. High cholesterol absorption efficiency and rapid biliary secretion of chylomicron remnant cholesterol enhance cholelithogenesis in gallstone-susceptible mice. *Biochim Biophys Acta* 1733:90-99.

[31] Portincasa, P., Moschetta, A., Puglisi, F., and Wang, D. 2008. *Medical treatment of gallstone disease*. Milano: Springer Italia S.r.l. 9 pp.

[32] Lammert, F., and Miquel, J.F. 2008. Gallstone disease: from genes to evidence-based therapy. *J Hepatol* 48 Suppl 1:S124-135.

[33] Sherlock, S., Dooley, J., and . 2002. *Diseases of the liver and biliary system.* Oxford: Blackwell Science.

[34] Portincasa, P., Moschetta, A., Petruzzelli, M., Palasciano, G., Di Ciaula, A., and Pezzolla, A. 2006. Gallstone disease: Symptoms and diagnosis of gallbladder stones. *Best Pract Res Clin Gastroenterol* 20:1017-1029.

[35] Ammon, H.V., and Hofmann, A.F. 1983. The Langenbuch paper. I. An historical perspective and comments of the translators. *Gastroenterology* 85:1426-1433.

[36] Langenbuch, C. 1882. Ein fall von exstirpation der gallenblase wegen chronischer cholelithiasis. *Heilung. Berlin Klin Wochenschr* 19:3.

[37] Schiff, M. 1873. Il coleinato di soda nella cura dei calcoli biliari. *L'Imparziale* 13:2.

[38] Dabney, W. 1876. The use of choleate of soda to prevent the formation of gallstones. *Am J Med Sci* 71.

[39] Rewbridge, A. 1937. The disappearance of gallstone shadows following the prolonged admnistration of bile acids. *Surgery* 1:6.

[40] Danzinger, R.G., Hofmann, A.F., Schoenfield, L.J., and Thistle, J.L. 1972. Dissolution of cholesterol gallstones by chenodeoxycholic acid. *N Engl J Med* 286:1-8.

[41] Hou, R., and Goldberg, A.C. 2009. Lowering low-density lipoprotein cholesterol: statins, ezetimibe, bile acid sequestrants, and combinations: comparative efficacy and safety. *Endocrinol Metab Clin North Am* 38:79-97.

[42] Istvan, E.S., and Deisenhofer, J. 2001. Structural mechanism for statin inhibition of HMG-CoA reductase. *Science* 292:1160-1164.

[43] Zhu, Y., Li, F., and Guo, G.L. 2011. Tissue-specific function of farnesoid X receptor in liver and intestine. *Pharmacol Res* 63:259-265.

[44] Hofmann, A.F., Amelsberg, A., and vanSonnenberg, E. 1993. Pathogenesis and treatment of gallstones. *N Engl J Med* 328:1854-1855.

[45] Tait, N., and Little, J.M. 1995. The treatment of gall stones. *BMJ* 311:99-105.

[46] Johnston, D.E., and Kaplan, M.M. 1993. Pathogenesis and treatment of gallstones. *N Engl J Med* 328:412-421.

[47] Gibney, E.J. 1990. Asymptomatic gallstones. *Br J Surg* 77:368-372.

[48] Jorgensen, T. 1989. Abdominal symptoms and gallstone disease: an epidemiological investigation. *Hepatology* 9:856-860.

[49] Festi, D., Sottili, S., Colecchia, A., Attili, A., Mazzella, G., Roda, E., and Romano, F. 1999. Clinical manifestations of gallstone disease: evidence from the multicenter Italian study on cholelithiasis (MICOL). *Hepatology* 30:839-846.

[50] Thistle, J.L., Cleary, P.A., Lachin, J.M., Tyor, M.P., and Hersh, T. 1984. The natural history of cholelithiasis: the National Cooperative Gallstone Study. *Ann Intern Med* 101:171-175.

[51] Friedman, G.D., Raviola, C.A., and Fireman, B. 1989. Prognosis of gallstones with mild or no symptoms: 25 years of follow-up in a health maintenance organization. *J Clin Epidemiol* 42:127-136.

[52] Gracie, W.A., and Ransohoff, D.F. 1982. The natural history of silent gallstones: the innocent gallstone is not a myth. *N Engl J Med* 307:798-800.

[53] Friedman, G.D. 1993. Natural history of asymptomatic and symptomatic gallstones. *Am J Surg* 165:399-404.

[54] Venneman, N.G., Renooij, W., Rehfeld, J.F., VanBerge-Henegouwen, G.P., Go, P.M., Broeders, I.A., and van Erpecum, K.J. 2005. Small gallstones, preserved gallbladder motility, and fast crystallization are associated with pancreatitis. *Hepatology* 41:738-746.

[55] Venneman, N.G., Buskens, E., Besselink, M.G., Stads, S., Go, P.M., Bosscha, K., van Berge-Henegouwen, G.P., and van Erpecum, K.J. 2005. Small gallstones are associated with increased risk of acute pancreatitis: potential benefits of prophylactic cholecystectomy? *Am J Gastroenterol* 100:2540-2550.

[56] Paumgartner, G., Carr-Locke, D., Dubois, F., Roda, E., and Thistle, J. 1993;. Strategies in the treatment of gallstone disease. Working team report. *Gastroenterol Int* 6::11.

[57] Brugge, W. 2000. *The silent gallstone*. New York: Marcel Dekker, Inc, . 8 pp.

[58] Keus, F., de Jong, J., Gooszen, H., van Laarhoven, C., Keus, F., and Jong., d. 2006. Small incision versus open cholecystectomy for patients with symptomatic cholecystolithiasis. In *Cochrane Database Syst Rev.*

[59] Keus, F., de Jong, J., Gooszen, H., and van Laarhoven, C. 2006. Laparoscopic versus open cholecystectomy for patients with symptomatic cholecystolithiasis. In *Cochrane Database Syst Rev.*

[60] Keus, F., de Jong, J., Gooszen, H., and van Laarhoven, C. 2006. Laparoscopic versus small-incision cholecystectomy for patients with symptomatic cholecystolithiasis. In *Cochrane Database Syst Rev.*

[61] Lammert, F., Neubrand, M.W., Bittner, R., Feussner, H., Greiner, L., Hagenmuller, F., Kiehne, K.H., Ludwig, K., Neuhaus, H., Paumgartner, G., et al. 2007. [S3-guidelines for diagnosis and treatment of gallstones. German Society for Digestive and Metabolic Diseases and German Society for Surgery of the Alimentary Tract]. *Z Gastroenterol* 45:971-1001.

[62] Giger, U.F., Michel, J.M., Opitz, I., Th Inderbitzin, D., Kocher, T., and Krahenbuhl, L. 2006. Risk factors for perioperative complications in patients undergoing laparoscopic cholecystectomy: analysis of 22,953 consecutive cases from the Swiss Association of Laparoscopic and Thoracoscopic Surgery database. *J Am Coll Surg* 203:723-728.

[63] Tuveri, M., and Tuveri, A. 2007. Laparoscopic cholecystectomy: complications and conversions with the 3-trocar technique: a 10-year review. *Surg Laparosc Endosc Percutan Tech* 17:380-384.

[64] Duca, S., Bala, O., Al-Hajjar, N., Lancu, C., Puia, I.C., Munteanu, D., and Graur, F. 2003. Laparoscopic cholecystectomy: incidents and complications. A retrospective analysis of 9542 consecutive laparoscopic operations. *HPB (Oxford)* 5:152-158.

[65] Pokorny, W.J., Saleem, M., O'Gorman, R.B., McGill, C.W., and Harberg, F.J. 1984. Cholelithiasis and cholecystitis in childhood. *Am J Surg* 148:742-744.

[66] Gumiero, A.P., Bellomo-Brandao, M.A., and Costa-Pinto, E.A. 2008. Gallstones in children with sickle cell disease followed up at a Brazilian hematology center. *Arq Gastroenterol* 45:313-318.

[67] Bogue, C.O., Murphy, A.J., Gerstle, J.T., Moineddin, R., and Daneman, A. 2010. Risk factors, complications, and outcomes of gallstones in children: a single-center review. *J Pediatr Gastroenterol Nutr* 50:303-308.

[68] Chan, S., Currie, J., Malik, A.I., and Mahomed, A.A. 2008. Paediatric cholecystectomy: Shifting goalposts in the laparoscopic era. *Surg Endosc* 22:1392-1395.

[69] Amaral, J.F., and Thompson, W.R. 1985. Gallbladder disease in the morbidly obese. *Am J Surg* 149:551-557.

[70] Sleisenger, M., 2006. *Gastrointestinal disease: pathophysiology, diagnosis, management.* Philadelphia: W.B. Saunders.

[71] 1988. The epidemiology of gallstone disease in Rome, Italy. Part II. Factors associated with the disease. The Rome Group for Epidemiology and Prevention of Cholelithiasis (GREPCO). *Hepatology* 8:907-913.

[72] Lowenfels, A.B., Lindstrom, C.G., Conway, M.J., and Hastings, P.R. 1985. Gallstones and risk of gallbladder cancer. *J Natl Cancer Inst* 75:77-80.

[73] Randi, G., Franceschi, S., and La Vecchia, C. 2006. Gallbladder cancer worldwide: geographical distribution and risk factors. *Int J Cancer* 118:1591-1602.

[74] Ashur, H., Siegal, B., Oland, Y., and Adam, Y.G. 1978. Calcified ballbladder (porcelain gallbladder). *Arch Surg* 113:594-596.

[75] Bonatsos, G., Birbas, K., Toutouzas, K., and Durakis, N. 2001. Laparoscopic cholecystectomy in adults with sickle cell disease. *Surg Endosc* 15:816-819.

[76] Thistle, J.L., May, G.R., Bender, C.E., Williams, H.J., LeRoy, A.J., Nelson, P.E., Peine, C.J., Petersen, B.T., and McCullough, J.E. 1989. Dissolution of cholesterol gallbladder stones by methyl tert-butyl ether administered by percutaneous transhepatic catheter. *N Engl J Med* 320:633-639.

[77] Sauerbruch, T., Delius, M., Paumgartner, G., Holl, J., Wess, O., Weber, W., Hepp, W., and Brendel, W. 1986. Fragmentation of gallstones by extracorporeal shock waves. *N Engl J Med* 314:818-822.

[78] Vergunst, H., Brakel, K., Nijs, H.G., Lameris, J.S., Ten Kate, F.J., Schroder, F.H., and Terpstra, O.T. 1994. Methyl tert-butyl ether improves the efficacy of extracorporeal shock wave lithotripsy of human gallstones implanted in pigs. *Eur J Surg* 160:619-625.

[79] Sackmann, M., Niller, H., Klueppelberg, U., von Ritter, C., Pauletzki, J., Holl, J., Berr, F., Neubrand, M., Sauerbruch, T., and Paumgartner, G. 1994. Gallstone recurrence after shock-wave therapy. *Gastroenterology* 106:225-230.

[80] Pauletzki, J., Holl, J., Sackmann, M., Neubrand, M., Klueppelberg, U., Sauerbruch, T., and Paumgartner, G. 1995. Gallstone recurrence after direct contact dissolution with methyl tert-butyl ether. *Dig Dis Sci* 40:1775-1781.

[81] Makino, I., Shinozaki, K., Yoshino, K., and Nakagawa, S. 1975. [Dissolution of cholesterol gallstones by long-term administration of ursodeoxycholic acid]. *Nihon Shokakibyo Gakkai Zassh* 72:13.

[82] van Erpecum, K.J., Portincasa, P., Stolk, M.F., van de Heijning, B.J., van der Zaag, E.S., van den Broek, A.M., van Berge Henegouwen, G.P., and Renooij, W. 1994. Effects of bile salt and phospholipid hydrophobicity on lithogenicity of human gallbladder bile. *Eur J Clin Invest* 24:744-750.

[83] Van Erpecum, K.J., Portincasa, P., Gadellaa, M., Van de Heijning, B.J., Van Berge Henegouwen, G.P., and Renooij, W. 1996. Effects of bile salt hydrophobicity on crystallization of cholesterol in model bile. *Eur J Clin Invest* 26:602-608.

[84] Portincasa, P., van Erpecum, K.J., Jansen, A., Renooij, W., Gadellaa, M., and vanBerge-Henegouwen, G.P. 1996. Behavior of various cholesterol crystals in bile from patients with gallstones. *Hepatology* 23:738-748.

[85] Wang, D.Q., and Carey, M.C. 1996. Complete mapping of crystallization pathways during cholesterol precipitation from model bile: influence of physical-chemical variables of pathophysiologic relevance and identification of a stable liquid crystalline state in cold, dilute and hydrophilic bile salt-containing systems. *J Lipid Res* 37:606-630.

[86] Kupfer, R.M., Maudgal, D.P., and Northfield, T.C. 1982. Gallstone dissolution rate during chenic acid therapy. Effect of bedtime administration plus low cholesterol diet. *Dig Dis Sci* 27:1025-1029.

[87] Lanzini, A., Facchinetti, D., and Northfield, T.C. 1988. Maintenance of hepatic bile acid secretion rate during overnight fasting by bedtime bile acid administration. *Gastroenterology* 95:1029-1035.

[88] Hardison, W.G., and Grundy, S.M. 1984. Effect of ursodeoxycholate and its taurine conjugate on bile acid synthesis and cholesterol absorption. *Gastroenterology* 87:130-135.

[89] Uchida, K., Akiyoshi, T., Igimi, H., Takase, H., Nomura, Y., and Ishihara, S. 1991. Differential effects of ursodeoxycholic acid and ursocholic acid on the formation of biliary cholesterol crystals in mice. *Lipids* 26:526-530.

[90] Wang, D.Q., Tazuma, S., Cohen, D.E., and Carey, M.C. 2003. Feeding natural hydrophilic bile acids inhibits intestinal cholesterol absorption: studies in the gallstone-susceptible mouse. *Am J Physiol Gastrointest Liver Physiol* 285:G494-502.

[91] van de Heijning, B.J., van de Meeberg, P.C., Portincasa, P., Doornewaard, H., Hoebers, F.J., van Erpecum, K.J., and Vanberge-Henegouwen, G.P. 1999. Effects of ursodeoxycholic acid therapy on in vitro gallbladder contractility in patients with cholesterol gallstones. *Dig Dis Sci* 44:190-196.

[92] Guarino, M.P., Cong, P., Cicala, M., Alloni, R., Carotti, S., and Behar, J. 2007. Ursodeoxycholic acid improves muscle contractility and inflammation in symptomatic gallbladders with cholesterol gallstones. *Gut* 56:815-820.

[93] Xiao, Z.L., Rho, A.K., Biancani, P., and Behar, J. 2002. Effects of bile acids on the muscle functions of guinea pig gallbladder. *Am J Physiol Gastrointest Liver Physiol* 283:G87-94.

[94] Stolk, M.F., Van de Heijning, B.J., Van Erpecum, K.J., Verheem, A., Akkermans, L.M., and Van Berge-Henegouwen, G.P. 1996. Effect of bile salts on in vitro gallbladder motility: preliminary study. *Ital J Gastroenterol* 28:105-110.

[95] Paumgartner, G., Pauletzki, J., and Sackmann, M.e.o. 1994. Ursodeoxycholic acid treatment of cholesterol gallstone diseas. *Scand J Gastroenter* Suppl ; 204:5.

[96] Leopold, G.R., Amberg, J., Gosink, B.B., and Mittelstaedt, C. 1976. Gray scale ultrasonic cholecystography: a comparison with conventional radiographic techniques. *Radiology* 121:445-448.

[97] Portincasa, P., Di Ciaula, A., Palmieri, V., Vendemiale, G., Altomare, E., and Palasciano, G. 1994. Sonographic evaluation of gallstone burden in humans. *Ital J Gastroenterol* 26:141-144.

[98] Everson, G.T., Braverman, D.Z., Johnson, M.L., and Kern, F., Jr. 1980. A critical evaluation of real-time ultrasonography for the study of gallbladder volume and contraction. *Gastroenterology* 79:40-46.

[99] Portincasa, P., Moschetta, A., Colecchia, A., Festi, D., and Palasciano, G. 2003. Measurements of gallbladder motor function by ultrasonography: towards standardization. *Dig Liver Dis* 35 Suppl 3:S56-61.

[100] Pauletzki, J., Althaus, R., Holl, J., Sackmann, M., and Paumgartner, G. 1996. Gallbladder emptying and gallstone formation: a prospective study on gallstone recurrence. *Gastroenterology* 111:765-771.

[101] Portincasa, P., van Erpecum, K.J., van De Meeberg, P.C., Dallinga-Thie, G.M., de Bruin, T.W., and van Berge-Henegouwen, G.P. 1996. Apolipoprotein E4 genotype and gallbladder motility influence speed of gallstone clearance and risk of recurrence after extracorporeal shock-wave lithotripsy. *Hepatology* 24:580-587.

[102] Venneman, N.G., vanBerge-Henegouwen, G.P., Portincasa, P., Stolk, M.F., Vos, A., Plaisier, P.W., and van Erpecum, K.J. 2001. Absence of apolipoprotein E4 genotype, good gallbladder motility and presence of solitary stones delay rather than prevent gallstone recurrence after extracorporeal shock wave lithotripsy. *J Hepatol* 35:10-16.

[103] Festi, D., Frabboni, R., Bazzoli, F., Sangermano, A., Ronchi, M., Rossi, L., Parini, P., Orsini, M., Primerano, A.M., Mazzella, G., et al. 1990. Gallbladder motility in cholesterol gallstone disease. Effect of ursodeoxycholic acid administration and gallstone dissolution. *Gastroenterology* 99:1779-1785.

[104] Portincasa, P., Di Ciaula, A., Baldassarre, G., Palmieri, V., Gentile, A., Cimmino, A., and Palasciano, G. 1994. Gallbladder motor function in gallstone patients: sonographic and in vitro studies on the role of gallstones, smooth muscle function and gallbladder wall inflammation. *J Hepatol* 21:430-440.

[105] Pereira, S.P., Veysey, M.J., Kennedy, C., Hussaini, S.H., Murphy, G.M., and Dowling, R.H. 1997. Gallstone dissolution with oral bile acid therapy. Importance of pretreatment CT scanning and reasons for nonresponse. *Dig Dis Sci* 42:1775-1782.

[106] Pereira, S.P., Hussaini, S.H., Kennedy, C., and Dowling, R.H. 1995. Gallbladder stone recurrence after medical treatment. Do gallstones recur true to type? *Dig Dis Sci* 40:2568-2575.

[107] Hussaini, S.H., Pereira, S.P., Murphy, G.M., Kennedy, C., Wass, J.A., Besser, G.M., and Dowling, R.H. 1995. Composition of gall bladder stones associated with octreotide: response to oral ursodeoxycholic acid. *Gut* 36:126-132.

[108] Sackmann, M., Eder, H., Spengler, U., Pauletzki, J., Holl, J., Paumgartner, G., and Sauerbruch, T. 1993. Gallbladder emptying is an important factor in fragment disappearance after shock wave lithotripsy. *J Hepatol* 17:62-66.

[109] Senior, J.R., Johnson, M.F., DeTurck, D.M., Bazzoli, F., and Roda, E. 1990. In vivo kinetics of radiolucent gallstone dissolution by oral dihydroxy bile acids. *Gastroenterology* 99:243-251.

[110] Jazrawi, R.P., Pigozzi, M.G., Galatola, G., Lanzini, A., and Northfield, T.C. 1992. Optimum bile acid treatment for rapid gall stone dissolution. *Gut* 33:381-386.

[111] Paumgartner, G. 1996. *Therapeutic options and choice of appropriate treatment.* Dordrecht: Kluwer Academic Publishers. 6 pp.

[112] Lanzini, A., Jazrawi, R.P., Kupfer, R.M., Maudgal, D.P., Joseph, A.E., and Northfield, T.C. 1986. Gallstone recurrence after medical dissolution. An overestimated threat? *J Hepatol* 3:241-246.

[113] Rabenstein, T., Radespiel-Troger, M., Hopfner, L., Benninger, J., Farnbacher, M., Greess, H., Lenz, M., Hahn, E.G., and Schneider, H.T. 2005. Ten years experience with piezoelectric extracorporeal shockwave lithotripsy of gallbladder stones. *Eur J Gastroenterol Hepatol* 17:629-639.

[114] Bateson, M., Bouchier, I., Trash, D., Maudgal, D., and Northfield, T. 1981. Calcification of radiolucent gall stone during treatment with ursodeoxycholic acid. *Br Med J (Clin Res Ed)* 283:2.

[115] Sackmann, M., Ippisch, E., Sauerbruch, T., Holl, J., Brendel, W., and Paumgartner, G. 1990. Early gallstone recurrence rate after successful shock-wave therapy. *Gastroenterology* 98:392-396.

[116] Villanova, N., Bazzoli, F., Taroni, F., Frabboni, R., Mazzella, G., Festi, D., Barbara, L., and Roda, E. 1989. Gallstone recurrence after successful oral bile acid treatment. A 12-year follow-up study and evaluation of long-term postdissolution treatment. *Gastroenterology* 97:726-731.

[117] Petroni, M.L., Jazrawi, R.P., Pazzi, P., Zuin, M., Lanzini, A., Fracchia, M., Facchinetti, D., Alvisi, V., Ferraris, R., Bland, J.M., et al. 2000. Risk factors for the development of gallstone recurrence following medical dissolution. The British-Italian Gallstone Study Group. *Eur J Gastroenterol Hepatol* 12:695-700.

[118] Petroni, M.L., Jazrawi, R.P., Lanzini, A., Zuin, M., Pazzi, P., Fracchia, M., Boga, E., Facchinetti, D., Alvisi, V., Galatola, G., et al. 1996. Repeated bile acid therapy for the long-term management of cholesterol gallstones. *J Hepatol* 25:719-724.

[119] O'Leary, D.P., and Johnson, A.G. 1993. Future directions for conservative treatment of gallbladder calculi. *Br J Surg* 80:143-147.

[120] Gilat, T., and Konikoff, F. 2000. Pregnancy and the biliary tract. *Can J Gastroenterol* 14 Suppl D:55D-59D.

[121] Sugerman, H.J., Brewer, W.H., Shiffman, M.L., Brolin, R.E., Fobi, M.A., Linner, J.H., MacDonald, K.G., MacGregor, A.M., Martin, L.F., Oram-Smith, J.C., et al. 1995. A multicenter, placebo-controlled, randomized, double-blind, prospective trial of prophylactic ursodiol for the prevention of gallstone formation following gastric-bypass-induced rapid weight loss. *Am J Surg* 169:91-96; discussion 96-97.

[122] Tint, G.S., Salen, G., Colalillo, A., Graber, D., Verga, D., Speck, J., and Shefer, S. 1982. Ursodeoxycholic acid: a safe and effective agent for dissolving cholesterol gallstones. *Ann Intern Med* 97:351-356.

[123] Meredith, T.J., Williams, G.V., Maton, P.N., Murphy, G.M., Saxton, H.M., and Dowling, R.H. 1982. Retrospective comparison of 'Cheno' and 'Urso' in the medical treatment of gallstones. *Gut* 23:382-389.

[124] Tomida, S., Abei, M., Yamaguchi, T., Matsuzaki, Y., Shoda, J., Tanaka, N., and Osuga, T. 1999. Long-term ursodeoxycholic acid therapy is associated with reduced risk of biliary pain and acute cholecystitis in patients with gallbladder stones: a cohort analysis. *Hepatology* 30:6-13.

[125] Venneman, N.G., Besselink, M.G., Keulemans, Y.C., Vanberge-Henegouwen, G.P., Boermeester, M.A., Broeders, I.A., Go, P.M., and van Erpecum, K.J. 2006. Ursodeoxycholic acid exerts no beneficial effect in patients with symptomatic gallstones awaiting cholecystectomy. *Hepatology* 43:1276-1283.

[126] Kallien, G., Lange, K., Stange, E.F., and Scheibner, J. 1999. The pravastatin-induced decrease of biliary cholesterol secretion is not directly related to an inhibition of cholesterol synthesis in humans. *Hepatology* 30:14-20.

[127] Duane, W.C., Hunninghake, D.B., Freeman, M.L., Pooler, P.A., Schlasner, L.A., and Gebhard, R.L. 1988. Simvastatin, a competitive inhibitor of HMG-CoA reductase, lowers cholesterol saturation index of gallbladder bile. *Hepatology* 8:1147-1150.

[128] Loria, P., Bertolotti, M., Cassinadri, M.T., Dilengite, M.A., Bozzoli, M., Carubbi, F., Concari, M., Guicciardi, M.E., and Carulli, N. 1994. Short-term effects of simvastatin on bile acid synthesis and bile lipid secretion in human subjects. *Hepatology* 19:882-888.

[129] Hanson, D.S., and Duane, W.C. 1994. Effects of lovastatin and chenodiol on bile acid synthesis, bile lipid composition, and biliary lipid secretion in healthy human subjects. *J Lipid Res* 35:1462-1468.

[130] Saunders, K.D., Cates, J.A., Abedin, M.Z., and Roslyn, J.J. 1993. Lovastatin and gallstone dissolution: a preliminary study. *Surgery* 113:28-35.

[131] Smit, J.W., Van Erpecum, K.J., Portincasa, P., Renooij, W., Erkelens, D.W., and Van Berge-Henegouwen, G.P. 1995. Effects of simvastatin and cholestyramine on bile lipid composition and gall bladder motility in patients with hypercholesterolaemia. *Gut* 37:654-659.

[132] Tazuma, S., Hatsushika, S., Aihara, N., Sagawa, H., Yamashita, G., Sasaki, M., Sasaki, H., Mizuno, S., Tao, S., and Kajiyama, G. 1992. Inhibitory effects of pravastatin, a competitive inhibitor of hydroxymethylglutaryl coenzyme A reductase, on cholesterol gallstone formation in prairie dogs. *Digestion* 51:179-184.

[133] Abedin, M.Z., Narins, S.C., Park, E.H., Smith, P.R., and Kirkwood, K.S. 2002. Lovastatin alters biliary lipid composition and dissolves gallstones: a long-term study in prairie dogs. *Dig Dis Sci* 47:2192-2210.

[134] Davis, K.G., Wertin, T.M., and Schriver, J.P. 2003. The use of simvastatin for the prevention of gallstones in the lithogenic prairie dog model. *Obes Surg* 13:865-868.

[135] Tsai, C.J., Leitzmann, M.F., Willett, W.C., and Giovannucci, E.L. 2009. Statin use and the risk of cholecystectomy in women. *Gastroenterology* 136:1593-1600.

[136] Bodmer, M., Brauchli, Y.B., Krahenbuhl, S., Jick, S.S., and Meier, C.R. 2009. Statin use and risk of gallstone disease followed by cholecystectomy. *JAMA* 302:2001-2007.

[137] Erichsen, R., Froslev, T., Lash, T.L., Pedersen, L., and Sorensen, H.T. 2011. Long-term statin use and the risk of gallstone disease: A population-based case-control study. *Am J Epidemiol* 173:162-170.

[138] Chapman, B.A., Burt, M.J., Chisholm, R.J., Allan, R.B., Yeo, K.H., and Ross, A.G. 1998. Dissolution of gallstones with simvastatin, an HMG CoA reductase inhibitor. *Dig Dis Sci* 43:349-353.

[139] Porsch-Ozcurumez, M., Hardt, P.D., Schnell-Kretschmer, H., von Bergmann, K., Darui, C., Nonhoff, J., Abletshauser, C., and Klor, H.U. 2001. Effects of fluvastatin on biliary lipids in subjects with an elevated cholesterol saturation index. *Eur J Clin Pharmacol* 56:873-879.

[140] Smith, J.L., Roach, P.D., Wittenberg, L.N., Riottot, M., Pillay, S.P., Nestel, P.J., and Nathanson, L.K. 2000. Effects of simvastatin on hepatic cholesterol metabolism, bile lithogenicity and bile acid hydrophobicity in patients with gallstones. *J Gastroenterol Hepatol* 15:871-879.

[141] Wilson, I.R., Hurrell, M.A., Pattinson, N.R., and Chapman, B.A. 1994. The effect of simvastatin and bezafibrate on bile composition and gall-bladder emptying in female non-insulin-dependent diabetics. *J Gastroenterol Hepatol* 9:447-451.

[142] Smit, J.W., van Erpecum, K.J., Renooij, W., Stolk, M.F., Edgar, P., Doornewaard, H., and Vanberge-Henegouwen, G.P. 1995. The effects of the 3-hydroxy, 3-methylglutaryl coenzyme A reductase inhibitor pravastatin on bile composition and nucleation of cholesterol crystals in cholesterol gallstone disease. *Hepatology* 21:1523-1529.

[143] Miettinen, T.E., Kiviluoto, T., Taavitsainen, M., Vuoristo, M., and Miettinen, T.A. 1998. Cholesterol metabolism and serum and biliary noncholesterol sterols in gallstone patients during simvastatin and ursodeoxycholic acid treatments. *Hepatology* 27:649-655.

[144] Sharma, B.C., Agarwal, D.K., Baijal, S.S., and Saraswat, V.A. 1997. Pravastatin has no effect on bile lipid composition, nucleation time, and gallbladder motility in persons with normal levels of cholesterol. *J Clin Gastroenterol* 25:433-436.

[145] Caroli-Bosc, F.X., Le Gall, P., Pugliese, P., Delabre, B., Caroli-Bosc, C., Demarquay, J.F., Delmont, J.P., Rampal, P., and Montet, J.C. 2001. Role of fibrates and HMG-CoA reductase inhibitors in gallstone formation: epidemiological study in an unselected population. *Dig Dis Sci* 46:540-544.

[146] Gonzalez-Perez, A., and Garcia Rodriguez, L.A. 2007. Gallbladder disease in the general population: association with cardiovascular morbidity and therapy. *Pharmacoepidemiol Drug Saf* 16:524-531.

[147] Wang, D.Q. 2007. Regulation of intestinal cholesterol absorption. *Annu Rev Physiol* 69:221-248.

[148] Davis, H.R., and Veltri, E.P. 2007. Zetia: inhibition of Niemann-Pick C1 Like 1 (NPC1L1) to reduce intestinal cholesterol absorption and treat hyperlipidemia. *J Atheroscler Thromb* 14:99-108.

[149] Ge, L., Wang, J., Qi, W., Miao, H.H., Cao, J., Qu, Y.X., Li, B.L., and Song, B.L. 2008. The cholesterol absorption inhibitor ezetimibe acts by blocking the sterol-induced internalization of NPC1L1. *Cell Metab* 7:508-519.

[150] Davis, H.R., Jr., Zhu, L.J., Hoos, L.M., Tetzloff, G., Maguire, M., Liu, J., Yao, X., Iyer, S.P., Lam, M.H., Lund, E.G., et al. 2004. Niemann-Pick C1 Like 1 (NPC1L1) is the intestinal phytosterol and cholesterol transporter and a key modulator of whole-body cholesterol homeostasis. *J Biol Chem* 279:33586-33592.

[151] Altmann, S.W., Davis, H.R., Jr., Zhu, L.J., Yao, X., Hoos, L.M., Tetzloff, G., Iyer, S.P., Maguire, M., Golovko, A., Zeng, M., et al. 2004. Niemann-Pick C1 Like 1 protein is critical for intestinal cholesterol absorption. *Science* 303:1201-1204.

[152] Davies, J.P., Scott, C., Oishi, K., Liapis, A., and Ioannou, Y.A. 2005. Inactivation of NPC1L1 causes multiple lipid transport defects and protects against diet-induced hypercholesterolemia. *J Biol Chem* 280:12710-12720.

[153] Wang, H.H., and Wang, D.Q. 2005. Reduced susceptibility to cholesterol gallstone formation in mice that do not produce apolipoprotein B48 in the intestine. *Hepatology* 42:894-904.

[154] Di Ciaula, A., Wang, D.Q., Wang, H.H., Bonfrate, L., and Portincasa, P. 2010. Targets for current pharmacologic therapy in cholesterol gallstone disease. *Gastroenterol Clin North Am* 39:245-264, viii-ix.

[155] Mangelsdorf, D.J., Thummel, C., Beato, M., Herrlich, P., Schutz, G., Umesono, K., Blumberg, B., Kastner, P., Mark, M., Chambon, P., et al. 1995. The nuclear receptor superfamily: the second decade. *Cell* 83:835-839.

[156] Janowski, B.A., Willy, P.J., Devi, T.R., Falck, J.R., and Mangelsdorf, D.J. 1996. An oxysterol signalling pathway mediated by the nuclear receptor LXR alpha. *Nature* 383:728-731.

[157] Parks, D.J., Blanchard, S.G., Bledsoe, R.K., Chandra, G., Consler, T.G., Kliewer, S.A., Stimmel, J.B., Willson, T.M., Zavacki, A.M., Moore, D.D., et al. 1999. Bile acids: natural ligands for an orphan nuclear receptor. *Science* 284:1365-1368.

[158] Makishima, M., Okamoto, A.Y., Repa, J.J., Tu, H., Learned, R.M., Luk, A., Hull, M.V., Lustig, K.D., Mangelsdorf, D.J., and Shan, B. 1999. Identification of a nuclear receptor for bile acids. *Science* 284:1362-1365.

[159] Repa, J.J., and Mangelsdorf, D.J. 2002. The liver X receptor gene team: potential new players in atherosclerosis. *Nat Med* 8:1243-1248.

[160] Kalaany, N.Y., and Mangelsdorf, D.J. 2006. LXRS and FXR: the yin and yang of cholesterol and fat metabolism. *Annu Rev Physiol* 68:159-191.

[161] Modica, S., Murzilli, S., Salvatore, L., Schmidt, D.R., and Moschetta, A. 2008. Nuclear bile acid receptor FXR protects against intestinal tumorigenesis. *Cancer Res* 68:9589-9594.

[162] Moschetta, A., Bookout, A.L., and Mangelsdorf, D.J. 2004. Prevention of cholesterol gallstone disease by FXR agonists in a mouse model. *Nat Med* 10:1352-1358.

[163] Liu, Y., Binz, J., Numerick, M.J., Dennis, S., Luo, G., Desai, B., MacKenzie, K.I., Mansfield, T.A., Kliewer, S.A., Goodwin, B., et al. 2003. Hepatoprotection by the farnesoid X receptor agonist GW4064 in rat models of intra- and extrahepatic cholestasis. *J Clin Invest* 112:1678-1687.

[164] Uppal, H., Zhai, Y., Gangopadhyay, A., Khadem, S., Ren, S., Moser, J.A., and Xie, W. 2008. Activation of liver X receptor sensitizes mice to gallbladder cholesterol crystallization. *Hepatology* 47:1331-1342.

[165] Turley, S.D., and Dietschy, J.M. 1981. The contribution of newly synthesized cholesterol to biliary cholesterol in the rat. *J Biol Chem* 256:2438-2446.

[166] Wang, H.H., Afdhal, N.H., and Wang, D.Q. 2006. Overexpression of estrogen receptor alpha increases hepatic cholesterogenesis, leading to biliary hypersecretion in mice. *J Lipid Res* 47:778-786.

[167] Mendez-Sanchez, N., Zamora-Valdes, D., Chavez-Tapia, N.C., and Uribe, M. 2007. Role of diet in cholesterol gallstone formation. *Clin Chim Acta* 376:1-8.

[168] Zhu, X., Zhang, S., and Huang, Z. 1995. The trend of the gallstone disease in China over the past decade. *Zhonghua Wai Ke Za Zhi* 33:7.

[169] Huang, Y., Zhang, X., and Yang, R. 1984. Changes in cholelithiasis in Tianjin in the past 30 years. *Chin Med J* 97:3.

[170] 1987. [Characteristic features of cholelithiasis in China. A nationwide survey of 11342 surgical cases 1983-1985]. *Zhonghua Wai Ke Za Zhi* 25:321-329, 380.

[171] Nagase, M., Tanimura, H., Setoyama, M., and Hikasa, Y. 1978. Present features of gallstones in Japan. A collective review of 2,144 cases. *Am J Surg* 135:788-790.

[172] Nakayama, F., and Miyake, H. 1970. Changing state of gallstone disease in Japan. Composition of the stones and treatment of the condition. *Am J Surg* 120:794-799.

[173] Carey, M.C. 1978. Critical tables for calculating the cholesterol saturation of native bile. *J Lipid Res* 19:945-955.

[174] Wang, D.Q., Paigen, B., and Carey, M.C. 1997. Phenotypic characterization of Lith genes that determine susceptibility to cholesterol cholelithiasis in inbred mice: physical-chemistry of gallbladder bile. *J Lipid Res* 38:1395-1411.

[175] Wang, D.Q., Lammert, F., Paigen, B., and Carey, M.C. 1999. Phenotypic characterization of lith genes that determine susceptibility to cholesterol cholelithiasis in inbred mice. Pathophysiology Of biliary lipid secretion. *J Lipid Res* 40:2066-2079.

[176] Wang, D.Q., and Carey, M.C. 2003. Measurement of intestinal cholesterol absorption by plasma and fecal dual-isotope ratio, mass balance, and lymph fistula methods in the mouse: an analysis of direct versus indirect methodologies. *J Lipid Res* 44:1042-1059.

[177] Duan, L.P., Wang, H.H., and Wang, D.Q. 2004. Cholesterol absorption is mainly regulated by the jejunal and ileal ATP-binding cassette sterol efflux transporters Abcg5 and Abcg8 in mice. *J Lipid Res* 45:1312-1323.

[178] Wang, H.H., Afdhal, N.H., Gendler, S.J., and Wang, D.Q. 2006. Evidence that gallbladder epithelial mucin enhances cholesterol cholelithogenesis in MUC1 transgenic mice. *Gastroenterology* 131:210-222.

[179] Wang, D.Q., Lammert, F., Cohen, D.E., Paigen, B., and Carey, M.C. 1999. Cholic acid aids absorption, biliary secretion, and phase transitions of cholesterol in murine cholelithogenesis. *Am J Physiol* 276:G751-760.

[180] Buhman, K.K., Accad, M., Novak, S., Choi, R.S., Wong, J.S., Hamilton, R.L., Turley, S., and Farese, R.V., Jr. 2000. Resistance to diet-induced hypercholesterolemia and gallstone formation in ACAT2-deficient mice. *Nat Med* 6:1341-1347.

[181] Amigo, L., Quinones, V., Mardones, P., Zanlungo, S., Miquel, J.F., Nervi, F., and Rigotti, A. 2000. Impaired biliary cholesterol secretion and decreased gallstone formation in apolipoprotein E-deficient mice fed a high-cholesterol diet. *Gastroenterology* 118:772-779.

[182] Davis, H.R., Jr., Compton, D.S., Hoos, L., and Tetzloff, G. 2001. Ezetimibe, a potent cholesterol absorption inhibitor, inhibits the development of atherosclerosis in ApoE knockout mice. *Arterioscler Thromb Vasc Biol* 21:2032-2038.

[183] Portincasa, P., Di Ciaula, A., and vanBerge-Henegouwen, G.P. 2004. Smooth muscle function and dysfunction in gallbladder disease. *Curr Gastroenterol Rep* 6:151-162.

[184] van Erpecum, K.J., Wang, D.Q., Moschetta, A., Ferri, D., Svelto, M., Portincasa, P., Hendrickx, J.J., Schipper, M., and Calamita, G. 2006. Gallbladder histopathology

during murine gallstone formation: relation to motility and concentrating function. *J Lipid Res* 47:32-41.

[185] Mathur, A., Walker, J.J., Al-Azzawi, H.H., Lu, D., Swartz-Basile, D.A., Nakeeb, A., and Pitt, H.A. 2007. Ezetimibe ameliorates cholecystosteatosis. *Surgery* 142:228-233.

[186] 1980. Efficacy and indications of ursodeoxycholic acid treatment for dissolving gallstones. A multicenter double-blind trial. Tokyo Cooperative Gallstone Study Group. *Gastroenterology* 78:542-548.

[187] Temel, R.E., Tang, W., Ma, Y., Rudel, L.L., Willingham, M.C., Ioannou, Y.A., Davies, J.P., Nilsson, L.M., and Yu, L. 2007. Hepatic Niemann-Pick C1-like 1 regulates biliary cholesterol concentration and is a target of ezetimibe. *J Clin Invest* 117:1968-1978.

[188] de Bari, O., Neuschwander-Tetri, B., Liu, M., Portincasa, P., and Wang, D. 2012. Ezetimibe: its novel effects on the prevention and the treatment of cholesterol gallstones and nonalcoholic fatty liver disease. *J Lipids* 2012:17.

[189] Lammert, F., and Wang, D.Q. 2005. New insights into the genetic regulation of intestinal cholesterol absorption. *Gastroenterology* 129:718-734.

[190] Manhas, A., and Farmer, J.A. 2004. Hypolipidemic therapy and cholesterol absorption. *Curr Atheroscler Rep* 6:89-93.

[191] Insull, W., Jr., Koren, M., Davignon, J., Sprecher, D., Schrott, H., Keilson, L.M., Brown, A.S., Dujovne, C.A., Davidson, M.H., McLain, R., et al. 2001. Efficacy and short-term safety of a new ACAT inhibitor, avasimibe, on lipids, lipoproteins, and apolipoproteins, in patients with combined hyperlipidemia. *Atherosclerosis* 157:137-144.

[192] Grundy, S.M., Cleeman, J.I., Merz, C.N., Brewer, H.B., Jr., Clark, L.T., Hunninghake, D.B., Pasternak, R.C., Smith, S.C., Jr., and Stone, N.J. 2004. Implications of recent clinical trials for the National Cholesterol Education Program Adult Treatment Panel III Guidelines. *J Am Coll Cardiol* 44:720-732.

[193] Davidson, M.H., Maki, K., Umporowicz, D., Wheeler, A., Rittershaus, C., and Ryan, U. 2003. The safety and immunogenicity of a CETP vaccine in healthy adults. *Atherosclerosis* 169:113-120.

[194] Knopp, R.H., Dujovne, C.A., Le Beaut, A., Lipka, L.J., Suresh, R., and Veltri, E.P. 2003. Evaluation of the efficacy, safety, and tolerability of ezetimibe in primary hypercholesterolaemia: a pooled analysis from two controlled phase III clinical studies. *Int J Clin Pract* 57:363-368.

[195] Dujovne, C.A., Bays, H., Davidson, M.H., Knopp, R., Hunninghake, D.B., Stein, E.A., Goldberg, A.C., Jones, P., Lipka, L.J., and Cuffie-Jackson, C. 2001. Reduction of LDL cholesterol in patients with primary hypercholesterolemia by SCH 48461: results of a multicenter dose-ranging study. *J Clin Pharmacol* 41:70-78.

[196] Bays, H.E., Moore, P.B., Drehobl, M.A., Rosenblatt, S., Toth, P.D., Dujovne, C.A., Knopp, R.H., Lipka, L.J., Lebeaut, A.P., Yang, B., et al. 2001. Effectiveness and tolerability of ezetimibe in patients with primary hypercholesterolemia: pooled analysis of two phase II studies. *Clin Ther* 23:1209-1230.

[197] Dujovne, C.A., Ettinger, M.P., McNeer, J.F., Lipka, L.J., LeBeaut, A.P., Suresh, R., Yang, B., and Veltri, E.P. 2002. Efficacy and safety of a potent new selective cholesterol absorption inhibitor, ezetimibe, in patients with primary hypercholesterolemia. *Am J Cardiol* 90:1092-1097.

[198] Ballantyne, C.M. 2004. Role of selective cholesterol absorption inhibition in the management of dyslipidemia. *Curr Atheroscler Rep* 6:52-59.

[199] Jia, L., Ma, Y., Liu, G., and Yu, L. 2010. Dietary cholesterol reverses resistance to diet-induced weight gain in mice lacking Niemann-Pick C1-Like 1. *J Lipid Res* 51:3024-3033.

[200] Jia, L., Ma, Y., Rong, S., Betters, J.L., Xie, P., Chung, S., Wang, N., Tang, W., and Yu, L. 2010. Niemann-Pick C1-Like 1 deletion in mice prevents high-fat diet-induced fatty liver by reducing lipogenesis. *J Lipid Res* 51:3135-3144.

[201] van Heek, M., Farley, C., Compton, D.S., Hoos, L.M., Smith-Torhan, A., and Davis, H.R. 2003. Ezetimibe potently inhibits cholesterol absorption but does not affect acute hepatic or intestinal cholesterol synthesis in rats. *Br J Pharmacol* 138:1459-1464.

[202] Rosenblum, S.B., Huynh, T., Afonso, A., Davis, H.R., Jr., Yumibe, N., Clader, J.W., and Burnett, D.A. 1998. Discovery of 1-(4-fluorophenyl)-(3R)-[3-(4-fluorophenyl)-(3S)-hydroxypropyl]-(4S)-(4 -hydroxyphenyl)-2-azetidinone (SCH 58235): a designed, potent, orally active inhibitor of cholesterol absorption. *J Med Chem* 41:973-980.

[203] Burnett, D.A., Caplen, M.A., Davis, H.R., Jr., Burrier, R.E., and Clader, J.W. 1994. 2-Azetidinones as inhibitors of cholesterol absorption. *J Med Chem* 37:1733-1736.

[204] Clader, J.W. 2004. The discovery of ezetimibe: a view from outside the receptor. *J Med Chem* 47:1-9.

[205] Kosoglou, T., Statkevich, P., Johnson-Levonas, A.O., Paolini, J.F., Bergman, A.J., and Alton, K.B. 2005. Ezetimibe: a review of its metabolism, pharmacokinetics and drug interactions. *Clin Pharmacokinet* 44:467-494.

[206] Sudhop, T., and von Bergmann, K. 2002. Cholesterol absorption inhibitors for the treatment of hypercholesterolaemia. *Drugs* 62:2333-2347.

[207] Gagne, C., Gaudet, D., and Bruckert, E. 2002. Efficacy and safety of ezetimibe coadministered with atorvastatin or simvastatin in patients with homozygous familial hypercholesterolemia. *Circulation* 105:2469-2475.

[208] Davidson, M.H. 2003. Ezetimibe: a novel option for lowering cholesterol. *Expert Rev Cardiovasc Ther* 1:11-21.

[209] Jandacek, R.J., Heubi, J.E., and Tso, P. 2004. A novel, noninvasive method for the measurement of intestinal fat absorption. *Gastroenterology* 127:139-144.

[210] Labonte, E.D., Camarota, L.M., Rojas, J.C., Jandacek, R.J., Gilham, D.E., Davies, J.P., Ioannou, Y.A., Tso, P., Hui, D.Y., and Howles, P.N. 2008. Reduced absorption of saturated fatty acids and resistance to diet-induced obesity and diabetes by ezetimibe-treated and Npc1l1-/- mice. *Am J Physiol Gastrointest Liver Physiol* 295:G776-783.

[211] van Heek, M., Compton, D.S., and Davis, H.R. 2001. The cholesterol absorption inhibitor, ezetimibe, decreases diet-induced hypercholesterolemia in monkeys. *Eur J Pharmacol* 415:79-84.

[212] Havel, R.J. 2000. Remnant lipoproteins as therapeutic targets. *Curr Opin Lipidol* 11:615-620.

[213] Catapano, A. 2001. Ezetimibe: a selective inhibitor of cholesterol absorpti. *European Heart Journal Supplemen* 3:5.

[214] Repa, J.J., Dietschy, J.M., and Turley, S.D. 2002. Inhibition of cholesterol absorption by SCH 58053 in the mouse is not mediated via changes in the expression of mRNA for ABCA1, ABCG5, or ABCG8 in the enterocyte. *J Lipid Res* 43:1864-1874.

[215] Carstea, E.D., Morris, J.A., Coleman, K.G., Loftus, S.K., Zhang, D., Cummings, C., Gu, J., Rosenfeld, M.A., Pavan, W.J., Krizman, D.B., et al. 1997. Niemann-Pick C1 disease gene: homology to mediators of cholesterol homeostasis. *Science* 277:228-231.

[216] Loftus, S.K., Morris, J.A., Carstea, E.D., Gu, J.Z., Cummings, C., Brown, A., Ellison, J., Ohno, K., Rosenfeld, M.A., Tagle, D.A., et al. 1997. Murine model of Niemann-Pick C disease: mutation in a cholesterol homeostasis gene. *Science* 277:232-235.

[217] Davies, J.P., Levy, B., and Ioannou, Y.A. 2000. Evidence for a Niemann-pick C (NPC) gene family: identification and characterization of NPC1L1. *Genomics* 65:137-145.

[218] Chang, T.Y., and Chang, C. 2008. Ezetimibe blocks internalization of the NPC1L1/cholesterol complex. *Cell Metab* 7:469-471.

[219] Drover, V.A., Nguyen, D.V., Bastie, C.C., Darlington, Y.F., Abumrad, N.A., Pessin, J.E., London, E., Sahoo, D., and Phillips, M.C. 2008. CD36 mediates both cellular uptake of very long chain fatty acids and their intestinal absorption in mice. *J Biol Chem* 283:13108-13115.

[220] Nassir, F., Wilson, B., Han, X., Gross, R.W., and Abumrad, N.A. 2007. CD36 is important for fatty acid and cholesterol uptake by the proximal but not distal intestine. *J Biol Chem* 282:19493-19501.

[221] Wang, D.Q., Cohen, D.E., and Carey, M.C. 2009. Biliary lipids and cholesterol gallstone disease. *J Lipid Res* 50 Suppl:S406-411.

[222] Mazer, N.A., and Carey, M.C. 1983. Quasi-elastic light-scattering studies of aqueous biliary lipid systems. Cholesterol solubilization and precipitation in model bile solutions. *Biochemistry* 22:426-442.

[223] Somjen, G.J., and Gilat, T. 1983. A non-micellar mode of cholesterol transport in human bile. *FEBS Lett* 156:265-268.

[224] van Erpecum, K.J. 2005. Biliary lipids, water and cholesterol gallstones. *Biol Cell* 97:815-822.

[225] Wang, H.H., Portincasa, P., Afdhal, N.H., and Wang, D.Q. 2010. Lith genes and genetic analysis of cholesterol gallstone formation. *Gastroenterol Clin North Am* 39:185-207, vii-viii.

[226] Valasek, M.A., Repa, J.J., Quan, G., Dietschy, J.M., and Turley, S.D. 2008. Inhibiting intestinal NPC1L1 activity prevents diet-induced increase in biliary cholesterol in Golden Syrian hamsters. *Am J Physiol Gastrointest Liver Physiol* 295:G813-822.

[227] Chiang, D.J., Pritchard, M.T., and Nagy, L.E. 2011. Obesity, diabetes mellitus, and liver fibrosis. *Am J Physiol Gastrointest Liver Physiol* 300:G697-702.

[228] Fassio, E., Alvarez, E., Dominguez, N., Landeira, G., and Longo, C. 2004. Natural history of nonalcoholic steatohepatitis: a longitudinal study of repeat liver biopsies. *Hepatology* 40:820-826.

[229] Angulo, P. 2007. Obesity and nonalcoholic fatty liver disease. *Nutr Rev* 65:S57-63.

[230] Hubscher, S.G. 2006. Histological assessment of non-alcoholic fatty liver disease. *Histopathology* 49:450-465.

[231] Kleiner, D.E., Brunt, E.M., Van Natta, M., Behling, C., Contos, M.J., Cummings, O.W., Ferrell, L.D., Liu, Y.C., Torbenson, M.S., Unalp-Arida, A., et al. 2005. Design and validation of a histological scoring system for nonalcoholic fatty liver disease. *Hepatology* 41:1313-1321.

[232] Tiniakos, D., Vos, M., and Brunt, E. 2010. Nonalcoholic fatty liver disease: pathology and pathogenesis. *Annual Review of Pathology: Mechanisms of Disease* 5:27.

[233] Day, C.P., and James, O.F. 1998. Steatohepatitis: a tale of two "hits"? *Gastroenterology* 114:842-845.

[234] Soeters, P.B., and Grimble, R.F. 2009. Dangers, and benefits of the cytokine mediated response to injury and infection. *Clin Nutr* 28:583-596.

[235] Lackner, C. 2011. Hepatocellular ballooning in nonalcoholic steatohepatitis: the pathologist's perspective. Expert Review 16. *Journal of Lipids of Gastroenterology & Hepatology* 5:9.

[236] Neuschwander-Tetri, B.A. 2010. Hepatic lipotoxicity and the pathogenesis of nonalcoholic steatohepatitis: the central role of nontriglyceride fatty acid metabolites. *Hepatology* 52:774-788.

[237] Adams, L.A., and Angulo, P. 2005. Recent concepts in non-alcoholic fatty liver disease. *Diabet Med* 22:1129-1133.

[238] Angulo, P. 2005. Nonalcoholic fatty liver disease. *Revista de Gastroenterolog´ıa de Mexico* 70, supplement 3:5.

[239] Zheng, S., Hoos, L., Cook, J., Tetzloff, G., Davis, H., Jr., van Heek, M., and Hwa, J.J. 2008. Ezetimibe improves high fat and cholesterol diet-induced non-alcoholic fatty liver disease in mice. *Eur J Pharmacol* 584:118-124.

[240] Oosterveer, M., van Dijk, T., and Tietge, U.e.a. 2009. High fat feeding induces hepatic fatty acid elongation in mice. *PLoS One* 4.

[241] Utzschneider, K.M., and Kahn, S.E. 2006. Review: The role of insulin resistance in nonalcoholic fatty liver disease. *J Clin Endocrinol Metab* 91:4753-4761.

[242] Donnelly, K.L., Smith, C.I., Schwarzenberg, S.J., Jessurun, J., Boldt, M.D., and Parks, E.J. 2005. Sources of fatty acids stored in liver and secreted via lipoproteins in patients with nonalcoholic fatty liver disease. *J Clin Invest* 115:1343-1351.

[243] Tendler, D., Lin, S., Yancy, W.S., Jr., Mavropoulos, J., Sylvestre, P., Rockey, D.C., and Westman, E.C. 2007. The effect of a low-carbohydrate, ketogenic diet on nonalcoholic fatty liver disease: a pilot study. *Dig Dis Sci* 52:589-593.

[244] Gronbaek, H., Thomsen, K.L., Rungby, J., Schmitz, O., and Vilstrup, H. 2008. Role of nonalcoholic fatty liver disease in the development of insulin resistance and diabetes. *Expert Rev Gastroenterol Hepatol* 2:705-711.

[245] Shulman, G.I. 2000. Cellular mechanisms of insulin resistance. *J Clin Invest* 106:171-176.

[246] Chen, G., Liang, G., Ou, J., Goldstein, J.L., and Brown, M.S. 2004. Central role for liver X receptor in insulin-mediated activation of Srebp-1c transcription and stimulation of fatty acid synthesis in liver. *Proc Natl Acad Sci U S A* 101:11245-11250.

[247] Uyeda, K., and Repa, J.J. 2006. Carbohydrate response element binding protein, ChREBP, a transcription factor coupling hepatic glucose utilization and lipid synthesis. *Cell Metab* 4:107-110.

[248] Dentin, R., Pegorier, J.P., Benhamed, F., Foufelle, F., Ferre, P., Fauveau, V., Magnuson, M.A., Girard, J., and Postic, C. 2004. Hepatic glucokinase is required for the synergistic action of ChREBP and SREBP-1c on glycolytic and lipogenic gene expression. *J Biol Chem* 279:20314-20326.

[249] Repa, J.J., Liang, G., Ou, J., Bashmakov, Y., Lobaccaro, J.M., Shimomura, I., Shan, B., Brown, M.S., Goldstein, J.L., and Mangelsdorf, D.J. 2000. Regulation of mouse sterol regulatory element-binding protein-1c gene (SREBP-1c) by oxysterol receptors, LXRalpha and LXRbeta. *Genes Dev* 14:2819-2830.

[250] Shehadi, W.H. 1979. The biliary system through the ages. *Int Surg* 64:63-78.

[251] 1993. National Institutes of Health Consensus Development Conference Statement on Gallstones and Laparoscopic Cholecystectomy. *Am J Surg* 165:390-398.

[252] Cross, C.E., Halliwell, B., Borish, E.T., Pryor, W.A., Ames, B.N., Saul, R.L., McCord, J.M., and Harman, D. 1987. Oxygen radicals and human disease. *Ann Intern Med* 107:526-545.

[253] Ahmed, A., Cheung, R.C., and Keeffe, E.B. 2000. Management of gallstones and their complications. *Am Fam Physician* 61:1673-1680, 1687-1678.

[254] Corradini, S.G., Elisei, W., Giovannelli, L., Ripani, C., Della Guardia, P., Corsi, A., Cantafora, A., Capocaccia, L., Ziparo, V., Stipa, V., et al. 2000. Impaired human gallbladder lipid absorption in cholesterol gallstone disease and its effect on cholesterol solubility in bile. *Gastroenterology* 118:912-920.

[255] Caroli-Bosc, F.X., Deveau, C., Peten, E.P., Delabre, B., Zanaldi, H., Hebuterne, X., Hastier, P., Viudes, F., Belanger, F., Caroli-Bosc, C., et al. 1998. Cholelithiasis and dietary risk factors: an epidemiologic investigation in Vidauban, Southeast France. General Practitioner's Group of Vidauban. *Dig Dis Sci* 43:2131-2137.

[256] Holzbach, R.T., Marsh, M., Olszewski, M., and Holan, K. 1973. Cholesterol solubility in bile. Evidence that supersaturated bile is frequent in healthy man. *J Clin Invest* 52:1467-1479.

[257] Jirsa, M., and Groen, A. 2001. Role of biliary proteins and non-protein factors in kinetics of cholesterol crystallisation and gallstone growth. . *Front Biosci* 6:14.

[258] Hoogerbrugge-vd Linden, N., de Rooy, F.W., Jansen, H., and van Blankenstein, M. 1990. Effect of pravastatin on biliary lipid composition and bile acid synthesis in familial hypercholesterolaemia. *Gut* 31:348-350.

[259] LaMorte, W.W., Brotschi, E.A., Scott, T.E., and Williams, L.F., Jr. 1985. Pigment gallstone formation in the cholesterol-fed guinea pig. *Hepatology* 5:21-27.

[260] Hussain, S.A. 2007. Effect of melatonin on cholesterol absorption in rats. *J Pineal Res* 42:267-271.

[261] Chan, T.Y., and Tang, P.L. 1995. Effect of melatonin on the maintenance of cholesterol homeostasis in the rat. *Endocr Res* 21:681-696.

[262] Hussain, S., Hussein, K., and Saieed, B.e.a. 2004. Improvement of the hypolipidemic effect of lovastatin with melatonin. *Iraqi Postgrad Med J* 3:4.

[263] Al-Mahabashy, H., Hussain, S., and Numan, N.e.a. 2006. The effects of melatonin on the oxidative stress, protein glycation, microalbuminuria and lipid profile in type 2 diabetes mellitus. *Iraqi J Pharm Sci* 15:6.

[264] Ismail, S., Hussain, S., and Numan, N.e.a. 2004. Hypolipidemic effect of melatonin in dyslipidemia associated with diabetes. *Iraqi Postgrad Med J* 3:4.

[265] Gomez-Pinilla, P.J., Camello-Almaraz, C., Moreno, R., Camello, P.J., and Pozo, M.J. 2006. Melatonin treatment reverts age-related changes in Guinea pig gallbladder neuromuscular transmission and contractility. *J Pharmacol Exp Ther* 319:847-856.

[266] Morales, S., Camello, P.J., Alcon, S., Salido, G.M., Mawe, G., and Pozo, M.J. 2004. Coactivation of capacitative calcium entry and L-type calcium channels in guinea pig gallbladder. *Am J Physiol Gastrointest Liver Physiol* 286:G1090-1100.

[267] Morales, S., Camello, P.J., Mawe, G.M., and Pozo, M.J. 2005. Characterization of intracellular Ca(2+) stores in gallbladder smooth muscle. *Am J Physiol Gastrointest Liver Physiol* 288:G507-513.

[268] Van Erpecum, K.J., and Van Berge-Henegouwen, G.P. 1999. Gallstones: an intestinal disease? *Gut* 44:435-438.

[269] Portincasa, P., van Erpecum, K.J., and Vanberge-Henegouwen, G.P. 1997. Cholesterol crystallisation in bile. *Gut* 41:138-141.

[270] Xu, Q.W., and Shaffer, E.A. 1996. The potential site of impaired gallbladder contractility in an animal model of cholesterol gallstone disease. *Gastroenterology* 110:251-257.

[271] Chen, Q., Amaral, J., Biancani, P., and Behar, J. 1999. Excess membrane cholesterol alters human gallbladder muscle contractility and membrane fluidity. *Gastroenterology* 116:678-685.

[272] Jaworek, J., Nawrot, K., Konturek, S.J., Leja-Szpak, A., Thor, P., and Pawlik, W.W. 2004. Melatonin and its precursor, L-tryptophan: influence on pancreatic amylase secretion in vivo and in vitro. *J Pineal Res* 36:155-164.

[273] Tan, D., Manchester, L.C., Reiter, R.J., Qi, W., Hanes, M.A., and Farley, N.J. 1999. High physiological levels of melatonin in the bile of mammals. *Life Sci* 65:2523-2529.

[274] Messner, M., Huether, G., Lorf, T., Ramadori, G., and Schworer, H. 2001. Presence of melatonin in the human hepatobiliary-gastrointestinal tract. *Life Sci* 69:543-551.

[275] Aust, S., Thalhammer, T., Humpeler, S., Jager, W., Klimpfinger, M., Tucek, G., Obrist, P., Marktl, W., Penner, E., and Ekmekcioglu, C. 2004. The melatonin receptor subtype MT1 is expressed in human gallbladder epithelia. *J Pineal Res* 36:43-48.

[276] von Gall, C., Stehle, J.H., and Weaver, D.R. 2002. Mammalian melatonin receptors: molecular biology and signal transduction. *Cell Tissue Res* 309:151-162.

[277] van Erpecum, K.J., Venneman, N.G., Portincasa, P., and Vanberge-Henegouwen, G.P. 2000. Review article: agents affecting gall-bladder motility--role in treatment and prevention of gallstones. *Aliment Pharmacol Ther* 14 Suppl 2:66-70.

[278] Chen, X., and Cai, J. 2003. The impact of selective cycloxygenase-2 inhibitor celecoxib on the formation of cholesterol gallstone. *Zhonghua Nei Ke Za Zhi* 42:3.

[279] Kourie, J.I. 1998. Interaction of reactive oxygen species with ion transport mechanisms. *Am J Physiol* 275:C1-24.

[280] Lee, S.P., and Scott, A.J. 1982. The evolution of morphologic changes in the gallbladder before stone formation in mice fed a cholesterol-cholic acid diet. *Am J Pathol* 108:1-8.

[281] Lee, S.P., LaMont, J.T., and Carey, M.C. 1981. Role of gallbladder mucus hypersecretion in the evolution of cholesterol gallstones. *J Clin Invest* 67:1712-1723.

[282] Scott, A.J. 1978. Epithelial cell proliferation in diverse models of experimental cholelithiasis. *Gut* 19:558-562.

[283] Lee, S.P., and Nicholls, J.F. 1986. Nature and composition of biliary sludge. *Gastroenterology* 90:677-686.

[284] Burnstein, M.J., Ilson, R.G., Petrunka, C.N., Taylor, R.D., and Strasberg, S.M. 1983. Evidence for a potent nucleating factor in the gallbladder bile of patients with cholesterol gallstones. *Gastroenterology* 85:801-807.

[285] Bouchier, I.A., Cooperband, S.R., and el-Kodsi, B.M. 1965. Mucous substances and viscosity of normal and pathological human bile. *Gastroenterology* 49:343-353.

[286] Kim, H.J., Lee, S.K., Kim, M.H., Seo, D.W., and Min, Y.I. 2003. Cyclooxygenase-2 mediates mucin secretion from epithelial cells of lipopolysaccharide-treated canine gallbladder. *Dig Dis Sci* 48:726-732.

[287] van Klinken, B.J., Dekker, J., van Gool, S.A., van Marle, J., Buller, H.A., and Einerhand, A.W. 1998. MUC5B is the prominent mucin in human gallbladder and is also expressed in a subset of colonic goblet cells. *Am J Physiol* 274:G871-878.

[288] Lee, K.T., and Liu, T.S. 2001. Altered mucin gene expression in stone-containing intrahepatic bile ducts and cholangiocarcinomas. *Dig Dis Sci* 46:2166-2172.

[289] Vilkin, A., Nudelman, I., Morgenstern, S., Geller, A., Bar Dayan, Y., Levi, Z., Rodionov, G., Hardy, B., Konikoff, F., Gobbic, D., et al. 2007. Gallbladder inflammation is associated with increase in mucin expression and pigmented stone formation. *Dig Dis Sci* 52:1613-1620.

[290] Nunes, D.P., Afdhal, N.H., and Offner, G.D. 1999. A recombinant bovine gallbladder mucin polypeptide binds biliary lipids and accelerates cholesterol crystal appearance time. *Gastroenterology* 116:936-942.

[291] Afdhal, N.H., Ostrow, J.D., Koehler, R., Niu, N., Groen, A.K., Veis, A., Nunes, D.P., and Offner, G.D. 1995. Interaction of bovine gallbladder mucin and calcium-binding protein: effects on calcium phosphate precipitation. *Gastroenterology* 109:1661-1672.

[292] LaMont, J.T., Smith, B.F., and Moore, J.R. 1984. Role of gallbladder mucin in pathophysiology of gallstones. *Hepatology* 4:51S-56S.

[293] Rhodes, M., Allen, A., Dowling, R.H., Murphy, G., and Lennard, T.W. 1992. Inhibition of human gall bladder mucus synthesis in patients undergoing cholecystectomy. *Gut* 33:1113-1117.

[294] Chapman, W.C., Peterkin, G.A., 3rd, LaMorte, W.W., and Williams, L.F., Jr. 1989. Alterations in biliary motility correlate with increased gallbladder prostaglandin synthesis in early cholelithiasis in prairie dog. *Dig Dis Sci* 34:1420-1424.

[295] Ho, S.B., Shekels, L.L., Toribara, N.W., Gipson, I.K., Kim, Y.S., Purdum, P.P., 3rd, and Cherwitz, D.L. 2000. Altered mucin core peptide expression in acute and chronic cholecystitis. *Dig Dis Sci* 45:1061-1071.

[296] Jansson, R., Steen, G., and Svanvik, J. 1978. Effects of intravenous vasoactive intestinal peptide (VIP) on gallbladder function in the cat. *Gastroenterology* 75:47-50.

[297] Shiesh, S.C., Chen, C.Y., Lin, X.Z., Liu, Z.A., and Tsao, H.C. 2000. Melatonin prevents pigment gallstone formation induced by bile duct ligation in guinea pigs. *Hepatology* 32:455-460.

[298] Mayo, J.C., Sainz, R.M., Tan, D.X., Hardeland, R., Leon, J., Rodriguez, C., and Reiter, R.J. 2005. Anti-inflammatory actions of melatonin and its metabolites, N1-acetyl-N2-formyl-5-methoxykynuramine (AFMK) and N1-acetyl-5-methoxykynuramine (AMK), in macrophages. *J Neuroimmunol* 165:139-149.

[299] Wu, K.K. 2005. Control of cyclooxygenase-2 transcriptional activation by pro-inflammatory mediators. *Prostaglandins Leukot Essent Fatty Acids* 72:89-93.

[300] Xie, Q.W., Whisnant, R., and Nathan, C. 1993. Promoter of the mouse gene encoding calcium-independent nitric oxide synthase confers inducibility by interferon gamma and bacterial lipopolysaccharide. *J Exp Med* 177:1779-1784.

[301] Lowenstein, C.J., Alley, E.W., Raval, P., Snowman, A.M., Snyder, S.H., Russell, S.W., and Murphy, W.J. 1993. Macrophage nitric oxide synthase gene: two upstream regions mediate induction by interferon gamma and lipopolysaccharide. *Proc Natl Acad Sci U S A* 90:9730-9734.

[302] Wadleigh, D.J., Reddy, S.T., Kopp, E., Ghosh, S., and Herschman, H.R. 2000. Transcriptional activation of the cyclooxygenase-2 gene in endotoxin-treated RAW 264.7 macrophages. *J Biol Chem* 275:6259-6266.

[303] Herschman, H.R. 1996. Prostaglandin synthase 2. *Biochim Biophys Acta* 1299:125-140.

[304] Dixit, V., and Mak, T.W. 2002. NF-kappaB signaling. Many roads lead to madrid. *Cell* 111:615-619.

[305] Conter, R.L., Washington, J.L., Liao, C.C., and Kauffman, G.L., Jr. 1992. Gallbladder mucosal blood flow increases during early cholesterol gallstone formation. *Gastroenterology* 102:1764-1770.

[306] Nash, S., Stafford, J., and Madara, J.L. 1987. Effects of polymorphonuclear leukocyte transmigration on the barrier function of cultured intestinal epithelial monolayers. *J Clin Invest* 80:1104-1113.

[307] Hale, W.B., Turner, B., and LaMont, J.T. 1987. Oxygen radicals stimulate guinea pig gallbladder glycoprotein secretion in vitro. *Am J Physiol* 253:G627-630.

[308] Lee, D.W., Gilmore, C.J., Bonorris, G., Cohen, H., Marks, J.W., Cho-Sue, M., Meiselman, M.S., and Schoenfield, L.J. 1985. Effect of dietary cholesterol on biliary lipids in patients with gallstones and normal subjects. *Am J Clin Nutr* 42:414-420.

[309] Holan, K.R., Holzbach, R.T., Hermann, R.E., Cooperman, A.M., and Claffey, W.J. 1979. Nucleation time: a key factor in the pathogenesis of cholesterol gallstone disease. *Gastroenterology* 77:611-617.

[310] Eder, M.I., Miquel, J.F., Jongst, D., Paumgartner, G., and von Ritter, C. 1996. Reactive oxygen metabolites promote cholesterol crystal formation in model bile: role of lipid peroxidation. *Free Radic Biol Med* 20:743-749.

[311] Weiss, S.J. 1989. Tissue destruction by neutrophils. *N Engl J Med* 320:365-376.

[312] Esterbauer, H., Schaur, R.J., and Zollner, H. 1991. Chemistry and biochemistry of 4-hydroxynonenal, malonaldehyde and related aldehydes. *Free Radic Biol Med* 11:81-128.

[313] Geetha, A. 2002. Evidence for oxidative stress in the gall bladder mucosa of gall stone patients. *J Biochem Mol Biol Biophys* 6:427-432.

[314] Hardeland, R., Reiter, R.J., Poeggeler, B., and Tan, D.X. 1993. The significance of the metabolism of the neurohormone melatonin: antioxidative protection and formation of bioactive substances. *Neurosci Biobehav Rev* 17:347-357.

[315] Reiter, R.J., Tan, D.X., Terron, M.P., Flores, L.J., and Czarnocki, Z. 2007. Melatonin and its metabolites: new findings regarding their production and their radical scavenging actions. *Acta Biochim Pol* 54:1-9.

[316] Ozturk, H., Yagmur, Y., and Uzunlar, A.K. 2006. Effects of melatonin administration on intestinal adaptive response after massive bowel resection in rats. *Dig Dis Sci* 51:333-337.

[317] Bilici, D., Suleyman, H., Banoglu, Z.N., Kiziltunc, A., Avci, B., Ciftcioglu, A., and Bilici, S. 2002. Melatonin prevents ethanol-induced gastric mucosal damage possibly due to its antioxidant effect. *Dig Dis Sci* 47:856-861.

[318] Qi, W., Tan, D.X., Reiter, R.J., Kim, S.J., Manchester, L.C., Cabrera, J., Sainz, R.M., and Mayo, J.C. 1999. Melatonin reduces lipid peroxidation and tissue edema in cerulein-induced acute pancreatitis in rats. *Dig Dis Sci* 44:2257-2262.

[319] Sener-Muratoglu, G., Paskaloglu, K., Arbak, S., Hurdag, C., and Ayanoglu-Dulger, G. 2001. Protective effect of famotidine, omeprazole, and melatonin against acetylsalicylic acid-induced gastric damage in rats. *Dig Dis Sci* 46:318-330.

[320] Sener, G., Goren, F.O., Ulusoy, N.B., Ersoy, Y., Arbak, S., and Dulger, G.A. 2005. Protective effect of melatonin and omeprazole against alendronat-induced gastric damage. *Dig Dis Sci* 50:1506-1512.

[321] Bubenik, G.A. 2002. Gastrointestinal melatonin: localization, function, and clinical relevance. *Dig Dis Sci* 47:2336-2348.

[322] Contuk, G., Ercan, F., Cetinel, S., Cikler, E., and Sener, G. 2005. Role of melatonin in reducing water avoidance stress-induced degeneration of the liver. *Dig Dis Sci* 50:738-744.

[323] Worthington, H.V., Hunt, L.P., McCloy, R.F., Maclennan, I., and Braganza, J.M. 1997. A pilot study of antioxidant intake in patients with cholesterol gallstones. *Nutrition* 13:118-127.

[324] Lin, C., Shen, T., Fu, X., and Zhou, X. 1996. The ability of bile to scavenge superoxide radicals and pigment gallstone formation in guinea pigs. *HPB Surg* 10:73-76; discussion 76-77.

[325] Vagner, E., Khlebnikov, V., Terekhina, N., and Palatova, L. 1997. Antioxidants in the treatment of cholelithiasis patients. *Vestn Khir Im II Grek* 156:4.

[326] Tan, D.X., Poeggeler, B., Reiter, R.J., Chen, L.D., Chen, S., Manchester, L.C., and Barlow-Walden, L.R. 1993. The pineal hormone melatonin inhibits DNA-adduct formation induced by the chemical carcinogen safrole in vivo. *Cancer Lett* 70:65-71.

[327] Arteaga, S., Carmona, A., Luis, J., Andrade-Cetto, A., and Cardenas, R. 2005. Effect of Larrea tridentata (creosote bush) on cholesterol gallstones and bile secretion in hamsters. *J Pharm Pharmacol* 57:1093-1099.

[328] Abou-Gazar, H., Bedir, E., Takamatsu, S., Ferreira, D., and Khan, I.A. 2004. Antioxidant lignans from Larrea tridentata. *Phytochemistry* 65:2499-2505.

[329] Lawrentschuk, N., Hewitt, P.M., and Pritchard, M.G. 2003. Elective laparoscopic cholecystectomy: implications of prolonged waiting times for surgery. *ANZ J Surg* 73:890-893.

[330] Olson, D.W., and de, G. 2002. How long do patients wait for elective general surgery? *Can J Surg* 45:31-33.

[331] Rutledge, D., Jones, D., and Rege, R. 2000. Consequences of delay in surgical treatment of biliary disease. *Am J Surg* 180:466-469.

[332] Salman, B., Yuksel, O., Irkorucu, O., Akyurek, N., Tezcaner, T., Dogan, I., Erdem, O., and Tatlicioglu, E. 2005. Urgent laparoscopic cholecystectomy is the best management for biliary colic. A prospective randomized study of 75 cases. *Dig Surg* 22:95-99.

[333] Berr, F., Mayer, M., Sackmann, M.F., Sauerbruch, T., Holl, J., and Paumgartner, G. 1994. Pathogenic factors in early recurrence of cholesterol gallstones. *Gastroenterology* 106:215-224.

[334] Bachrach, W.H., and Hofmann, A.F. 1982. Ursodeoxycholic acid in the treatment of cholesterol cholelithiasis. part I. *Dig Dis Sci* 27:737-761.

[335] Thistle, J.L., Larusso, N.F., Hofmann, A.F., Turcotte, J., Carlson, G.L., and Ott, B.J. 1982. Differing effects of ursodeoxycholic or chenodeoxycholic acid on biliary cholesterol saturation and bile acid metabolism in man. A dose-response study. *Dig Dis Sci* 27:161-168.

[336] Thistle, J.L., Hofmann, A.F., Yu, P.Y., and Ott, B. 1977. Effect of varying doses of chenodeoxycholic acid on bile lipid and biliary bile acid composition in gallstone patients: a dose-response study. *Am J Dig Dis* 22:1-6.

[337] Schoenfield, L.J., and Marks, J.W. 1993. Oral and contact dissolution of gallstones. *Am J Surg* 165:427-430.

[338] Anderson, H. 1914. The medical treatment of cholelithiasis. *Can Med Assoc J* 4:8.

[339] Lee, S. 2004. Gallstones: how do we translate an old story into future therapy? *Nat Clin Pract Gastroenterol Hepatol* 1:2-3.

[340] Strasberg, S.M. 1995. *Acute calculus cholecystitis*. Philadelphia: Saunders. 30 pp.

[341] Womack, N., and Bricker, E. 1944. Pathogenesis of cholecystitis. *Arch Surg* 44:1.

[342] Xiao, Z.L., Amaral, J., Biancani, P., and Behar, J. 2005. Impaired cytoprotective function of muscle in human gallbladders with cholesterol stones. *Am J Physiol Gastrointest Liver Physiol* 288:G525-532.

[343] Lane, J.R., Starbuck, E.M., Johnson, A.K., and Fitts, D.A. 1999. Effects of bile duct ligation and captopril on salt appetite and renin-aldosterone axis in rats. *Physiol Behav* 66:419-425.

[344] Canturk, N.Z., Canturk, Z., Ozbilim, G., and Yenisey, C. 2000. Protective effect of vitamin E on gastric mucosal injury in rats with biliary obstruction. *Can J Gastroenterol* 14:499-503.

[345] Montilla, P., Cruz, A., Padillo, F.J., Tunez, I., Gascon, F., Munoz, M.C., Gomez, M., and Pera, C. 2001. Melatonin versus vitamin E as protective treatment against oxidative stress after extra-hepatic bile duct ligation in rats. *J Pineal Res* 31:138-144.

[346] Polat, A., and Emre, M.H. 2006. Effects of melatonin or acetylsalicylic acid on gastric oxidative stress after bile duct ligation in rats. *J Gastroenterol* 41:433-439.

[347] Ohta, Y., Kongo, M., and Kishikawa, T. 2003. Therapeutic effect of melatonin on cholestatic liver injury in rats with bile duct ligation. *Adv Exp Med Biol* 527:559-565.

[348] Ohta, Y., Imai, Y., Matsura, T., Yamada, K., and Tokunaga, K. 2005. Successively postadministered melatonin prevents disruption of hepatic antioxidant status in rats with bile duct ligation. *J Pineal Res* 39:367-374.

[349] Ohta, Y., Kongo-Nishimura, M., Imai, Y., Matsura, T., Kitagawa, A., and Yamada, K. 2006. alpha-Tocopherol protects against alpha-naphthylisothiocyanate-induced hepatotoxicity in rats less effectively than melatonin. *Chem Biol Interact* 161:115-124.

[350] Vitetta, L., Sali, A., Little, P., and Mrazek, L. 2000. Gallstones and gall bladder carcinoma. *Aust N Z J Surg* 70:667-673.

[351] Nervi, F., Duarte, I., Gomez, G., Rodriguez, G., Del Pino, G., Ferrerio, O., Covarrubias, C., Valdivieso, V., Torres, M.I., and Urzua, A. 1988. Frequency of gallbladder cancer in Chile, a high-risk area. *Int J Cancer* 41:657-660.

[352] Serra, I., and Diehl, A.K. 2002. Number and size of stones in patients with asymptomatic and symptomatic gallstones and gallbladder carcinoma. *J Gastrointest Surg* 6:272-273; author reply 273.

[353] Lowenfels, A.B., Maisonneuve, P., Boyle, P., and Zatonski, W.A. 1999. Epidemiology of gallbladder cancer. *Hepatogastroenterology* 46:1529-1532.

[354] Lam, C.M., Yuen, A.W., Wai, A.C., Leung, R.M., Lee, A.Y., Ng, K.K., and Fan, S.T. 2005. Gallbladder cancer presenting with acute cholecystitis: a population-based study. *Surg Endosc* 19:697-701.

[355] Abou-Saif, A., and Al-Kawas, F.H. 2002. Complications of gallstone disease: Mirizzi syndrome, cholecystocholedochal fistula, and gallstone ileus. *Am J Gastroenterol* 97:249-254.

[356] Tucker, L., and Tangedahl, T.N. 1979. Manifestations of gallstone disease. *Postgrad Med* 66:179-180, 183-174.

[357] Losanoff, J.E., Richman, B.W., and Jones, J.W. 2002. Complications of gallstone disease: gallstone ileus. *Am J Gastroenterol* 97:1843-1844; author reply 1844.

[358] Prevention, C.f.D.C.a. 2003. Trends in Aging—United States and worldwide. M.M. Mortal, and W. Rep, editors. 101–104,106.

[359] Wang, D.Q. 2002. Aging per se is an independent risk factor for cholesterol gallstone formation in gallstone susceptible mice. *J Lipid Res* 43:1950-1959.

[360] Karasek, M. 2004. Melatonin, human aging, and age-related diseases. *Exp Gerontol* 39:1723-1729.

[361] Karasek, M., and Winczyk, K. 2006. Melatonin in humans. *J Physiol Pharmacol* 57 Suppl 5:19-39.

[362] Diehl, A.K., Schwesinger, W.H., Holleman, D.R., Jr., Chapman, J.B., and Kurtin, W.E. 1994. Gallstone characteristics in Mexican Americans and non-Hispanic whites. *Dig Dis Sci* 39:2223-2228.

[363] Puppala, S., Dodd, G.D., Fowler, S., Arya, R., Schneider, J., Farook, V.S., Granato, R., Dyer, T.D., Almasy, L., Jenkinson, C.P., et al. 2006. A genomewide search finds major susceptibility loci for gallbladder disease on chromosome 1 in Mexican Americans. *Am J Hum Genet* 78:377-392.

[364] Mann, S. 2003. Melatonin for ulcerative colitis? *Am J Gastroenterol* 98:232-233.

[365] Maldonado, M.D., Murillo-Cabezas, F., Terron, M.P., Flores, L.J., Tan, D.X., Manchester, L.C., and Reiter, R.J. 2007. The potential of melatonin in reducing morbidity-mortality after craniocerebral trauma. *J Pineal Res* 42:1-11.

[366] Tan, D.X., Manchester, L.C., Terron, M.P., Flores, L.J., and Reiter, R.J. 2007. One molecule, many derivatives: a never-ending interaction of melatonin with reactive oxygen and nitrogen species? *J Pineal Res* 42:28-42.

[367] Manda, K., Ueno, M., and Anzai, K. 2007. AFMK, a melatonin metabolite, attenuates X-ray-induced oxidative damage to DNA, proteins and lipids in mice. *J Pineal Res* 42:386-393.

[368] Cuzzocrea, S., and Reiter, R.J. 2002. Pharmacological actions of melatonin in acute and chronic inflammation. *Curr Top Med Chem* 2:153-165.

[369] Rodriguez, M.I., Escames, G., Lopez, L.C., Lopez, A., Garcia, J.A., Ortiz, F., and Acuna-Castroviejo, D. 2007. Chronic melatonin treatment reduces the age-dependent inflammatory process in senescence-accelerated mice. *J Pineal Res* 42:272-279.

[370] Nosal'ova, V., Zeman, M., Cerna, S., Navarova, J., and Zakalova, M. 2007. Protective effect of melatonin in acetic acid induced colitis in rats. *J Pineal Res* 42:364-370.

[371] Gitto, E., Karbownik, M., Reiter, R.J., Tan, D.X., Cuzzocrea, S., Chiurazzi, P., Cordaro, S., Corona, G., Trimarchi, G., and Barberi, I. 2001. Effects of melatonin treatment in septic newborns. *Pediatr Res* 50:756-760.

[372] Gitto, E., Reiter, R.J., Sabatino, G., Buonocore, G., Romeo, C., Gitto, P., Bugge, C., Trimarchi, G., and Barberi, I. 2005. Correlation among cytokines, bronchopulmonary dysplasia and modality of ventilation in preterm newborns: improvement with melatonin treatment. *J Pineal Res* 39:287-293.

[373] Gitto, E., Reiter, R.J., Cordaro, S.P., La Rosa, M., Chiurazzi, P., Trimarchi, G., Gitto, P., Calabro, M.P., and Barberi, I. 2004. Oxidative and inflammatory parameters in respiratory distress syndrome of preterm newborns: beneficial effects of melatonin. *Am J Perinatol* 21:209-216.

[374] Klupinska, G., Poplawski, T., Drzewoski, J., Harasiuk, A., Reiter, R.J., Blasiak, J., and Chojnacki, J. 2007. Therapeutic effect of melatonin in patients with functional dyspepsia. *J Clin Gastroenterol* 41:270-274.

[375] Cutando, A., Gomez-Moreno, G., Arana, C., Escames, G., and Acuna-Castroviejo, D. 2007. Melatonin reduces oxidative stress because of tooth removal. *J Pineal Res* 42:419-420.

Chapter VI

Future Work and Conclusion

Portincassa et al. indicated in 2006 that two nuclear receptors in hepatocytes, the bile acid receptor or farnesoid X receptor (FXR) and the oxysterol receptors or liver X receptors (LXRs) play important roles in transcriptional regulation of the genes encoding these proteins (Portincasa, 2006). The expression of *ABCB11*and *ABCB4* is under FXR control, while *ABCG5* and *ABCG8* are target genes of LXRs. Through the quantitative trait loci approach, Paigen has identified genetic defects and described several *lith* genes in mice that are susceptible to cholesterol gallstones. Description of candidate *lith* genes in the mouse will eventually help in the identification of the human *LITH* genes. Several family and twin studies, including haplotype analysis, have indicated the role of a few genes (*ABCG5*, *ABCG8*, *FXR*, *LDLR*, *CYP7A1*, *Apolipoprotein B-100*, *APOE*, *CCKAR*) as common genetic determinants for cholesterol gallstone diseases in humans (Miquel, 1998). Amigo et al's study in 2006 indicated that modulation of *Mttp (*Microsomal triglyceride transfer protein) expression in the liver affects hepatic lipid synthesis and storage as well as biliary lipid secretion (Amigo et al., 2006). Their findings further indicated that inhibition of hepatic MTTP activity decreases the risk of experimental cholelithiasis by favoring phospholipid output into the bile. Jiang et al found in 2007 that up-regulation of *ABCG5/ABCG8* in gallstone patients - possibly mediated by increased *LXRα* - may contribute to the cholesterol supersaturation of bile (Cirillo, 2005). Their data were consistent with the possibility that increased amounts of biliary cholesterol may originate from plasma HDL cholesterol by enhanced transfer via SRBI.

In this doctorate dissertation and thesis, we have explored the whole aspect of gallstone diseases from the micro world of the genetic profiles of cholesterol gallstone patients and the crystallographic study of calcium carbonate gallbladder stones to the macro world of clinical pathophysiologically mechanistic gallbladder volume changes of gallstone patients and therapeutic aspects of gallstone diseases.

The future work may focus on other genes related to cholesterol and pigment gallstones, such as megalin and cubilin expressions in GB mucosa, mRNA expression levels of genes related to enterohepatic circulation in the ileal epithelium (OSTα-OSTβ) and genes related to cholesterol and pigment gallstones, such as UGT1A1.

In conclusion, the study on gallstone diseases is an active, time-honored, and exciting field of research. It has gone from the study of bile physiology by Admirand and Carey et al.

in the 1960's through the study on the motor function and crystal behaviors of cholesterol by Portincasa et al. in the 1990's, then moved on to the genetic study heralded by the Gpbar1 knockout study in mice by Vassileva et al. in 2006. The future is sure to encompass many of these genetic studies on gallstone disease. We surely hope we can be part of this great era.

The Future

The true frequency of gallstone disease at any point in time (i.e., prevalence) has advanced with the use of ultrasonographic surveys as opposed to clinical and necropsy studies. These studies have better defined important risk factors and ethnic differences. Cholelithiasis is rampant in American Indians and Hispanics, fostering the concept of a genetic basis for the racial differences. There is also an increased heritability in those who develop cholelithiasis early in life. The complicated pathogenesis of gallstone formation renders identification of genes causing stones difficult. Well defined monogenic forms of gallstone disease affecting the ABC transporters are rare, or if more common, such as the ABCG8 19H gene variant (responsible for hepatic cholesterol secretion), exhibit an attributable risk that only reaches 11%. Future epidemiologic studies should, therefore, clarify genetic susceptibility factors and their frequency, leading to new means for risk assessment, prevention, and treatment. Identifying gene variants for the gallstone phenotype would then require action: better defining the role of diagnostic imaging (ultrasonography to detect stone development), strategies for prevention (like ursodeoxycholic acid for LPAC syndrome), and the value of modifying environmental factors. The implications of changing environmental risk factors predict an increase in the numbers of individuals with gallstones. An aging population plus the rising epidemic of obesity and the metabolic syndrome are certain to aggravate the frequency and complications of gallstone disease. Identifying risk factors that can be altered (i.e., extreme obesity, rapid weight loss, sedentary lifestyle, and key dietary factors) will provide an opportunity for the prevention of cholelithiasis.

Index

#

A

B

C

D

E

H

I

J

K

L

M

N

O

P

Q

R

S

T

U

V

W

X

Y

Z